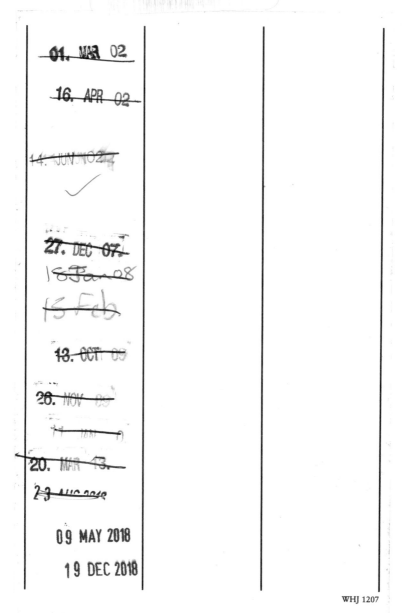
Books should be returned to the SDH Library on or before
the date stamped above unless a renewal has been arranged.

Salisbury District Hospital Library

Telephone: Salisbury (01722) 336262   extn. 4432 / 33
Out of hours answer machine in operation

Head and Neck Oncology Nursing

Head and Neck Oncology Nursing

Edited by

TRICIA FEBER

RGN, Cert. Cancer Nursing, Dip. Nursing Studies,
Macmillan Nurse Specialist, Head and Neck Oncology

Yorkshire Centre for Clinical Oncology, Cookridge Hospital,
Leeds

W

WHURR PUBLISHERS LTD
LONDON AND PHILADELPHIA

© 2000 Whurr Publishers Ltd
First published 2000 by
Whurr Publishers Ltd
19b Compton Terrace, London N1 2UN UK and
325 Chestnut Street, Philadelphia PA 19106 USA

British Library Cataloguing-in-Publication Data
A catalogue record for this book is available from the British Library.

ISBN 1 86156 147 4

Printed and bound in Great Britain by Athenæum Press Ltd, Gateshead, Tyne & Wear.

Contents

Section Two   87
Acute nursing management in head and neck cancer

Chapter 2.1   89
Airway management

Chapter 2.2   121
Mouth care

Chapter 2.3   147
Eating and swallowing problems

Dedication

This book is dedicated to the memory of my father-in-law, Derek Feber, my aunt, Marion Shaw, and my colleague Ann Haley, who died whilst it was being written. They were all people of tremendous courage who have unforgettably contributed to the world in their own very unique ways.

Contributors

Julie Batty BSc, SRD, Senior Oncology Dietitian, Yorkshire Centre for Clinical Oncology, Cookridge Hospital, Leeds

Graham Buckley, MSc, FRCS, Otolaryngologist-Head and Neck Surgeon, Leeds Teaching Hospitals NHS Trust

Jacqui Campbell, RGN, Cert. Cancer Nursing, Dip. Nursing Studies, Cert. Counselling, Macmillan Radiotherapy Clinical Nurse Specialist, Yorkshire Centre for Clinical Oncology, Cookridge Hospital, Leeds

Steven Edwards DCR(T), MSc Professional Studies, Cert. Counselling, Macmillan Radiographer Specialist, Yorkshire Centre for Clinical Oncology, Cookridge Hospital, Leeds

Tricia Feber, RGN, Cert. Cancer Nursing, Dip. Nursing Studies, Macmillan Nurse Specialist, Head and Neck Oncology, Cookridge Hospital, Leeds

Maria Harvey, BSc Hons Sp.Sci, MRCSLT, Senior Speech and Language Therapist, Leeds Teaching Hospitals NHS Trust

Claire Jones, RGN, DipNursing, ENT and Maxillofacial Ward and Outpatient Department Manager, York District Hospital

Debbie Robinson, MIOT, Senior Operating Department Assistant, York District Hospital

The publishers are grateful to the following companies for their support of this project:

Janssen-Cilag,
Harrogate

Merck Biomaterial,
Alton, Hampshire

Kapitex Healthcare,
Wetherby, West Yorks

Nycomed Amersham,
Birmingham.

Acknowledgements

My deepest gratitude to all the good friends and colleagues who have given me help and encouragement during the writing of this book. Especial thanks to the contributors, who have worked hard to produce some excellent chapters, as well as offering help and advice on my own chapters, and to Jane Garrud and Graham Buckley for their illustrations. Also especial thanks to Theresa Foxglove RGN, Dr Catherine Coyle, Consultant in Clinical Oncology, Dr Jane Adam, Consultant in Palliative Medicine, Dr Diana Dickson, Consultant Anaesthetist (Pain Specialist) and Alex Clarke, Clinical Psychologist, for their indispensable expert advice. Thanks to Mr David Mitchell, Consultant Maxillofacial Surgeon, for his knowledgeable and fatherly advice.

My grateful thanks to the sponsors: Nycomed Amersham, Kapitex Healthcare, Janssen-Cilag and Merck Biomaterials.

None of this book would have been written without the incredible support of my husband Ian, who has tolerated my unsociable behaviour, and learnt how to cook and shop. He is now a very good housewife and I recommend his cuisine. He has also provided excellent IT support, as well as paying the Internet bill. Our cat, Katkins, has helpfully provided company throughout the long hours on the computer, overseeing every word that has been typed.

Thank you everyone

Preface

This book aims to give nurses the evidence on which to plan effective care and services for people with head and neck cancer. In order to try and identify all the relevant information available, I undertook comprehensive searches on MEDLINE, CINAHL, CANCERLIT and PSYCHLIT, as well as hand-searching relevant journals and collecting information from relevant organizations, companies, expert professionals and colleagues. I have attempted to organize this information into a form which nurses will be able to use practically in their work. As I trawled the literature to write this book, it became evident that there are many gaps in our knowledge about nursing people with head and neck cancer, and that there is much work to be done to fill these gaps. The area is ripe for those keen to research and develop practice.

The unique role of the nurse in head and neck cancer is not only to ensure the patient's physical survival of the treatment modalities but also to give the patient the inner strength to survive. This is achieved through effective supportive interventions, as well as genuine care and attention, aimed towards promoting optimum health and wellbeing. However, it would be wrong to suggest that the nurse is solely responsible for the patient's recovery and wellbeing, as head and neck cancer patients require the full support of the whole multidisciplinary team in order to recover. It would also be wrong to suggest that patients are the passive recipients of care; they and their families are very active participants in their treatment and recovery. The key to successful rehabilitation is that this team works well together. This approach is very much reflected in this book, which contains contributions by the key members of such a team.

The following passage was written by a man who underwent a total laryngectomy for recurrence of a laryngeal cancer initially treated by radiotherapy.

Helping cancer patients is about *helping* — to confront, overcome and keep going.

When cancer has been diagnosed and communicated by the doctor/consultant to the patient, the next immediate steps should be a structured system of help, information and general support.

The individual reaction to being told that you have cancer is difficult to gauge. It can, I suppose, range from absolute terror and powerlessness to a determination to accept that one has to die some time, and make what one can of whatever remains of life. I suspect that, given the progress made in combating cancer, most people opt for the latter solution. Whatever end of this spectrum the individual purpose is, they need help and information, particularly before treatment/surgery — and after.

Nurses have an important role in helping individuals to face up to cancer. Doctors and consultants are OK for medical and technical information but nurses need to deal with the personal problems and these are important to the individual. The nurse should be a confidant and an enabler, listen and respond positively. She or he should also prompt even if it may not be taken up. This can be a formal or informal process, a mixture of the two works well, and a specialist nurse who is knowledgeable on head and neck cancer and able to coordinate and be readily available is essential. This pre-operation introduction was vital in obtaining information and advice about the operation and the recovery process.

The laryngectomy operation is not only the biggest operation that most people have experienced but is also an extremely traumatic event especially if the voice box is removed to say nothing of a hole in one's neck. At this time fears about the cancer tend to be replaced by the recovery process and the need to communicate. Small events like being taken for a bath on the morning after the operation by the nurse meant a lot in terms of coming out of the operation process.

The suggestion of using a 'Magic Slate', made by a former patient, and the writing up of a daily progress report to show to visitors are remembered as small things which helped to recover one's communication abilities and personality. Later on, a few days before discharge, the biggest psychological boost came on the occasion of the visit of the speech therapist. The discussion and the video presentation was a revelation of what could be done to produce speech, particularly the way that speech produced through valves retained the intonation of the natural speech which existed before the operation. Discharge from hospital was becoming a time for hope rather than despair. It was a time to face life again and it needed determination. Not everything was possible, lots of things were but in a restricted form. After a while, surprisingly enough, much more was possible than had been thought. The 'voice' and the need by other people to listen carefully became normal and even the stoma, whilst causing daily cleaning problems, was not the subject of too much curiosity.

It is seven years since cancer was first diagnosed. Looking back it is amazing to feel that in overcoming cancer I am actually getting more out of life than if I had not had this experience. That is due to the skill and dedication of the head and neck cancer doctors and nurses, the speech therapists, the ENT outpatients department and last but not least my colleagues and their partners and relatives who are members of the Leeds Laryngectomee Club, and its sub-section, the swimming club.

There is an old saying that you only get out of life what you put into it. In my case it is what collectively has been put in which has made the difference.

Jack Tinsdale 1998

Jack provides an ideal demonstration of how the team, including himself and fellow patients, can work to help with not only physical survival from cancer, but also the achievement of optimum psychosocial and emotional wellbeing. This book hopes to provide evidence and direction on which to base practice for achieving similarly good outcomes for all patients experiencing the challenges of head and neck cancer.

Tricia Feber 1999

Introduction

Nurses spend more time with patients than any other professional group, and their presence and care, in the therapeutic relationship which is developed, can contribute significantly to recovery. Due to the effects of their disease and medical treatment, head and neck cancer patients often need a high level of input from nurses; from 24-hour nursing care in hospital, to outpatient and community nursing support.

Sometimes it is very difficult for nurses to describe their therapeutic role to other professionals, as it is wide-ranging, encompassing many different roles including physical and technical care, advocacy, information-giving and health education, as well as complex psychological and emotional support. This seemingly vast toolbox of skills is often needed by nurses working in head and neck oncology. Frequently, these skills cannot easily be described in terms of concrete outcomes. Sometimes it is not what is said or done, but the very presence of the nurse that counts. Patients themselves value this tremendously. 'It's good to know that you're always there if we need help' is a common comment from families. Winnie the Pooh and Piglet provide a good demonstration of this phenomenon, as this extract from *The World of Pooh* shows:
"Piglet sidled up to Pooh from behind. 'Pooh' he whispered. 'Yes, Piglet?' 'Nothing,' said Piglet, taking Pooh's paw. 'I just wanted to be sure of you'" (Milne 1957, p. 261). However nurses must, to some extent at least, be able to know themselves, and to demonstrate to others, that their interventions are effective.

Most nurses work with the intention of delivering the best care possible to their patients. In order to achieve this, practice must be constantly refined and improved, in part by incorporating research evidence into practice. This book is intended to provide a package of evidence-based information that can be applied in the clinical setting to enhance support and care for people with head and neck cancer. Research provides answers for many questions of direct relevance to patient care (Cullum, 1998) such as:

- Which interventions are effective?
- Which interventions are ineffective or harmful?
- How do patients experiencing ill health feel about their health and their care?
- How can we organize care in a way that is efficient and benefits patients?

This book aims to try and answer some of these questions for nurses working in head and neck oncology and thus help in the improvement and refinement of care. It also aims to provide information from which standards can be set, in order that interventions can be measured. Chapter 3.1, which deals with quality of life, shows specifically how patient outcomes might be measured.

The philosophy

Nursing is the cornerstone of care for people with head and neck cancer and is concerned with the management of the actual and potential responses of patients to their cancer and its treatment. Nursing is also concerned with the rehabilitation of patients back into normal life.

In oncology more than anywhere, the limits of medicine are obvious and patients tend to seek help from other quarters. They often feel alienated from their bodies and can be tremendously traumatized, both psychologically and spiritually. People facing death and disfigurement are struggling to understand spiritual and emotional dimensions in themselves of which they were previously unaware. We therefore need a framework allowing sensitive, therapeutic healing of the whole person, their changed body function and image, the consequent changes in their environment, their experiences of the past and their beliefs for the future, in order to give effective help.

The underpinning philosophy of this book is taken from Rogers' *Science of Unitary Human Beings* (Rogers, 1990). This works on the following concepts:

- the purpose of nursing is to promote optimum health and well-being for all persons
- a person exists as an energy field which has infinite dimensions, including past, present and future
- the person's wholeness is irreducible and this wholeness continues into the environment which is an integral part of the person
- people are forever changing and moving onward, becoming more complex as they grow towards their potential
- there is no decline or decay of a person, only constant evolution and innovation
- the nurse acts through a mutual nurse–patient process, to facilitate the forward movement of the patient towards optimum health.

These concepts can be used to underpin creative, holistic nursing that will help the person to evolve through his or her cancer experience in a positive way.

How to use this book

This book is divided into five sections.

Section One provides a foundation for the rest of the book. The aim of this section is to give an understanding of head and neck cancer from its very origins in the social environment to its eventual diagnosis. The nurse should thus gain an understanding of the person with head and neck cancer, their past and present, and the environment in which they live. This section also provides information about the effective use of health promotion and sources of support within the community. This has very important implications for the patient's future care; nurses must be able to create an optimum and positive environment in the community for the patient and family.

Section Two addresses the acute physical aspects of nursing care for people during their cancer experience and aims to give detailed, up-to-date information. The chapters in this section strive to provide

comprehensively researched information and expert clinical guidance. The information covers all aspects of care, from acute to palliative and community settings. This section can be used to find
evidence-based strategies for nursing patients with head and neck
cancer.

Section Three addresses the psychosocial and emotional care of
people with head and neck cancer. The first chapter outlines the
major findings in quality of life studies over the last decade. It also
outlines tools that can be used to assess quality of life. The following
chapters on psychosocial and emotional problems and care aim to
help nurses to make sense of the complex effects of cancer, disfigurement and dysfunction on their patients and empower them to make
appropriate interventions.

Section Four acts as a specific guide to the different treatments. It
describes the surgical and oncological treatment modalities used in
head and neck cancer. This information can be used to inform and
develop practice, and also to help when giving patients accurate
information. As will be discussed in the first section of this book,
information given in an appropriate, supportive way helps to
empower patients and families to make informed, appropriate
choices for their future as well as to prepare them for the journey
ahead.

Section Five covers thyroid cancer in detail, as this topic requires
particular treatment and care, and did not fit easily into the other
sections.

Whilst nursing care must be evidence-based, the limitations of
research in describing the experience of the patient and the role of
the nurse is acknowledged. Van Dusen (1967) explained the difficulties in using research to describe the human experience:

> The person is translated into a fixed pre-determined protocol which is then data
> processable to arrive at some general statements of people. The protocol is fash-
> ioned to note certain given aspects, although many don't even do this reliably or
> validly. The individual's life, spread through time, and different under different
> circumstances, is the original complete protocol. In this form it can barely be
> read, let alone statistically processed. Moreover, it is a protocol in its own
> unique language, having a unique frame of reference.

For this reason, short vignettes of patient experiences, case examples and patients' comments are used throughout the book in order
to demonstrate more clearly exactly what patients experience. The

patients' names and personal details have been changed in order to maintain confidentiality. Although research is vital to provide a basis for our practice, we should never forget to include patients and their carers at every step as the concept underpinning clinical effectiveness is to improve the quality of life, and health, of the patient.

In summary, this book aims to provide a review of the literature and expert clinical guidance to act as a resource, an educational tool, and a sound evidence base for nurses, as well as to stimulate the development of excellence in nursing practice and care for people with head and neck cancer. Sadly, head and neck cancer care has not traditionally attracted the resources and research that more glamorous specialties enjoy. Nurses working in this area have an absolutely key role in ensuring that patients receive optimum, evidence-based care. This may involve both changing 'the way things are done' and fighting for resources. To quote a patient's view: "I have listened to nurses say 'I can't change anything, I'm just a nurse'. That is the equivalent of 'I was only following orders', a much used excuse at the Nuremberg trials" (Pembroke, 1998).

Section One
Core issues in head and neck cancer nursing

Chapter 1.1
Head and neck cancer: aetiology, epidemiology and health promotion

The person cannot be seen in isolation from their environment as they exist in a dynamic relationship with it.

Martha Rogers, 1990

Introduction

This chapter gives an overview of the causes, incidence and staging of head and neck cancer, including issues of delayed diagnosis and health promotion. As more than 90% of head and neck cancers are squamous cell carcinomas (Carew & Shah, 1998), and they therefore present the greatest health problems and issues for nurses working in this area, they will be the major focus of this chapter.

What is head and neck cancer?

Cancer is a complex group of diseases characterized by uncontrolled growth and spread of immature cells. Normal cells develop to a specific set of instructions in their DNA, which tells them what they are — for example, skin cells, mucosal cells, muscle cells or nerve cells — and their function (differentiation). They grow by cell division (mitosis). Their instructions also tell them to 'switch off' and stop dividing when they have fulfilled the body's need for new or replacement tissue. Due to complex genetic and cellular mechanisms still not fully understood, cancer cells have lost their 'switch off' mechanism and continue to grow beyond the body's need, invading and damaging adjacent tissues and organs. They also lose their ability to develop a specific identity and to function as mature cells.

3

Cancer cells that are easy to recognize under the microscope are referred to as well differentiated; cells that have lost their morphology are described as poorly differentiated or undifferentiated (anaplastic). Poorly differentiated cancer cells usually grow much faster and metastasize more easily than well-differentiated cells. This description of cancer biology is greatly oversimplified; for more detailed information, the reader is referred to the several good textbooks on the subject. The information here is based on the book by Souhami and Tobias (1995).

Cancers of the head and neck are themselves a complex group of cancers. They represent the sixth most common form of cancer worldwide (Carew & Shah, 1998). The International Classification of Diseases system defines them as occurring at the following sites: lip, tongue, floor of mouth, gum, other oral cavity sites, salivary glands, oropharynx, nasopharynx, hypopharynx, larynx, nose and sinuses, ear and thyroid.

The cells most commonly involved in head and neck cancer are squamous epithelial cells (Souhami & Tobias, 1995). These are the cells that line the upper respiratory and gastrointestinal tract. Tumours arising from the epithelium are called carcinomas, and therefore the most common malignant tumours in the head and neck are *squamous cell carcinomas*. A variant of squamous cell carcinoma, *lymphoepithelial carcinoma*, commonly arises in the lymphoid tissue of the nasopharynx and Waldeyer's ring (Fletcher, 1995). *Adenocarcinomas* arise from glandular tissue and are the predominant type in the salivary glands and thyroid gland. Glandular tissue is distributed throughout the head and neck epithelium and so adenocarcinoma can be found at most sites. Other carcinomas occurring in the head and neck are: *mucoepidermoid carcinoma, acinic cell carcinoma, adenoid cystic carcinoma* and *pleomorphic adenoma*. These are all seromucinous glandular cells arising from the mucous membrane and salivary glands. They occur much less frequently than squamous cell carcinomas, and their aetiology is uncertain. *Lymphomas* may occur in the cervical lymph nodes as well as other sites. They are usually treated by radiotherapy or chemotherapy. *Connective tissue sarcomas* are uncommon tumours that occur at most head and neck sites. Another group of carcinomas, the *thyroid carcinomas*, arise from follicular, papillary or medullary thyroid cells and are discussed separately in Chapter 5.1. Malignant head and neck tumours are usually primary but metastases from other sites like breast, kidney and prostate also occur occasionally.

Precancerous conditions

Before cells become malignant they undergo several changes which make their appearance abnormal (dysplastic). The degree of dysplasia present can be classified as mild, moderate or severe. Precancerous lesions are most commonly identified in the oral mucosa or on the vocal cords; both sites where the symptoms of cancer alert the patient and healthcare professional early. Precancerous lesions are seen as leukoplakia (a whitish patch) or erythroplakia (a bright red patch) (Fletcher, 1995). These lesions are usually removed by an excisional biopsy. Causes of the precancerous condition should be identified and education given to the patient about cause and prevention. The condition will often resolve if the patient stops smoking, or if dietary deficiencies are corrected. It is therefore vital that nurses working in clinics where precancerous conditions are diagnosed are skilled in helping patients to review their lifestyle and behaviours and helping them to create new, more healthy life patterns for the future.

There is a fine line between diagnosing severe dysplasia and carcinoma in situ. Carcinoma in situ describes a situation where dysplastic cells encompass the full thickness of the epithelial layer (Fletcher, 1995).

When a pathologist examines a tumour sample under the microscope, he/she can collect information about where the cancer originates from, how differentiated the cells are, and how they are behaving in terms of aggressive invasion (see Table 1.1.1). This information is vitally important to the surgical and medical team when choosing the optimum treatment regime.

Table 1.1.1: Histopathological grading (UICC, 1997)

GX	Grade of differentiation cannot be assessed
G1	Well differentiated
G2	Moderately differentiated
G3	Poorly differentiated
G4	Undifferentiated

Tumour stage

Staging of tumours is used to make treatment decisions, predict prognosis and to facilitate comparison of treatment between different centres. The TNM system is standard for carcinomas (UICC,

1997). The 'T' stage refers to the primary tumour and ranges from T1 to T4 (see Table 1.1.2). It is based on maximum surface diameter for some sites (e.g. oral cavity) and extent of anatomical invasion at others (e.g. larynx). It is becoming increasingly apparent that the tumour volume or depth of invasion may be more important predictors of prognosis, and attempts to measure these features radiologically are being made in some centres. Treatment will depend on the size and site of the tumour. As a general rule in head and neck cancer, T1 and T2 tumours are often treated with single-modality therapy consisting of radiotherapy or surgery, with local control rates that are equivalent at most sites. The choice of treatment depends on the anticipated functional outcome and the morbidity of the treatment. The standard treatment of advanced tumours is multimodality therapy (Carew & Shah, 1998). Chances of survival decrease the more advanced a cancer is. For more information on treatment modalities see Section Four.

Table 1.1.2: Primary tumour stage for lip and oral cavity carcinoma (UICC, 1997) (T staging varies for each site)

TX	Primary tumour cannot be assessed
T0	No evidence of primary tumour
Tis	Carcinoma in situ
T1	Tumour 2 cm or less in greatest dimension
T2	Tumour more than 2 cm but not more than 4 cm in greatest dimension
T3	Tumour more than 4 cm in greatest dimension
T4	Tumour invades adjacent structures

Nodal stage

Cancer cells may break off from the original tumour and travel in the bloodstream or lymphatic system to other parts of the body where they lodge in a small vessel and continue to divide, invading local structures. These new tumours are called secondaries or metastases. In head and neck cancer, most metastasizing cells are caught in the lymphatic nodes in the neck. Many patients present with lumps in the neck. The 'N' in TNM stands for node, and regional lymph node involvement is staged from 1 to 3 (see Table 1.1.3). This nodal stage is also an important determinant of treatment options and prognosis. The likelihood of survival is more closely related to the

N-stage than the T-stage. Most patients with nodal involvement will usually have surgery to remove the cervical nodes, if they are fit to undergo surgery (see Chapter 4.1). They will also require postoperative irradiation of the neck.

Table 1.1.3: Regional lymph node staging (UICC, 1997)

NX	Regional lymph nodes cannot be assessed
N0	No regional lymph node metastasis
N1	Metastasis in a single ipsilateral lymph node, 3 cm or less in greatest dimension
N2a	Metastasis in a single ipsilateral lymph node, more than 3 cm but not more than 6 cm in greatest dimension
N2b	Metastasis in multiple ipsilateral lymph nodes, none more than 6 cm in greatest dimension
N2c	Metastasis in bilateral or contralateral lymph nodes, none more than 6 cm in greatest dimension
N3	Metastasis in a lymph node more than 6 cm in greatest dimension

Distant metastases

Finally, the 'M' in TNM stands for distant metastases (Table 1.1.4). Because the lymphatic nodes in the neck do such an excellent job of filtering out metastatic cells, it is relatively rare to see a head and neck cancer cause distant metastases. The presence of distant metastases precludes curative treatment for most tumour sites. However, with improving treatment to the primary tumour, increasing numbers of patients now live long enough to develop distant metastases, which are usually in the lungs. The next most common site is the bones, and a few patients may develop liver metastases. Other possible sites are skin, brain and bone marrow.

Table 1.1.4: Distant metastases (UICC, 1997)

MX	Presence of distant metastasis cannot be assessed
M0	No distant metastasis
M1	Distant metastasis

Prognosis

Prognosis in head and neck cancer depends very much on tumour site and stage, as well as the nodal status. To give an example, the overall 5-year survival rate for laryngeal cancer is as follows: stage 1 or 2 disease 5-year survival rates range from 78% to 91%, whilst stage 3 and 4 rates range from 42% to 67% (Carew & Shah, 1998). However, survival is most profoundly affected by the nodal status of the patient; patients with N0 disease have 5-year survival rates of 72.1% to 87.5% even with advanced stage laryngeal tumours. In contrast, patients with nodal disease have a 5-year survival of 46.2% for all T stages (Carew & Shah, 1998). Prognosis also, unfortunately, depends on where in the world the affected individual lives and what access they have to healthcare. Even within the UK there are regional variations in prognosis of cancer depending on whether the patient has access to a site-specialist cancer treatment team (Calman & Hine, 1994).

Incidence

The most recent figures on incidence of head and neck cancer in the UK at the time of writing are shown in Figure 1.1.1. Although head and neck cancer accounted for only 3.8% of all female malignancies and 1.6% of all male malignancies (Office for National Statistics, 1997), it is such a debilitating, disfiguring disease with high costs in terms of treatment and disease morbidity, that it should be classified as a major cancer site (Yuska, 1989).

Signs and symptoms

The symptoms of head and neck cancer are often insidious, and similar to symptoms experienced from minor ailments: blocked nose, sore throat, hoarse voice, earache, mouth ulcers, swollen lymph glands. These are commonly interpreted as minor infections and patients may treat themselves with homemade remedies, or remedies from the pharmacist. The general practitioner sees hundreds of patients with similar symptoms who do not have head and neck cancer and it is easy to see how a cancer diagnosis might be missed in the early stages of the disease. However, any symptom persisting for more than 2 weeks should be investigated (Boyle et al, 1995).

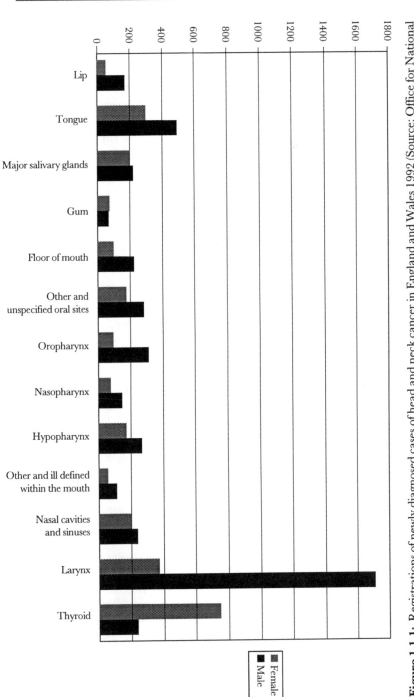

Figure 1.1.1: Registrations of newly diagnosed cases of head and neck cancer in England and Wales 1992 (Source: Office for National Statistics, 1998)

Causes

Who are the high-risk individuals?

The following information is relevant mainly to the common, squamous cell carcinomas. The salivary gland and thyroid cancers have a different pathology and are therefore exceptions to this group. Salivary gland cancer is a rare disease with a largely unknown origin. There is limited evidence to suggest that radiation and ultraviolet exposure may be implicated as a causative factor (Spitz et al, 1988). Tobacco and alcohol use are unrelated to salivary gland cancer (Muscat & Wynder, 1998). Risk factors for thyroid cancer are discussed in Chapter 5.1

Data from several studies on squamous cell carcinoma of the head and neck serve to confirm that high-risk patients have the following characteristics:

- male, average age 65
- disadvantaged socioeconomic groups
- history of occupational exposure to dust, fumes or chemicals
- use of tobacco and alcohol
- a low level of awareness of the serious nature of the symptoms
- presentation with advanced tumours.

Tobacco use

Tobacco use is the primary risk factor for squamous cell carcinoma. There are several carcinogenic agents in tobacco smoke: polycyclic aromatic hydrocarbons, benzo[a]pyronene, nitrosamines, vinyl chloride, polonium 210, nickel and cadmium (Wynder & Hoffman, 1982). Linear dose response effects of tobacco as a carcinogen have been consistently demonstrated in studies (Cohen et al, 1971; Rothman et al, 1980; Bofetta et al, 1992). Relative risk, disease onset and presentation will depend on the daily amount consumed, the duration of the habit and the types and manner in which tobacco is used (Bofetta et al, 1992). Tobacco is most commonly used by smoking cigarettes and may also be used via cigars, pipes, snuff and chewing. There is an association between the site of tobacco placement and the site of tumour occurrence. For example, cigarette smokers tend to have tumours of the larynx and lung, whereas pipe smokers have lip and oral cavity tumours. Snuff users have an increased risk of cheek and gum malignancies. In Asia, betel-nut quid chewing (areca, palm seed, shell or slaked lime, and tobacco rolled in betel leaf) has been shown to cause cheek, gum and oral cavity cancers (Winn et al, 1981; World Health Organization, 1984; US Department of Health and Human Services, 1986). In the Sudan, people chew a local tobacco species with high levels of nicotine and nornicotine ground into a paste with sodium bicarbonate and water. This is called *toombak* and is kept in the oral cavity for several hours. This causes tumours at the site of contact with the oral mucosa (Idris et al, 1994).

It is therefore important that nurses are conversant with nicotine addiction and smoking cessation strategies and this subject is dealt with in depth in Chapter 1.3.

Alcohol use

Alcohol is a solvent and an irritant. It has been shown to shut off DNA synthesis, thus creating a vulnerable cellular environment for invasion of carcinogens (Hsu & Furlong, 1991). Excessive consumption has been shown to increase the risk of oral cancer (Blot et al, 1998), with concomitant tobacco and alcohol consumption increasing the risk by 44.5% (Craddock, 1993). There is a high incidence of oral cancer in regions where alcohol consumption is high (Johnson & Warnakulasuriya, 1993), and the incidence of cancer of the head and neck is four times higher in male alcoholics than in the general population (Schmidt & Popham, 1981). Use of alcohol-based mouthwashes has also been implicated in oral cancers, although we cannot be sure whether they contributed to cancer initiation, or were being used to relieve symptoms (Blot et al, 1983).

Helping people with alcohol problems is discussed in Chapter 1.3.

Occupation

There is evidence that occupational exposures to high levels of dusts (wood, coal, textiles, cement, metals) and chemicals are implicated in squamous cell head and neck cancer (Goldbold & Tompkins, 1979; Maier et al, 1991). A study in Leeds showed that 69% of patients with head and neck cancer had occupations that involved exposure to dust, chemicals or fumes, the most common being textiles, the motor trade (including lorry driving), the building trade, mining and engineering (Feber et al, 1997).

There is some evidence that certain occupations expose individuals to agents which may increase the risk of developing salivary gland cancer. Zheng et al (1996) found that occupational exposure to silica dust was linked to a 2.5-fold increased risk of salivary gland cancer. Swanson & Burns (1997) found significantly elevated odds ratios for women who worked as hairdressers and recommend research to assess dyes and sprays that may act as inhaled carcinogens. Horn-Ross et al (1997) found increased risk in people with occupational exposure to X-rays, nickel compounds/alloys, and those working in the rubber industry.

Diet and nutrition

Case control analyses in the literature have indicated that diets high in fruits and vegetables and vitamins A and C may protect against oral cancer. In a meta-analysis of the literature, the Department of Health concludes that there is limited, moderately consistent evidence that higher intakes of fruits and vegetables are associated with reduced risk of laryngeal cancer, weakly consistent evidence that high fruit consumption is associated with reduced risk of oropharyngeal cancer, and inconsistent evidence that high vegetable consumption is associated with reduced risk of oropharyngeal cancer (Department of Health, 1998). Dietary sources of vitamins A and C are shown in Table 1.1.5.

Deficiency of vitamin A (retinol) in particular is associated with an increased risk of head and neck cancer (Johnson & Warnakula-suriya, 1993). Deficiency and excess of retinol cause marked changes in epithelial tissues, and epithelial cells are believed to be one of the major targets for the physiological action of retinol in vertebrates (Lotan et al, 1991). Low levels of retinol leave the cell vulnerable to invasion by oncogenes and eventually an abnormality in DNA structure occurs, leading to rapid cellular replication. The DNA appears to lose its ability to repair and then attempts to correct the abnormal growth process with gross replication of oncogenic infused cells. Administration of retinoid therapy has been shown to reverse this process and trials are being carried out to assess its value in chemo-prevention of precancerous conditions (Lippman & Spitz, 1991).

Chinese salted fish consumption, particularly during childhood, is consistently associated with a higher risk of nasopharyngeal cancer in case control studies (Department of Health, 1998).

Iron deficiency produces marked atrophy of the oral mucosa and this atrophy may make cells susceptible to entry by carcinogens

Table 1.1.5: Vitamins A, C and iron

Nutrient	Sources	Function
Vitamin A (retinol)	Dairy produce, eggs, margarine, dark green vegetables, yellow vegetables; e.g. carrots, oranges, apricots, peaches, red peppers, spinach, parsley, watercress, broccoli	Maintains skin, eyes, hair, nails, mucous membranes, the immune system
Vitamin C (ascorbic acid)	Found in virtually all fresh fruit and vegetables. Deteriorates during cooking and over time. Good sources: leafy vegetables, tomatoes, potatoes, strawberries, blackcurrants, oranges, kiwi fruit	Maintains the immune system, speeds tissue repair, and is important for the absorption of iron
Iron	Meat, fish, pulses, grains, nuts, seeds, dark green leafy vegetables, dried fruit, egg yolk	Important in the manufacture of red blood cells

(Lamey, 1993). It is known that people with Plummer–Vinson syndrome, an iron deficiency anaemia, have an increased risk for cancers of the tongue, hypopharynx and oesophagus (Schleper, 1989).

Many studies have shown that poverty is linked to poor diet, and whilst it is appropriate that nurses give information on improving diet, the issue of poverty must be addressed, and work done with community groups and councils to explore ways of accessing deprived communities to affordable supplies of fresh food.

Green tea is the most widely consumed beverage in the world, next to water, and is especially popular in the Far East. A major constituent of green tea is epigallocatechin-3-gallate (EGCG), which has demonstrated chemopreventive activity in a variety of cancers (Yang & Wang, 1993). Khafif et al (1998) demonstrated that EGCG inhibited the growth of premalignant and malignant oral squamous carcinoma cells in vitro. They recommend further investigation for the potential of green tea in oral cancer chemoprevention trials.

Genetic factors

Whilst some cancers have been shown to be hereditary (for example breast and colorectal cancers), there is no evidence to suggest that head and neck cancers are hereditary, with the exception of medullary thyroid carcinomas (see Chapter 5.1). There is, however, increasing evidence that certain individuals may have a genetic predisposition to be more susceptible to carcinogens than others.

Viral causes

There is evidence that some viruses can initiate head and neck cancer. Viruses commonly implicated are the Epstein–Barr virus, human papilloma virus and herpes simplex virus (Shillitoe, 1987). The viruses are thought to activate cellular gene types and thus provoke a malignant disorder in the cellular pathway. Nasopharyngeal cancer is particularly associated with the Epstein–Barr virus and there is a high incidence in areas where Epstein–Barr virus is prevalent; South-east China, the Philippines, Malaysia, Greenland, North Africa and the Mediterranean Basin (Fletcher, 1995).

Immunity and cancer

The immune system is thought to be responsible for the destruction of abnormal cells occurring in the body throughout our lives. Therefore a healthy immune system will reduce the chances of a cancer developing. Poor immune function will result from several of the above factors (poor nutrition, use of tobacco and alcohol). People who are immunosuppressed, for example transplant patients, have been shown to have increased incidence of cancer (Schleper, 1989). Human immunodeficiency virus (HIV) has been shown to accelerate the development of head and neck cancer in patients with significant risk factors (tobacco and alcohol use); HIV also had a detrimental effect on cure rates (Singh et al, 1996). There is also some interesting research on the negative effect of stress on the immune system, showing signs of an interrelationship between the mind and body in the fight against cancer (Lewis et al, 1994). This is important information; evidence shows that psychological interventions to support people with cancer may have a positive effect on prognosis and outcomes of the disease.

General health

Funk et al (1997) compared the general health status of patients recently diagnosed with head and neck cancer with age-matched US population normative data. They found that the newly diagnosed patients had significantly worse overall general health profiles than the general population. This was true for both physical and mental functioning. Prout et al (1990) similarly found that 73% of a sample of 124 head and neck cancer patients reported using medical care regularly prior to their diagnosis. A survey of 188 head and neck cancer patients in Leeds (Feber et al, 1997) found that 54% of the sample reported existing health problems: 41% had lung disease (chronic obstructive airways disease, asthma, emphysema), 32% reported heart disease and 23% reported vascular disease. This information points to the fact that this group do not experience optimum wellbeing throughout their lives and nurses may already be in regular contact with them for other reasons.

Social factors

The Black Report highlighted the evidence that poverty causes ill health in the 1980s, but the government in power at the time did everything it could to suppress this fact and blame the 'victims'. People at risk of head and neck cancer fall very much into this group of vulnerable people. The rates of these smoking-related cancers have been shown to be consistently higher in deprived areas. They are particularly high in the most deprived areas (Yorkshire Cancer Organization, 1994). Patients are usually in the over-65 age group, and smoking and drinking are elements of value systems that have deep social meaning for them. People at risk of head and neck cancer are among the most vulnerable groups of society: the poor, homeless, elderly, immigrants, chronically sick and disabled. Nurses must not, therefore, focus on head and neck cancer as a disease 'caused by tobacco or alcohol'. People with head and neck cancer must be seen from a holistic point of view; head and neck cancer is often a result of a variety of stressors in the environment and cultural and societal problems may be implicated just as much as tobacco use. These factors will also continue to affect the diagnosis and outcomes of the disease.

Late diagnosis

Studies on referral patterns and diagnosis in head and neck cancer suggest that patients are likely to delay seeking medical advice (Scully et al, 1986; Schnetler, 1992; Kowalski et al, 1994). This is shown to be due to patient ignorance and neglect of symptoms and also to misdiagnosis by professionals. Kowalski et al (1994) showed that two of the most important consequences of advanced-stage presentation were a conspicuous increase in treatment costs and a longer hospital stay. Advanced head and neck cancer is significantly more expensive to treat, needing lengthy surgery, intensive care and hospital stays. Radical radiotherapy is also lengthy and expensive. Even patients requiring only palliative care tend to have significant problems requiring a high input from community nursing services and often prolonged inpatient palliative care (hospice or nursing home). Although these patients do not account for a large proportion of cancers, they do account for a large drain on health resources and severe disability if they present late rather than early.

Delay is therefore a significant problem (Scully et al, 1986). However, most of the literature focuses on the professional's role in delay, rather than factors contributing to the patient's role in delay. The data shows that patients have very low levels of awareness of head and neck cancer, and that this may be a major contributing factor to presenting with advanced head and neck cancer. There was also a low level of awareness factor in some healthcare professionals, but professional delay in referral was much less significant than patient delay in seeking help. If any significant improvements in early diagnosis are to be made, it is vital that the issue of patient delay is addressed.

Whilst public awareness of breast cancer, skin cancer and lung cancer is now quite good due to extensive media publicity, knowledge about head and neck cancer is extremely low. Research from the Health Education Authority shows that most people do not know that smoking and drinking account for 90% of all cases of oral cancer in the UK. Out of nearly 2,000 adults questioned, half had never heard of oral cancer, a quarter incorrectly identified car exhaust fumes as a risk factor, and one in 10 thought dental fillings were implicated. Only one in five identified alcohol with oral cancer (Health Education Authority, 1996a). We can therefore assume that knowledge about other head and neck cancers is also low; oral cancer is the only site that has been reported in the literature.

In a survey of 188 patients in Leeds, patients' levels of awareness of their cancer symptoms were explored. They had all experienced classic signs and symptoms of head and neck cancer, but there was a low awareness of the warning signs. Only 4.2% connected their symptoms with cancer (see Table 1.1.6). This lack of awareness meant that the average delay for first seeking help was 16 weeks. Fifty-seven patients (29.8%) experienced delays in diagnosis of more than 5 weeks, with half of these (29 patients) not seeking help for 9 weeks to 6 months. This is a typical picture, corroborated by several studies (Horowitz et al, 1996).

Table 1.1.6: Patients' perceptions of their cancer symptoms

Nothing to worry about	23.9%
Infection	14.1%
Sore throat	9.2%
Other minor ailment	32.4%
Abscess	2.8%
Caused by dental treatment	2.1%
Mouth ulcer	11.3%
Cancer	4.2%

Health promotion

Head and neck cancer is not a high-profile disease in terms of preventive activity. It is not an issue central to the mass media prevention campaigns, nor a visible component of preventive programmes for tobacco and alcohol related diseases (Izquierdo & Rozier, 1996). An expert panel in the United States considered that high on the list of priorities for goals in oral and dental health should be investigations of public health solutions for low prevalence but high morbidity and mortality disease such as oral cancer (Downer, 1993). Nurses are ideally placed to develop expertise in health promotion, because of their skills and closeness to their clients. However, health promotion can become a 'victim blaming' activity in which people are considered to be culpable for their own problems and individuals are made responsible for their own health, rather than government and society. Health promotion strategy should understand its clients as social beings and move away from 'victim blaming' to empowerment and facilitation (Buxton, 1996).

Screening

The purpose of screening is to interrupt the natural history of the disease by identifying it at its early asymptomatic stage and thus prevent its progression to advanced disease and death (Chamberlain, 1993).

Screening for head and neck cancer is almost entirely discussed in the dental literature. However, patients are much more likely to present to their general practitioner (GP) with their initial cancer symptoms (Yellowitz & Goodman, 1995). Ninety-two per cent of patients in the Leeds survey presented to the GP with their initial cancer symptoms. Of the 62 patients (17%) who had never seen a dentist, 76% had regular contact with their GP. Prout et al (1990) found that of a sample of 124 patients, 73% had been seeing their GP regularly in the 24 months prior to their diagnosis, whilst only 19% reported regular dental visits. Seventy-seven percent of Prout et al's sample were late-stage cases and they conclude that systematic examinations for oral cancer had not occurred and that the visits to their healthcare provider represented missed opportunities for early detection. Thus, although dentists may be the ideal professional to perform oral examinations, early detection falls largely to GPs and practice nurses, who do not have a high level of awareness.

Delay in referral by the healthcare professional to the head and neck cancer service occurred in several studies, showing a possible low level of awareness in some professionals. Yellowitz et al (1992) found that 18% of physicians screened for oral cancer, against 83.4% of dentists. There was a statistically significant relationship between physicians' perceived lack of training, and perceived lack of oral cancer knowledge, and their infrequent performance of an oral examination. There is no literature on healthcare professionals' knowledge of other (non-oral) head and neck cancers, which is a matter for concern because laryngeal cancers account for the greatest percentage of head and neck cancers. It is important that these are not ignored by dentists, doctors and nurses screening high-risk patients, and that public awareness of all head and neck cancers is addressed.

Educational programmes for the primary healthcare team have been shown to be successful in breast cancer, where a low-cost seminar programme demonstrated an increase in professionals' knowledge about breast cancer and screening (Reding et al, 1995). An educational programme to promote screening for head and neck cancer was targeted to providers of care for high-risk patients at seven inner city healthcare sites in Boston, USA. This resulted in a large increase in screening for these cancers (Prout et al, 1992). In a later evaluation of this screening, the authors conclude that primary care-based screening strategies can reach large numbers of at-risk individuals in busy inner city practice settings and that a focused approach to head and neck cancer screening in high-risk individuals is a valuable activity (Prout et al, 1997).

In a demonstration project for the American Cancer Society, education representatives made 1-hour visits to family physician surgeries to provide training to the whole team. This resulted in a 35% increase in the adoption of cancer prevention and screening procedures in the surgeries (Williams et al, 1994). These simple procedures could be performed easily and quickly on patients in high-risk groups. They could form part of the routine annual health checks in the elderly. An audit of these activities by GPs and practice nurses may be indicated, as well as further study on raising the primary healthcare team's awareness. Another group of healthcare professionals who may be useful in education and screening are mental health professionals working within addiction, who most frequently come into contact with those very high-risk patients who both smoke and drink.

What are the costs of screening?

Screening for head and neck cancer does not require expensive equipment or laboratory tests, as breast, cervical and prostate screening do — it is a visual and manual examination, and therefore the main cost is in professionals' time. Unless a suspicious symptom is identified, there is no waiting for results of tests for the patient, thus no potential psychological costs.

Primary prevention

The most common primary prevention programmes are those targeted at reducing smoking and alcohol consumption. Safe sun practices are also important as solar damage can contribute to squamous cell carcinoma and melanoma of the head and neck. Giving information about dietary factors in cancer prevention is important, as head and neck cancer has been associated with low consumption of fresh fruit and vegetables. Primary prevention can be carried out in schools, the workplace and the community, but is a long-term investment in health for the future. Employers must realize that by introducing effective worksite cancer prevention and screening programmes they cannot only fulfil their social responsibility, but also achieve reductions in healthcare costs (Kurtz et al, 1994). No-smoking policies can be implemented in the workplace, along with such actions as providing fresh fruit in vending machines and canteens. Educational material in the workplace has been shown to be effective; a brief educational intervention on breast cancer to women employees at diverse worksites showed positive results for the entire group of women who participated — raised awareness of screening importance and increased discussions of breast cancer at work (Kurtz et al, 1994). Similar material on head and neck cancer should be targeted at workplaces of high-risk groups; occupational health nurses would play a key role here. As the majority of people are over 65 when head and neck cancer is diagnosed, the workplace is not the best place to target with health promotion for immediate results, but it can be seen as an investment for the future.

Whilst primary prevention may have an important role to play, low income and poverty act as key health hazards, increasing exposure to other health hazards such as poor housing, pollution and poor social support networks. Evidence suggests that social and material circum-stances influence health to a greater extent than health knowledge and attitudes, and most evaluations of projects that attempt to change health behaviours show that health advice has only a minor influence. Health promotion activities that fail to address economic disadvantage may increase inequalities by improving the health of high-income groups and doing little to change the health of low-income groups (Blackburn, 1994). As discussed earlier in this chapter, smoking and drinking in this group are elements of value systems that have deep social meaning. Within these cultural systems, adoption of 'healthy lifestyles' is very unlikely, and health promotion activities of this kind are likely to be ineffective (Davison, 1994). Indeed, they are likely to cause more harm than good by fostering guilt and low self-esteem, contra-indicators to change (Buchmann, 1997). Primary prevention does not, therefore, appear to be an effective way of tackling head and neck cancer; this ideology of 'individual responsibility' tends to obscure relevant societal and larger contextual realities (Rush, 1997). Nurses therefore need to explore additional, less traditional strategies.

Raising awareness: empowerment in the community

People with head and neck cancer are generally the precontemplaters in the Model of Change (Prochaska & de Clemente, 1985). (For more information on the stages of the Model of Change see Chapter 1.3.) Precontemplaters are people who have no desire whatsoever to change their current behaviours and cannot be coerced into contemplating changing their damaging addictions. However, harm minimization strategies can be used to support them. Nurses need to explore ways in which high-risk groups can be empowered to detect head and neck cancer at an early stage and seek the appropriate help (harm minimization) that is available in the form of expert head and neck oncology teams within cancer centres (Calman & Hine, 1994). If an individual is empowered to have his or her head and neck cancer diagnosed and treated early and successfully, their feeling of self-efficacy may then ultimately motivate them to adopt a more healthy lifestyle.

For initiatives to have real impact, there is a need to develop multi-agency and multi-sectoral alliances (Buxton, 1996). Links with community groups, trade unions, schools, etc., may prove very successful. Involving the community and the client in health promotion planning is central to success, and the client should be allowed to define his or her own needs (Peckham & Winters, 1996). One of the main problems identified in public health projects is 'short-termism'. Short-termism presents a number of difficulties in community development projects: insufficient time to develop credibility in the community, inability to plan for long-term gains, inadequate time to demonstrate health outcomes and inadequate building of infrastructures to maintain activity in the community when the project ends. The difficulty of building strong intersectoral and inter-agency links is a further issue, arising from the predominance of the medical model and the structural restrictiveness of the NHS (Peckham & Winters, 1996). Community-based approaches to public health are even more marginalized and frequently seen as a luxury, with the money put into incentives for numbers in screening programmes for GPs.

Targeting awareness campaigns

In the Leeds study, 81% of the sample were not working — 20% on long-term sick leave, 73% retired. Those in the retired group experienced the longest delays in presenting for help (average 20 weeks). Older people often delay seeking treatment and are less likely than younger age groups to participate in screening and self-examination practices (Joseph, 1988). The reasons for this have been determined as: inadequate knowledge about cancer, low economic status and fear of cancer and its treatment (Weinrich & Weinrich, 1986). This information is important for planning head and neck cancer awareness programmes for this group.

One method of raising awareness could be to supply information specific to head and neck cancer to areas frequented by these patients, such as the Post Office (collection of benefits and pensions), social service offices and GP surgeries. In Leeds, 53% of patients attended the Working Men's Club regularly — would it be viable to use a head and neck cancer education programme in these areas? There is no doubt that health promotion for this group has to be community-based and that we need to understand people's health and life beliefs and values for it to have any effect. Further exploration is needed in the community, perhaps with the use of client focus groups. An innovative and effective awareness programme will incorporate the 'users' of the service in a creative way.

Ethnic minorities

The Asian populations in the UK are known to be at risk from head and neck cancer due to betel-quid chewing. The Bangladeshi community is particularly vulnerable (Bedi, 1996). Betel-quid chewing is seen as a sign of entering adulthood with those who do not chew being seen as deviant by the community. The sale of betel-quid is commonplace in these communities and there is very little perception of it as a health risk (Bedi, 1996). People within ethnic minorities are also vulnerable because of poor education, low levels of knowledge about cancer, low incomes and poor access to healthcare. There is also a language barrier for many elderly people from these groups. They therefore also require carefully designed community programmes to raise awareness of health risks and symptoms, and to educate them about the curability of cancer — many Asians consider cancer to be a death sentence and a taboo, and may be too frightened to seek help.

Summary

The literature review in this section demonstrates the need for inter-disciplinary and interprofessional healthcare delivery approaches aimed at reducing head and neck cancer mortality, improving quality of life and reducing healthcare costs. Consideration should be given to including head and neck cancer screening in routine health checks for the elderly, as well as low-cost education programmes for primary healthcare teams, in the workplace and in the community. Current resources available for use in raising awareness of head and neck cancer are shown in Table 1.1.7.

However, nurses should examine not only the motives of the client, but also their own motives in health promotion. Are professional agendas and screening quotas being chased, with clients coerced to conform? Or are clients being empowered to question the roots of their disease-causing poverty and their tobacco addiction? Vast amounts of NHS research monies may be poured into treating people with tobacco-related disease once it is too late, rather than

Table 1.1.7: Head and neck cancer awareness literature

Literature	Source
Tell me about Mouth Cancer	British Dental Health Foundation Eastlands Court St Peter's Road Rugby CV21 3QP Tel: 01788 546365 www.dentalhealth.org.uk
Mouth Cancer. How to Reduce Your Risk	Cancer Research Campaign Education Department 10 Cambridge Terrace London NW1 4JL
Oral Cancer — Prevent It! (for professionals) Mouth Cancer — Prevent It! (for the public: English and Bengali)	Oral Health and Ethnicity Unit Leeds Dental Institute Clarendon Way Leeds LS2 9LU (or contact your local oral and maxillofacial department to find out what information they provide)

tackling the source of the problem — poverty and the power of the tobacco companies to advertise and sell a lethal and addictive substance to the young. One million of today's children will die in middle age if current smoking trends continue (Imperial Cancer Research Fund, 1994).

A health promotion strategy should empower clients to recognize symptoms and seek help quickly, but this will be ineffective if the professionals whose help is sought are themselves unaware of the disease and treatment. Therefore an innovative, two-pronged strategy needs developing, to address effective empowerment for patients and health professionals alike.

All this information paints a picture of an extremely vulnerable population at risk of head and neck cancer. It must be remembered that there are also notable exceptions to the rule, and that some individuals who have never abused tobacco and alcohol will also unfortunately present with head and neck cancer. However, this chapter has focused on the majority, who exist in an environment of deprivation that causes stress and anxiety, which in turn affects physiological, psychological and social functioning. Tobacco and alcohol are used to cope with these stressors and have become an important part of their culture. Occupations tend to involve exposure to carcinogens. Poor education leads to a low level of awareness and poor use of healthcare services. Head and neck cancer may develop as a direct result of this environment.

People in poor socioeconomic environments and people from ethnic minorities are particularly vulnerable to poor health, but paradoxically they may have poor access to healthcare and poor knowledge of disease prevention (Aday, 1993). The links between low income and poor health are well documented, as well as the links with increased use of drugs (Rachlis & Kusner, 1989; Aday, 1993). In addition, people with head and neck cancer are mainly elderly, and are thus also more vulnerable because they experience a decrease in physical abilities at a time when they have a reduced income and fewer social support resources. Nurses need to be very aware of their patients' past life patterns and environment, in order to plan support, give health education and to be aware of the high risk for poor treatment tolerance and morbidity in this group, considering that they will be undergoing major surgery and radiotherapy in many cases.

It is also important that nurses are aware of the complex social issues surrounding head and neck cancer. The current ideology in healthcare is of 'individual responsibility' and it is very easy to 'blame' head and neck cancer patients for abusing their bodies. However, head and neck cancer — along with many other cancers — is a result of social inequality, class and political factors. So this is a disease whose causes go well beyond individual responsibility, and it is important that the inextricable roles of culture, society and the environment are acknowledged.

Chapter 1.2
Cancer diagnosis and the pre-treatment phase

Introduction

The patient's cancer journey usually begins in the outpatient department and it is therefore outpatient nurses who carry the major responsibility of caring for the patient and family in the diagnostic phase. This chapter is based on the principle that nursing acts to guide the patient and family through the emotional turmoil of head and neck cancer diagnosis using a teaching and coaching function (Benner, 1984). In order to support the patient from the outset, the nurse should understand something about the medical diagnostic procedures and investigations that the patient may undergo. This chapter also examines how the outpatient nurse is in a key position to influence the psychosocial outcomes for the patient and family by:

- facilitating a therapeutic environment for the medical team to break bad news
- following this up with a comprehensive assessment and facilitation of coping skills
- initiating nurse led preoperative and pre-treatment educational programmes
- accessing the patient to other members of the supportive therapy team.

Cancer diagnosis and stress

A cancer diagnosis creates a specific stress to the patient and family. In a study of quality of life in head and neck cancer patients throughout the treatment trajectory, Hodder et al (1997) found particularly high levels of distress during the diagnostic phase. According to Lazarus & Folkman (1984), a primary appraisal takes place in such a situation; this involves mental activity asking 'What is the threat?'. A threat can be seen in terms of actual harm or loss, threatened harm or loss, or challenge. Actual harm or loss involves illness, injury or damage to the person or social esteem, or loss of a loved one. The most damaging life events are those in which central and extensive commitments are lost. A threatened harm or loss has not yet taken place but causes stress because of concerns about the anticipated event. An existing harm or loss is always fused with a threat because every loss has negative implications for the future. A threat permits anticipatory coping; it can be planned for and worked through in advance. It will have an affective (emotional) component (fear, anxiety, anger, grief). A challenge is similar to a threat, but the cognitive and affective components are positive; appraisal focuses on the potential for gain or growth and is accompanied by pleasurable emotions (excitement, eagerness).

The primary appraisal is followed by a secondary appraisal which involves the mobilization of coping efforts: 'What can be done about it?'. The coping outcome will depend on the person's feeling of self-efficacy in this situation, their evaluation of the consequences of their coping strategy, and the personal stake at risk. Emotion increases if the person has a high stake. In the case of cancer diagnosis this is life or death. Stress increases if the person feels low self-efficacy; that is, helpless. A high stake coupled with helplessness can be devastating for the person. Additionally, a person with a deficiency in coping resources is much more psychologically vulnerable.

Reappraisal of a threat can also occur over time. The initial appraisal is changed on the basis of new information and an effort is made to reinterpret it more positively, or view the threat or harm in a less damaging way. People who appraise situations as challenges rather than threats have better morale, better quality of functioning and better somatic health than people who are easily threatened.

Lazarus and Folkman (1984) describe studies in which subjects were exposed to stress under different circumstances. Some of this data shows that longer periods of uncertainty about whether and when the harm would occur caused greater stress. If subjects were allowed sufficient time to reappraise the situation, they could considerably mitigate the stress effects. Personality and cognitive styles also have an effect on coping. Denial-orientated people do best with

denial-like appraisal modes, and intellectualizers are best with intel-
lectualizing modes.

From this important psychological theory, we can see how
patients may be helped to cope with cancer diagnosis, surgery and
radiotherapy (threats of loss and harm to the person, family, social
life, future etc.) by careful coaching from the nurse. This coaching
aims to:

- facilitate a positive secondary appraisal
- help the patient and family to mitigate stress via anticipatory
  work (e.g. preoperative preparation) and giving a time schedule to
  reduce uncertainty
- guide the patient and family towards suitable coping strategies
- promote self-efficacy by coaching the patient and family to
  achieve goals, manage problems and avert crises. This prevents
  helplessness
- enable the nurse to identify negative appraisals and give information to facilitate a more positive reappraisal of the situation.

Lazarus and Folkman (1984) state: 'people usually want to know
what is happening and what it means for their wellbeing, while, at
the same time, they usually prefer to put a positive light on things'.

To do this effectively, the nurse must correctly identify the
patient's and family members' personality and cognitive styles, and
constantly review their cognitive processes and affective states, as
well as their progress towards effective appraisal and coping.

At the same time, the patient may have a huge amount of new
information and experience to absorb, as a whole gamut of tests and
investigations are arranged. Whilst some of the information in this
chapter on breaking bad news and pre-treatment information is not
specific to head and neck cancer alone, it is so crucial to the patient's
whole experience that it cannot be omitted.

Medical diagnostic procedures the patient may undergo

Initial clinical examination

Careful inspection of the primary site will be made, with measurement of the tumour dimensions and examination for direct extension into adjacent tissues and local lymph node areas. In outpatients,

mirror techniques can be used to examine the upper airways (indirect laryngoscopy and nasopharyngoscopy), whilst fibre-optic nasendoscopy is also commonly used to give a better view. Routine blood screening, including liver function tests, will be performed. Fine needle aspiration cytology (FNAC) is increasingly useful for the diagnosis of cervical lymphadenopathy and for thyroid and salivary gland tumours (Gharib et al, 1993; Van den Brekel, 1996; Al-Khafaji et al, 1998). A narrow-gauge needle is used to aspirate cells from the tumour. Staining and cytological assessment can be carried out in approximately 30 minutes, which facilitates decision-making in the outpatient clinic.

Examination under anaesthetic

After the initial consultation the majority of patients will require endoscopic examination to assess the local extent and size of the tumour and to take a biopsy for histological examination. There is a high incidence of synchronous and metachronous primary tumours in patients with squamous carcinoma (McGuirt, 1982; Fitzpatrick et al, 1984). Endoscopy therefore includes an examination of the oral cavity, larynx, pharynx and oesophagus. This is usually carried out using rigid endoscopes under general anaesthesia. This technique allows some assessment of tumour mobility and the use of the microscope for endoscopic removal of some small tumours. A recent refinement is the use of vital staining of tumours combined with contact rigid endoscopy. This gives a high-power view of the tumour and surrounding epithelium, which allows a microscopic assessment.

Radiological investigations

Radiological examination is used to assess the primary tumour and to look for metastatic disease. Chest X-ray is a useful screen to exclude metastatic disease or a synchronous primary lung cancer. Chest computerized tomography (CT) scanning is used for higher risk tumours and can be carried out with a scan of the primary tumour. Sectional imaging of the tumour is used for anatomical localization and to assess invasion of adjacent structures. CT and magnetic resonance imaging (MRI) are both used; each has advantages and they provide complementary information in the assessment of some tumours. CT scanning is particularly good at bone imaging. The use of spiral CT scanning allows very rapid image acquisition. This is particularly useful for laryngeal tumours because it reduces image degradation due to movement (Castelijns et al, 1996; Zharen et al, 1997). MRI is better at assessing soft tissue spread and in differentiating tumour from surrounding tissue. Imaging can also be carried out in sagittal and coronal planes, making it particularly helpful in assessing tumours of the sinuses and tongue base. Ultrasound scanning is useful in the detection of thyroid tumours and cervical lymph nodes, particularly when combined with image-guided FNAC. The latter technique offers equivalent accuracy to CT and MR in the assessment of metastatic disease in the cervical nodes (Van den Brekel, 1992). The newer techniques of positron emission tomography (PET) and single-photon emission computerized tomography (SPECT) assess metabolic activity and have the potential to offer increased accuracy in identification of recurrent and cervical nodal disease. At present, however, these techniques do not offer any significant advantages over conventional imaging (Wang et al, 1996). An oral pantogram may be performed to exclude invasion of the mandible or maxilla in oral lesions. This also provides a detailed survey of the teeth to allow planning of dental care prior to radiotherapy treatment.

Referral to a tertiary (specialist) head and neck cancer centre

A diagnosis of head and neck cancer by the local medical team means that referral to a head and neck cancer treatment centre should now be made. Head and neck cancer has been designated as an uncommon cancer which will have better outcomes from both a survival and functional point of view if treated by a medical team with a high degree of expertise (Calman & Hine, 1994). This expertise can only be gained by frequent practice and it is therefore better for one central team to see all patients, rather than many teams in different areas performing surgery and treatment sporadically. Centralization also means that expensive services can be used more efficiently.

Treatment decision

The final part of the diagnostic phase is for the medical team to explain the full implications of the cancer to the patient and discuss treatment options. Generally speaking, early tumours are treated either by radiotherapy or by surgery with local control rates that are equivalent at most sites. The choice of treatment depends on the anticipated functional outcome and the morbidity of the treatment. The standard treatment of advanced tumours, on the other hand, is a combination of surgery and radiotherapy. Adenocarcinomas, including salivary and thyroid tumours, are less radiosensitive and the first-line treatment is surgery. Radiotherapy has an adjunctive role for high-grade or advanced disease. Sarcoma and melanoma are much rarer tumours that are usually treated surgically. Head and neck lymphoma is usually treated with radiotherapy or chemotherapy.

Cervical node metastases, whether overt or microscopic, are an important factor in determining treatment. Squamous carcinoma initially spreads to the regional cervical lymph nodes and then to distant sites. Although nodal metastases indicate a worse prognosis, tumours are potentially still curable at this stage.

Their presence is dependent principally on the site of the tumour. At some sites, notably the pharynx, more than half the patients have cervical node metastases at the time of presentation. Radiotherapy appears to be less effective on nodal disease than on the primary tumour, and removal by neck dissection is the first-line treatment. If the tumour deposit has spread beyond the capsule of the lymph node, or if several lymph nodes are involved, the use of postoperative radiotherapy improves the chance of tumour control.

This consultation entails complex information-giving and must be performed very carefully. Patients will be told about intricate surgical and reconstructive techniques, complicated aftercare, alterations to their mouth, speech and eating abilities, prosthetic equipment and postoperative radiotherapy — all in one consultation.

Pre-treatment dental care

Another important consideration in the pre-treatment phase is dental care for patients who will be undergoing radiotherapy as either primary or postoperative treatment. It is extremely important that any teeth with a poor prognosis are removed pre-treatment to avoid osteoradionecrosis of the mandible. Patients due to undergo surgery should have extractions performed at the same time as the operation (Doerr & Marunick, 1997). Patients due to have a beam direction mask made need to have extractions prior to their impression, in case later changes to the shape of their face alter the precise fit of the mask.

The nurse's role during investigations

The outpatient nurse plays a very important role during the diagnostic phase. She/he should give careful explanations to the patient prior to all tests and investigations. Giving comprehensive information (procedural and sensory) about each investigation will allow the patient to anticipate and deal with it effectively. It is important to ascertain any problems — for example, many patients experience claustrophobia whilst having a scan; the MRI scan in particular may cause problems as the head is enclosed and the scanner is noisy. The nurse can teach the patient relaxation techniques and suggest that the patient takes along a favourite audiotape to listen to whilst having the scan. The nurse can also liaise with the radiographer performing the scan if problems are anticipated.

The nurse's role in liaison between cancer units and cancer centres

The outpatient nurse can also provide a vital link for the patient between secondary (local district general hospital, or cancer unit) and tertiary (specialist cancer treatment centre) services, providing information to the patient about the next stage, helping the patient make travel arrangements and liaising with the nursing staff in the tertiary centre. Nurses in both the cancer unit and cancer centre have a responsibility to develop links to facilitate this process.

The nurse's role in breaking bad news

Nurses in the outpatient department have a key role to play in providing a suitable environment for the giving of bad news, even though the bad news itself is usually given by medical staff. Research shows that patients have a need for privacy, an unhurried interview that is not constantly interrupted, with a time for silence or being alone to take in information, and an opportunity to ask questions. They need to be reassured by the nurse that they will be able to cope and that help will be available if needed. They also need to be reassured that the nurse understands that they will not be able to take everything in, and offered further opportunities to ask more questions (Dear, 1995).

The bad news interview

The 'bad news interview' has a major impact on both the short- and long-term mental state of the patient and can influence the outcome of the disease (Fallowfield & Baum, 1989). The diagnosis will cause chaos and disorganization in the patient and family's life. It is therefore extremely important that the nurse understands the principles of good practice in breaking bad news and how good nursing practice can influence the outcomes for the patient.

Studies have shown that the way in which bad news is broken is extremely important and has a long-lasting effect on the patient. Professionals who have been trained to break bad news have been shown to have much better outcomes in terms of patient satisfaction and in terms of the anxiety and depression that patients experience in the long term (Fallowfield, 1993). Police officers receive more training than healthcare professionals on breaking bad news and interestingly a study of 150 bereaved parents whose children had died of various causes showed that parents rated police officers more highly than healthcare professionals. Guidance on good practice in breaking bad news can be found in Fallowfield (1993) and Buckman (1992).

The nurse should try to ensure that the patient brings a relative or friend with them into the consultation room; the presence of a trusted relative at this time has been shown to facilitate long-term adjustment to the diagnosis of breast cancer (Fallowfield et al, 1987). Information should be simple, clear and honest — it is important not to be falsely reassuring or unduly negative. Research shows that many patients express dissatisfaction with clinicians' information-giving: clinicians may withhold information which they find distressing and underestimate the amount of information patients require. In a study of 101 patients, 94% wanted as much information as possible, whether good or bad (Fallowfield et al, 1995). Studies also show that patients forget up to 50% of the information given, even about simple procedures. When the diagnosis is cancer the information dropout may be more substantial (Buckman, 1992). Many patients are reluctant to ask questions (Audit Commission, 1993), and lack of information can cause uncertainty, anxiety and stress (Audit Commission, 1993). The nurse must be aware of all these points so that her/his supportive and educational interventions can be designed to correct any of these problems.

Nursing care after breaking bad news

The nurse plays a key role after the 'bad news consultation'; the patient should be taken into a quiet, private room where the nurse should allow time for the information to be assimilated, and allow the expression of emotions without criticism or defensiveness, being empathic and comforting as necessary. The nurse can then reinforce information about the disease, the reasons for certain treatments and procedures, expected side effects and strategies to cope with possible threats, to offer a sense of control in an otherwise chaotic situation.

A comprehensive nursing assessment of the patient and family is essential to allow implementation of the appropriate supportive interventions. Breitbart and Holland (1988) emphasize the importance of this in the preparation of the head and neck cancer patient for surgery. Assessment covers emotional and psychological state, beliefs and attitudes, key support figures, relationships, critical roles, educational background and language skills, previous experiences of cancer, previous experiences of hospitals and treatment, financial state, physical state and symptom control. The patient should also be screened for a past history of psychological problems, as well as existing anxiety and depression, as this is an important predictor of postoperative psychological symptoms (White, 1998). Such a comprehensive assessment will then allow the planning of strategies with the patient and family.

The importance of this intervention cannot be understated. McEleney (1996) quotes the experience of a woman with nasal carcinoma who described her experience at the head and neck clinic as follows:

> I shall never forget that day. The thought of losing my nose and being disfigured for life was appalling. However, I was taken into another room and the nurse talked to me in such a caring and practical manner that I began to feel more reconciled to the situation. I also knew that if I did not have surgery I could die.

Other strategies to consider in breaking bad news

- Studies have shown that providing patients with an audiotape of their consultation increases information retention and understanding. Giving patients tapes of their initial consultation resulted in 20% more patients asking for clarification of information at their second consultation and 22% fewer requests at the second consultation for details which they had already been told at the previous consultation (Ford et al, 1995).

- Other studies using educational interventions with patients to teach them to identify and ask questions all resulted in improved patient participation (Roter, 1984; Greenfield et al, 1985). A strategy to assess patients' desired level of participation, help identify questions and give support in obtaining information was successful incorporated into a busy oncology clinic (Neufeld et al, 1993).

Attitudes to cancer

At this point, it may be helpful to consider the impact of attitudes to cancer from both the nurse's and the patient's perspectives and reflect how they might affect communication.

The nurse

Studies have shown that although nurses have access to information about survival rates and knowledge of new and better treatments, their attitudes to cancer can be just as pessimistic as the general public. This leads to poor communication with the use of euphemisms such as 'tumour', 'growth', 'lump', 'wart' or 'polyp' rather than the word 'cancer'. Such indirect avoidance means that patients' psychological and emotional needs are never appreciated or dealt with (Purandare, 1997). Because nurses work intimately with patients they are frequently asked the most frightening and personal questions (Benner & Wrubel, 1989). It is therefore very important that nurses come to terms with cancer themselves before they can work effectively with patients. It is also important that they constantly update themselves professionally as well as develop skills through reflection.

The patient

The patient's previous experience of, attitudes and beliefs about cancer are particularly important — cancer is dreaded by the public and usually assumed to end in a painful, protracted death. Cancer treatment is assumed to involve extreme nausea and hair loss. It is important to identify and deal with such misconceptions. It is vital that the patient be encouraged to express all such fears, as undisclosed concerns cause information blocking (Maguire et al, 1996), which will impede the patient's participation in the treatment decision and preoperative education.

Facilitating coping strategies

Crisis disturbs normal daily life and can either enhance personal growth or damage and destroy self-esteem (Wright, 1993). Coping is defined as a series of cognitive and behavioural efforts to manage circumstances that evoke responses exceeding one's current personal resources, that is, a crisis (Lazarus & Folkman, 1984). The patient may experience emotions ranging from shock, disbelief, confusion and denial to anger, grief and the inner turmoil central to the experience of losing control over one's life and destiny (Murray Parkes, 1975; Saunders, 1990). Literature suggests that coping with a cancer diagnosis is a significant problem for patients and families, putting the family at risk of disintegration. Increasing the coping response of the family may profoundly affect the long-term psychological and physical outcome for the patient. Using counselling, teaching and social support skills, the nurse can initiate effective coping responses to a potentially devastating diagnosis which will begin to reintegrate body, mind and spirit and result in a smoother transition phase. Families who had a member diagnosed with cancer identified helpful nursing behaviours as listening, providing information, availability, sensitivity, empathy, respectfulness and honesty (Kumasaka & Dungan, 1993).

Nursing care should therefore be aimed at developing a therapeutic relationship with the family to help in the development of a coping strategy to deal with the situation. Benner surmises that nurses become experts in coaching patients through illness; they take what is foreign and fearful to the patient and make it familiar and less frightening. This process includes the following elements (from Benner, 1984, Chapter 5):

- timing: capturing the patient's readiness to learn
- assisting patients to integrate the implications of illness and treatment into their lifestyle
- eliciting and understanding the patient's interpretation of the illness
- providing an interpretation of the condition and giving a rationale for procedures
- coaching: making culturally avoided aspects of an illness approachable and understandable — this is particularly pertinent to patients with head and neck cancer as facial disfigurement, the

alaryngeal voice, the tracheostomy and eating difficulties, are socially taboo.

Once this initial important process of helping the patient cope with the diagnosis and understanding and agreeing to a mutually desirable treatment plan has been achieved, preoperative or pre-radiotherapy preparation can be initiated.

Preoperative and pre-radiotherapy preparation

Patient preparation for treatment

Preoperative preparation by nurses is vital for a number of well-established reasons. Patients who express dissatisfaction with pre-operative information also experience more clinically significant psychological symptoms (White, 1998). Good preoperative information helps to reduce anxiety and patients are likely to recover better if they have been well informed and had chance to discuss their concerns. Effective discharge planning for the patient's home and social needs can start even before they are admitted, and this has a positive effect on bed usage (Hayward, 1975; Devine & Cook, 1983; Hathaway, 1986). The King's Fund report on head and neck cancer care (Edwards, 1997) found that patients consistently reported how important preparatory information was for them; the report makes clear recommendations for improvements in information-giving.

Breitbart and Holland (1988) emphasize the importance of the preoperative period for head and neck cancer patients, many of whom will experience major fears about the procedure and the extent of the postoperative deficit. Individuals whose identity is dependent upon physical appearance or verbal communication skills will require special attention. In their studies on the psychosocial responses of head and neck cancer patients to treatment, Fiegenbaum (1981) and Strauss (1989) recommend more comprehensive preparation for surgery and its consequences in head and neck cancer patients. Moore et al (1996) studied quality of life in patients undergoing radiotherapy to the base of tongue and concluded that patients and families should be educated extensively regarding treatment effects on eating and speech. Stam et al (1991) completed a structured interview with 51 laryngectomees. Preoperative counselling proved to be a crucial factor in postoperative adjustment. They found that preoperative counselling, including visits by the speech therapist and fellow laryngectomees, strongly predicted later quality of life. A substantial number of authors have found that laryngectomees consistently report postoperatively that they wish they had more preoperative counselling (Minear & Lucente, 1979; Johnson et al, 1979; Natvig, 1983; Craven & West, 1987; Lehman & Krebs, 1991). All their studies underline the crucial importance of preoperative preparation, including a laryngectomee visitor. It is important not to forget to include the family in preoperative counselling; Blood et al (1994) found that laryngectomy created severe stress in caregivers and that spouses needed preoperative and postoperative counselling. Studies on preparation of patients for radiotherapy and chemotherapy show that such interventions similarly reduce anxiety and promote coping behaviours (Frith, 1991).

Timing of information

Pre-treatment preparation should begin at the outpatient visit. The patient will then have the intervening period at home to assimilate information and discuss it with the family. Giving the bulk of preoperative information on the day of admission for surgery is highly unsatisfactory — admission to hospital is a stressful experience, with the patient experiencing 'crushing vulnerability' (Morrison, 1994). This practice may also mean that the family misses out on information. Written information should be provided by the nurse and there are excellent resources available in the form of booklets, audiocassettes and videos (see Table 1.2.1). The nurse should offer patients the opportunity to speak to an ex-patient (Breitbart & Holland, 1988; BACUP, 1995). Information on establishing a buddy scheme is provided in Chapter 1.4. If the patient's psychological state is such that information blocking is occurring, the nurse should make an appointment to see the patient a few days later.

Type of information

Information can be described as falling into two categories: procedural and sensory. Procedural information orients the patient to the forthcoming event by giving concrete descriptions of what they can expect and do to help themselves. Sensory information helps the patient to create a mental picture of the procedure which aids their

Table 1.2.1: Patient Information Resources

Resource	Contact
National Association of Laryngectomy Clubs: numerous patient information booklets, emergency cards and car stickers, audiocassettes, video, information about swimming for laryngectomees	The National Association of Laryngectomy Clubs 6 Rickett Street, Fulham London SW6 1RU Tel 020 73819993 Fax 020 7810025
Booklet: Understanding Cancer of the Mouth and Throat Booklet: Understanding Thyroid Cancer	CancerBACUP 3 Bath Place Rivington Street London EC2A 3JR Tel 020 7613 2121 or 0808 800 1234 www.cancerbacup.org.uk
Booklets: Laryngectomy: Your Questions Answered After Your Laryngectomy: A Patient's Guide	Kapitex Healthcare Ltd Kapitex House 1 Sandbeck Way Wetherby West Yorks LS22 7GH Tel 01937 580211
Book: Laryngectomy is not a Tragedy (by Sydney Norgate)	Cancer Laryngectomee Trust National Association of Neck Breathers Claremount House Claremount Road Halifax HX3 6AW Tel 01422 364448
Patient information pack: colour brochures and information on tracheostomy and laryngectomy products (Buchanan protectors, cravats, shower shields, etc.)	Kapitex Healthcare Ltd Kapitex House 1 Sandbeck Way Wetherby West Yorks LS22 7GH Tel 01937 580211
Patient education visual aids — sketch pads and posters (laryngectomy) Brochure on laryngectomy products	Forth Medical Limited Forth House 42 Kingfisher Court Hambridge Road Newbury Berkshire RG14 5SJ Tel 01635 550100

(contd)

Table 1.2.1: (contd) .

Resource	Contact
Macmillan Cancer Relief Booklets:	Macmillan Cancer Relief
The Cancer Guide	Anchor House
Financial Help for People with Cancer	15–19 Britten Street
Help is There	London SW3 3TZ
Macmillan Nurses	Tel 020 7351 7811
Benefits information	Local Social Services Department
Help with prescription charges	Local Post Office
information	
Changing Faces	Changing Faces
Numerous booklets including:	1 & 2 Junction Mews
When Cancer Affects the Way	Paddington
You Look	London W2 1PN
Video: REACHOUT	Tel 020 7706 4234

interpretation of what is happening, reducing anxiety both before and during the procedure. Thus the patient becomes more familiar with events, feels less anxious and is able to cooperate with instructions during and after the event (Poroch, 1995).

Preoperative information

Hathaway's meta-analysis of preoperative instruction studies showed that preoperative teaching programmes by nurses had a beneficial effect on postoperative outcomes; preoperative instruction accounted for a 20% improvement in outcomes. The findings also suggest that nurses should adapt instruction according to the patient's level of fear/anxiety. When individuals display a low level of fear/anxiety, procedural aspects of care should be focused on, and when there is a high level of anxiety the focus should be on psychological content (Hathaway, 1986).

This principle is demonstrated by a study of patient preoperative information preferences about intensive care units. Patients rated as most helpful information which facilitated emotion-focused coping by allowing reinterpretation of the event as less of a threat (threats being to survival, bodily integrity and comfort). For example, knowing that pain and nausea would be controlled and one's mouth would be moistened, lessened the threat to comfort. The knowledge that one will have a urinary catheter inserted may ease worries about coping with a bottle or bedpan, but there may be other worries about the physical discomfort and indignity of having a catheter inserted. The knowledge that one would be closely monitored by a nurse was also important because it lessened the threat to survival. Patients were reported to find a preoperative visit to the ICU helpful.

Depondt & Gehanno (1995) describe the use of a video about the perioperative period and initial recovery for laryngectomy patients. Laryngectomy videos are available in the UK from the National Association of Laryngectomy Clubs, London.

Pre-radiotherapy information

Radiotherapy treatment usually takes place in an outpatient setting and patients can be taught self-care skills by the nurse to manage side effects and so enhance coping and feelings of control over the situation (Dodd, 1987). Fieler et al (1996) asked patients undergoing radiotherapy what they needed to know. The patients stated that essential knowledge included:

- what the side effects will be, when to expect them, and how long they will last;
- how treatment kills cancer cells.

Patients stated that information helped them to 'mentally prepare', 'take care of self', 'relieve anxiety', 'schedule activities' and 'keep me informed'. Their main complaint was conflicting advice from everyone 'from the surgeon, radiation oncologist, oncology fellow, nurses and treatment technicians'. Hinds et al (1995) interviewed 83 patients before and after radiotherapy and found that they preferred to have as much information as possible to help them cope and to reduce anxiety. These patients also said that they wanted information even if it is 'bad news'.

The planning process which takes place prior to radiotherapy (see Chapter 4.3) can be very stressful. The beam direction mask often induces anxiety and panic attacks which can be prevented and managed if the patient has been well prepared and by using cognitive behavioural strategies, neurolinguistic programming and relaxation techniques (see Chapter 3.3) The nurse should provide a written, visual and sensory information package. The mask in particular often causes misconceptions (the man in the iron mask is often mentioned!). Showing the patient a mask and allowing them to handle it as part of the education session will reassure them. A photo story is also helpful to explain the mask making process as many patients are extremely anxious about their impression appointment, anticipating that their face will be covered in plaster and that they will not be able to breathe. Patients who listened to audiotapes describing radiotherapy, its side effects and self-care activities to relieve them, were more knowledgeable about the treatment and practised more helpful self-care behaviours than a control group (Hagopian 1996), therefore this is an intervention which should be considered.

Structured support programmes

It is important that preoperative or pre-treatment education is carefully structured; ad hoc education is often incomplete and when compared to structured education programmes has much less satisfactory outcomes (Felton et al, 1976). When a structured preoperative preparation package for patients undergoing laryngectomy was used, patient satisfaction levels increased from 59% to 85% (Feber, 1998). The package consisted of a comprehensive outpatient nursing assessment, an education session with the patient and family in outpatients or at home (according to patient preference), provision of a comprehensive information pack, and a preoperative meeting with and assessment by the district nurse at home. Comments from patients before the support strategy was implemented were:

- very little information was available or no one was on hand to give it
- there was an out-of-date book about the operation
- we had to find out for ourselves
- (I would have liked) someone to help me from being afraid because I was on my own
- (I would have liked) someone to be available to discuss and answer questions particularly about the need for and the general outcome of the operation.

These comments compare to post-implementation comments:

- overall the care I received was first class and I could not wish for a better team
- from day one and still I feel the support we have had (my wife and I) has been truly first class.

Another nursing audit in Leeds examined the experience of 35 patients diagnosed with oral and maxillofacial cancers who had not benefited from a structured preoperative teaching programme. The majority of information was given on the day of admission to hospital for surgery. Only five felt that information-giving on the day of admission was satisfactory. Patients made comments on the timing and type of preoperative information-giving, such as:

- I would have liked a full explanation of every step of the operation which was to be performed on me before my admission to hospital — I wasn't told until my admission
- I would have liked some warning about losing my teeth
- I would have liked to meet someone who had already had the operation
- my appearance (after the operation) was a great shock to me and my family
- I would have liked charts, pictures, videos, showing the extent of scarring, stitching, etc.
- I think we really need to be more prepared and have a lot of confidence in ourselves.

Similar feelings were also reflected by the patients in the King's Fund head and neck cancer study (Edwards, 1997).

The importance of nursing liaison

Pre-treatment preparation should also include liaison with other healthcare professionals, for example the speech therapist and the district nurse, who should also meet the patient in the pre-treatment phase. This is especially important for patients who will have communication difficulties postoperatively (see Chapter 2.5). Social services may also be initiated by the nurse at this stage, firstly to avert any financial or family crisis during the treatment phase, and secondly in anticipation of discharge needs. The nurse can arrange for equipment such as telephone communication devices (e.g. the Claudius 2) and suction pumps to be installed in the patient's home so that the patient can learn how to use them before they arrive home after surgery in a more vulnerable state. Patients having nutritional problems will obviously need attention from the dietitian, as optimum nutritional status is extremely important to ensure good treatment outcomes (see Chapter 2.3).

Summary

In summary, the diagnostic phase is the most crucial time in the patient's cancer journey. Good, evidence-based nursing care at this time will improve both physical and psychological outcomes for the patient and family. Hospital stays will be shorter and, if crises are anticipated and prevented, fewer healthcare and social service resources may need to be used at a later date on crisis management. The patient and family will also be able to put all their emotional resources into positive coping strategies rather than crisis management. The importance of managing this phase well cannot be underestimated. For those interested in reading further, the following references are recommended: Carnevali & Reiner, 1990; Wright, 1993; Edwards, 1997.

Strategy for practice for outpatient nursing teams

- Provide a private, comfortable room in the outpatients department for bad news interviews.
- Provide a post bad news consultation nursing assessment and support session.
- Provide comprehensive patient education packages for each treatment modality (involve patients when developing information packages).
- Provide a full range of written, visual and auditory educational aids.
- Give patients access to the whole team (hospital and community) as early as possible.
- Include the family in all these interventions.

Chapter 1.3
Managing tobacco and alcohol addiction

Introduction

Many head and neck cancer patients have pre-existing psychological problems that have resulted in chronic abuse of alcohol and tobacco. The psychological sequelae can influence care and rehabilitation by the development of withdrawal states, continuation of drinking and dementia (Breitbart & Holland, 1988). The physical treatment of cancer is relatively straightforward in comparison to helping a patient unpick the web of his/her behaviour to overcome addiction. However, when faced with a life-threatening illness, patients are likely to be more motivated to change their behaviour. The evidence on smoking-related treatment complications also shows that it is beneficial for patients to stop smoking preoperatively or pre-radiotherapy. Bjordal et al (1995) found that 72% of head and neck cancer patients who smoked continued to smoke after treatment and concluded that 'a stop smoking programme may give a higher cost-benefit with regard to survival compared with the usual extensive investigations in order to detect relapse or secondary cancer'.

Assessment of addiction and application of interventions to support stopping are therefore very important as part of the care of the patient with head and neck cancer. As this needs to happen as early as possible before surgery or radiotherapy in order to have the maximum benefit, it is an important role for the outpatient nurse. As most patients will require help with smoking or drinking cessation or both, it is vital that all nurses, and particularly outpatient nurses, are appropriately skilled and have a knowledge of psychological theory in addiction. This chapter will give an overview of addiction and show how to use the theory of the Model of Change.

What is addiction?

Definition

Although the word 'addiction' is used in everyday language, it is very difficult to define. McMurran defines it as 'a degree of involvement in a behaviour that can function both to produce pleasure and to provide relief from discomfort, to the point where the costs outweigh the benefits'. She also emphasizes that 'there is no single explanation for addiction'; there are biological factors, psychological factors, cultural and social factors (McMurran, 1994).

Social background

The disease model or medical model of human behaviour became prominent in the nineteenth century. Medical, scientific concepts were applied to problems that had previously been regarded as within moral and spiritual domains. Thus, addiction became a disease needing treatment rather than an undesirable behaviour requiring punishment, although these two concepts still tend to exist alongside each other to a certain extent. It is interesting that people with addiction to drugs other than alcohol and nicotine (for example opiates) seem to be offered more in the way of treatment and resources. Even so, 'alcoholics' are also offered a fair amount of support by medical and psychiatric services in comparison with smokers, who have to deal with their nicotine addiction largely by themselves, having to fund their own pharmacological support to withdraw from nicotine. Alcoholism was a term invented in the nineteenth century. The disease model of alcoholism defines it as craving, a loss of control over substance use, and assumes it to be irreversible, despite evidence that this may not be the case. The debate over whether alcoholism is a genetic disease or a personality disorder continues (Jurd, 1992; Heather, 1992).

In society today, drug and alcohol addiction are stigmatizing, but nicotine addiction does not carry the same stigma; society's relationship with it is much more complex. In the earlier half of this century, the medical profession recommended smoking to patients for relief of anxiety and depression; soldiers in the Second World War were even provided with regular cigarette rations by the government. Today, the tobacco industry and taxation of tobacco are powerful reasons to allow nicotine to be consumed freely. A recent study showed that it would actually cost the health service more to maintain people in old age if they did not die early from tobacco-related illness, even when the costs of treating this illness are considered (Barendregt et al, 1997).

Dependence

Dependence is another term used to describe addictive behaviour (Edwards & Gross, 1976). It is a concept developed in the 1970s in alcohol studies, despite the lack of supporting evidence for its existence as a syndrome (McMurran, 1994). Edwards and Gross defined seven elements of dependence in relation to alcohol:

1. Narrowing of the drinking repertoire; the person drinks every day, irrespective of time or company.
2. Salience of drink-seeking behaviour; drinking takes priority over other activities.
3. Increased tolerance to alcohol.
4. Repeated withdrawal symptoms.
5. Relief or avoidance of withdrawal symptoms by further drinking.
6. Subjective awareness of compulsion to drink.
7. Reinstatement after abstinence; once drinking starts again after abstinence there is a rapid return to previous level of consumption.

Physical dependence can occur for many substances, including nicotine and alcohol. It can also be defined as a biochemical and physiological adaptation of an organism whereby normal functioning depends on the continued administration of a substance. It is physical dependence that results in withdrawal reactions after the abrupt cessation of a substance. Thus gradual withdrawal of a substance using a reducing regime can help to prevent unpleasant acute withdrawal symptoms.

Psychological theories of addiction

There are a number of theories about addictions based on psychological models that will help nurses to understand their patients' behaviours:

Classical conditioning
Pavlov 1849–1936

This theory describes how repeated behaviour leads to a conditioned response. Having a cigarette after every meal means that smoking becomes a conditioned response to eating a meal. Three meals per day with a cigarette afterwards for 40 years mean 43,800 conditioning episodes. These conditioned responses can be deprogrammed from the brain by providing the cue (e.g. a meal) but not allowing the response to take place. This is called extinction. However, they can spontaneously recur at a later date.

Operant conditioning
Skinner 1904–1990

Operant conditioning describes the relationship between behaviour and its consequences. Reinforcement increases the likelihood of a behaviour. Positive reinforcement rewards the behaviour directly (e.g. physical satisfaction from smoking a cigarette), whilst negative reinforcement rewards the behaviour by providing an escape from an aversive experience (e.g. relief from boredom or anxiety). Positive and negative punishment work in the same way. For a person smoking a cigarette, each inhalation causes positive reinforcement by stimulation of pleasure centres in the brain, and negative reinforcement by eliminating the unpleasant feeling of nicotine deprivation. Smoking 20 cigarettes per day at 10 puffs per cigarette thus leads to 200 reinforcements per day. A smoker of 40 years would therefore have had 292,000 reinforcements — no wonder the habit is so difficult to break!

Social learning theory
Bandura, 1977

This theory relates to the interaction of the person, environment and behaviour. A person can decide what to do in any situation by weighing up the outcomes of his/her actions. Everyone learns from other people's examples as well as their own experiences — this is called modelling. Behaviour is regulated by personal internal standards. Self-efficacy is important as it determines what we choose to do and how long we will persist at trying to do it. Low self-efficacy means that the person does not believe him/herself able to achieve a task successfully and therefore he/she will feel apprehension and avoid it. A person with high self-efficacy will perform their task in a relaxed way and will persist to overcome any obstacles. To have high self-efficacy about a task, a person must know what to do, have seen others achieve it, have previous personal experience of success, and feel relaxed enough to do it (Bandura, 1977). People with low self-efficacy may have learnt that smoking or drinking help them to cope with problems. As the person becomes more reliant on the substance, dependence may develop and the substance is used to avoid withdrawal effects. If alcohol is being used in this way, unreliability, poor work performance and breakdown of relationships may ensue. This loss of social support systems then leads to low self-esteem and further drinking and a vicious circle develops.

Expectancy theory
Goldman et al, 1987

An outcome expectancy is a belief that a person holds about substance use; if I drink or smoke, then a specific outcome will follow: I will relax, I will enjoy myself, etc. Conversely, if I don't drink or smoke I will become unpleasantly anxious and tense, I will not enjoy myself, etc.

Alcohol

The effects of alcohol

Alcohol is a psychotropic drug that can be legally used by adults in most societies. It is primarily used to enhance social intercourse. Different beverages contain different amounts of alcohol and the term unit of alcohol can be used as a measure of alcohol irrespective of the specific beverage (see Table 1.3.1).

Recommended units of alcohol per day are as follows:

men 3–4 units per day
women 2–3 units per day
(Health Education Authority, 1997)

Alcohol misuse can result in chronic and debilitating damage to the person (Health Education Authority, 1997), such as:

- Medical problems
  acute gastritis, pancreatitis, trauma, head injury, accidents, liver

cirrhosis, cancers of the upper digestive tract, oesophageal varices, gastrointestinal ulceration, vitamin deficiency, cardiomy-opathy, peripheral neuropathy, epilepsy and brain damage (Wernicke's encephalopathy, Korsakoff's psychosis).

• Social problems
   social isolation, aggressive behaviour, domestic violence, sexual and relationship problems, employment problems, financial debt.

• Legal problems
   driving or drunkenness offences, theft, shoplifting and assault.

• Psychological problems
   low self-esteem, depression and suicide attempts, phobias, anxiety, poor coping skills, cognitive impairment, poor self-efficacy, drinking to cope with stress. In a group of 47 head and neck cancer patients, depression and poor overall quality of life were associated with alcohol use prior to diagnosis (List et al, 1997).

Table 1.3.1: Units of alcohol in various drinks

Drink	Unit
Spirits — 1 pub measure, gin, whisky, vodka	1
1 glass fortified wine, sherry, Martini, port	1
1 glass table wine	1–2
1 pint beer/lager	2–3
1 pint low-alcohol beer	0.33
1 can beer/lager	1.5
1 bottle super/special lager	2.5
1 can super/special lager	4
1 pint regular cider	3
1 bottle strong cider	2.5
1 bottle of wine	7–12
1 litre bottle of wine	10–18
1 bottle fortified wine	14
1 bottle of spirits	30
1 glass/can alcoholic lemonade	2

Attitudes of healthcare professionals to patients with alcohol problems

Earlier in this chapter we discussed how nurses' attitudes towards cancer can have a detrimental effect on the way they communicate with patients. Personal awareness and challenging beliefs is also important when helping patients with addiction. Studies show that healthcare professionals tend to have negative attitudes towards people with alcohol problems (Cooper, 1994a; Riley, 1996), yet evidence shows that attitudes towards people with alcohol-related problems affect treatment outcomes (Leake & King, 1977). Nurses may spend long periods of time with head and neck patients and develop close, therapeutic relationships that can enhance treatment and management of alcohol-related problems. However, there is a common misconception that alcohol-related problems are the province of the mental health team, and that non-mental-health professionals are not in a position to help (Cooper, 1994a). Evidence shows that very few general nurses have received any education in alcohol-related problems (Cooper, 1994a). It is therefore important that the whole team are up to date with current thinking in the alcohol field and with change management strategies. The basics are given in this chapter, but nurses should consider contacting their local specialist alcohol service for in-service training, and also find out how their head and neck unit can link into their service.

Tobacco and smoking

Constituents of tobacco

The burning of tobacco yields mainstream and sidestream smoke. Mainstream smoke is generated in the burning cone and hot zones during puff-drawing, travels through the tobacco column and exits from the mouthpiece. Sidestream smoke forms in between puff-drawing and is emitted into the air freely from the smouldering tobacco product. Tobacco smoke contains more than 4,000 chemical constituents which are present in a gas or particulate phase. The particulate phase includes:

- nicotine, which is a very powerful and addictive drug. Nicotine reaches the central nervous system within seconds of being inhaled, activating the release of norepinephrine, dopamine and other neurotransmitters
- tar, which is a complex mixture of chemicals. Many of these are carcinogenic. It is a brown, treacly substance that is deposited in the respiratory tract and gradually absorbed
- benzene
- benzo(a)pyrene.

The gas phase includes:

- carbon monoxide, which binds to haemoglobin more readily than oxygen, meaning that the blood is less well oxygenated
- ammonia
- dimethylnitrosamine
- formaldehyde
- hydrogen cyanide
- acetone

(Health Education Authority, 1996b).

Major smoking-related illnesses

These include coronary heart disease, cerebrovascular disease, aortic aneurysm and athersclerotic peripheral vascular disease, chronic obstructive pulmonary disease, cancers of the lung, oral cavity, oesophagus and larynx, cancers of the bladder, kidney, pancreas, cervix, and gastrointestinal ulceration. The relative risk of dying from a smoking-related illness increases with the number of cigarettes smoked per day (Health Education Authority, 1996b).

Nicotine and depression

Smoking and depression are strongly linked. Smokers are more likely to have a history of major depression than non-smokers. Smokers with a history of depression are also more likely to be highly dependent on nicotine and have a lower likelihood of successfully quitting. When they do quit, depression is more apt to be a prominent symptom (Benowitz, 1997).

Smoking before surgery

Smoking diminishes proliferation of red blood cells, fibroblasts and macrophages. It also increases platelet adhesiveness, which causes microclots and decreases microperfusion, which in turn causes thrombotic microvascular occlusion and eventually tissue ischaemia. Nicotine produces cutaneous vasoconstriction due to the release of adrenal and peripheral catecholamines, which also increase heart rate, blood pressure and oxygen demand. These catecholamines also result in the release of hormones that undermine wound healing by retarding the rate of epithelialization. Carbon monoxide inhibits the binding of oxygen and thus reduces the amount of oxygen reaching the periphery. It also makes oxygen less able to dissociate from red blood cells and diffuse into the tissues. This leads to cellular hypoxia and diminished wound healing. Hydrogen cyanide inhibits the enzyme systems necessary for oxidative metabolism and oxygen transport at the cellular level (Silverstein, 1992). Smoking damages the ciliary function in the airways and increases mucous production by the goblet cells. It also alters the responsiveness of inflammatory cells in the lungs — more inflammatory cells are recruited as a response to the chemicals and these can degrade normal structures causing oedema, fibrosis and epithelial hyperplasia (McCusker, 1992). Smoking may reduce the effectiveness of some anaesthetic and analgesic drugs. Patients may also experience nicotine withdrawal when smoking is suddenly stopped on admission to hospital (see Table 1.3.3).

Thus postoperative complications in smokers include: impaired wound healing, wound infections, chest infections, cough, circulation and heart problems (stroke and myocardial infarction). In order to reduce these complications, cessation should be at least 24 hours (preferably 1 week, but ideally 6 weeks) prior to surgery (Haddock & Burrows, 1997). Haddock and Burrows found that educating presurgery smokers (leaflet, smoking diary and advice on nicotine replacement) about these risks, significantly increased the number of patients stopping or reducing smoking preoperatively, particularly in subjects who had been assessed as precontemplators (see section on Precontemplation, below).

Effects of smoking on head and neck cancer treatment

Specifically within the head and neck cancer field, smoking considerably increases the risks of serious postoperative complications (McCulloch et al, 1997). It adversely affects wound healing and the success of free tissue transfer reconstruction (Silverstein, 1992) as well as other techniques such as osseointegrated implants for prosthetic rehabilitation (McGhee et al, 1997). Smoking both exacerbates and delays healing of radiation mucositis (Rugg et al, 1990), and patients who continue to smoke have been shown to carry a higher risk of cancer recurrence than patients who stop (Browman et al, 1993a).

Helping people change

The Model of Change

Prochaska et al (1992) developed the 'Model of Change', which defines five stages through which a person moves from no motivation to change, to actively changing behaviour, to successfully dealing with the problem and maintaining the behaviour change (see Figure 1.3.1). This is a very useful model to help nurses assess their patients and plan interventions. Many studies show that this type of behavioural therapy is the most effective way of helping people with addiction problems (DiClemente et al, 1991; Prochaska et al, 1993; Velicer et al, 1993).

The patient's position in the change model can be assessed by the nurse, and nursing interventions can be aimed at this identified stage; different interventions are required for each stage. This model of motivational counselling has been defined as 'a directive, client-centred counselling style for helping the client explore and resolve ambivalence about behaviour change (Rollnick & Miller, 1995). A confrontational, 'lecturing' style should be avoided as it can cause resistance and denial (Miller, 1983).

To avoid repetition, this section will cover the issues of assessment and stages of the Model of Change for both alcohol and tobacco together. Very often, patients will be using both substances and therefore require assessment of both at the same time.

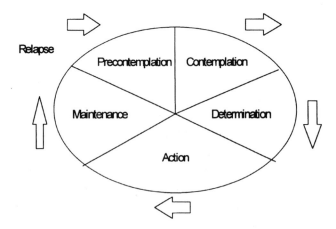

Figure 1.3.1: The Model of Change

Assessment of the patient's problem

Alcohol

It is important that nursing and medical staff know exactly how much a patient is drinking so that the appropriate action can be taken to avoid withdrawal symptoms when they are admitted to hospital. Alcohol withdrawal resulting from hospitalization and delirium tremens postoperatively carries major morbidity (delirium tremens mortality is 15%) (Breitbart & Holland, 1988). Breitbart and Holland (1988) recommend admission to hospital for detoxification preoperatively for patients actively drinking before surgery.

Cooper (1994b) suggests that a drinking profile should consist of:

- usual frequency and quantity of alcohol consumption
- details of last drinking occasion
- time of day the last alcohol consumption commenced
- whether alcohol is the first drink of the day
- where alcohol consumption takes place
- drinking preferences (alone or in company)
- where it is most difficult to control alcohol consumption
- attempts at previous control or abstinence.

The patient may feel embarrassed about his/her drinking levels or may worry about shocking the nurse or people around (e.g. other patients). They may not want their family to know about the extent of their alcohol use. Therefore, the nurse should ensure that the interview is carried out in a private area and that the patient knows confidentiality will be maintained. The nurse should help the patient feel at ease by being non-judgemental and by maintaining unconditional positive regard. It is helpful for the nurse to explain why she/he needs to know about drinking levels, as this will encourage the patient to be honest; saying, for example, 'I need to know how much alcohol you normally have in your blood because it is dangerous to stop drinking suddenly and we want to avoid you having any unpleasant withdrawal symptoms in hospital or any adverse reactions to the anaesthetic'.

It is important to ascertain what strength of alcohol the patient uses as well as the amount — e.g. if a patient drinks 10 cans of lager per day it should be ascertained whether it is normal or extra strong. It is important for nurses to be alert to recognize alcohol withdrawal symptoms. Assessment of the severity of withdrawal symptoms (see Table 1.3.2) can be made by asking 'how do you feel in the morn-

Table 1.3.2: Alcohol withdrawal symptoms

Symptom	Time scale
Sleep disturbance — withdrawal rouses Anxiety Irritable Dysphoria Cannot face people Tremor of hands Retching Sweating Tremor of face Tremor of body Perceptual disturbance — illusions, transient hallucinatory state	4–24 hours
Seizures	36 hours
Delirium	72 hours

ing?' (NB: People with severe alcohol dependency do not have hang-
overs — they have withdrawal symptoms.) If the patient does not
state how much they drink, Burns and Adams (1997) suggest factors
that increase patients' risk of experiencing withdrawal:

- previous episode of withdrawal
- alcohol intake of more than 10 standard drinks per day
- regular use of alcohol with other sedatives
- previous history of alcohol-related disease
- alcohol-related physical signs
- abnormal pathology
- confusion, anxiety, not attributable to other causes.

This information should be shared with the medical team, who
should prescribe the appropriate pharmacological support.

Tobacco

Rollnick et al (1997) suggest the following 'quick assessment' of the
patient's smoking habit:

- Establish rapport — 'What sort of smoker are you? Tell me a bit
  about your smoking'; 'You may well be a little fed up with people

lecturing you about smoking. I'm not going to do that, but it would help me if I understood how you really feel about your smoking.'

- Motivation to quit — 'If on a scale of 1 to 10, 1 is not motivated to give up smoking and 10 is 100% motivated, what number would you give yourself at the moment?'
- Confidence in ability to quit — 'If you were to decide to stop smoking now, how confident are you that you would succeed? If on a scale of 1 to 10, 1 means not at all confident and 10 means 100% confident, what number would you give yourself now?'

Assessment of the patient's level of nicotine addiction can be assessed by the following questions:

- 'How many cigarettes a day do you smoke?' 'Do you need a cigarette first thing in the morning?'. Heavily dependent smokers will start smoking within 20 minutes of waking, and may even be woken by withdrawal. They will smoke over 20 cigarettes per day.
- 'Can you stay in a No Smoking area for several hours without having to go outside for a cigarette?'. Heavily dependent smokers will report the need to go outside for a cigarette.
- Nicotine withdrawal symptoms are outlined in Table 1.3.3.

Table 1.3.3: Nicotine withdrawal symptoms

Symptom	Time scale
Craving	Usually starts within a few hours of the last cigarette and lasts 2 to 3 minutes
Negative mood Irritability Restlessness Tension Poor concentration Nervousness	Often worse on day 3 when the body has cleared itself of nicotine
Hunger Disturbed sleep Dreams Weight gain	Decrease after 4 weeks, but may continue longer
Cilia regrow in lungs and begin to clear out secretions; patient will experience an increase in coughing and expectoration of mucus	1 to 9 months

The precontemplation stage

The precontemplator is motivated to continue to drink/smoke; the benefits of drinking or smoking outweigh the costs in their perception. This may explain why Ostroff et al (1995) found that head and neck cancer patients with less severe disease who undergo less extensive treatment are particularly at risk for continued tobacco use. The patient may never move out of this phase, or may move out but return at a later date. As a sizeable group of patients may fall into this category it is particularly important that we can support the alcohol users effectively with harm-minimization strategies (Table 1.3.4). Information on the benefits of stopping smoking/drinking should be given in a non-judgemental way so that the patient can make an informed judgement about his/her behaviour.

The contemplation stage

Movement into the contemplation phase may often be precipitated by the diagnosis of a smoking-related cancer. Information should be given in a non-threatening, non-personalized way. Listen to the patient's own story about his or her drinking/smoking habit and build on any ambivalence the patient might have towards it. Avoid making the patient feel embarrassed or defensive. Give objective, non-personalized, non-threatening information about the adverse effects of alcohol/tobacco use. This introduces conflict in the patient's mind about the benefits versus the costs of drinking/smoking — the balance changes as the patient reconsiders and becomes motivated to change habits.

The patient can be prompted to think about the benefits versus the costs by answering the following questions:

'What are the good things about smoking/drinking for you?'
'What are the less good things about smoking/drinking for you?'

Sensitive counselling is essential and relatives may be enlisted to help in a therapeutic alliance. At this stage for alcohol-related problems, referral to the local addiction unit for expert help should be considered, with the patient's permission.

The determination stage

The patient makes a decision to change and moves into the 'determination phase' — he/she now believes that stopping will make a difference and feels confident that he/she has the ability to stop (self-

Table 1.3.4: Harm minimization strategies

Risk of harm	Harm minimization strategy
Sudden withdrawal — tremors, retching, anxiety, hallucinations, seizures, delirium	Assess degree of dependence and usual level of consumption Institute appropriate level of pharmacological support to detoxify patient via reducing regimen
Risk of long-term disease — neuropathy, cardiac atrophy, brain atrophy, liver disease, etc.	Attention to physical condition — nutritional advice Thiamine supplements (300 mg od vit B strong compound TDS, vit C 100 mg TDS)
Risk of depressive illness weight loss, mood fluctuation. A period of short-term abstinence (1 week detox + 2 weeks) may be required to distinguish diagnosis of depression from symptoms of alcoholism	Treatment of depression
Anxiety — can be confused with symptoms of withdrawal. May be using alcohol to deal with anxiety	Use anxiety-reducing strategies — information giving, encouraging expression of fears, relaxation therapy, complementary therapies
Low self-esteem — many alcoholics have low self-esteem. Relatives may also be affected Low self-esteem is a contraindication for change	Use strategies to promote self-esteem — giving information, encouraging participation in decision-making, treating with respect and dignity, encouraging positive self talk
Domestic violence	Assess social situation Give relatives information and support

efficacy). Good self-esteem is important for this to take place. Low self-esteem contraindicates change. The nurse can help the patient to brainstorm specific problem areas and choose options to deal with them. A drinking or smoking diary may help the patient to become more aware of his/her habit and weak areas. The patient can then be asked to choose the best options and generate an action plan. It helps to set a date for stopping to give the patient time to mentally prepare.

There are many books and leaflets available to help smokers quit, and the unit should have a good stock of these. Unfortunately there are not many self-help leaflets for patients with alcohol problems. It may be helpful for the patient to learn relaxation and meditation techniques in preparation for stopping and the unit should have a good stock of audiocassettes for loan to patients. See Table 1.3.5 for details of resources.

Table 1.3.5: Resources

Leaflets:	Distribution Department
Thinking about Stopping?	Health Education Authority
Stopping Smoking Made Easier	Hamilton House
	Mabledon Place
	London WC1H 9TX
	or your local Health Promotion Unit
Telephone helplines:	
Quitline	Tel 0800 00 22 00
Healthbox	Tel 0800 66 55 44
Books:	
How to Stop Smoking and Stay Stopped	From bookshops
for Good (Gillian Riley, Vermilion)	
The Quit for Life Programme	
(David Marks, The British Psychological	
Society)	
Alcohol services:	Contact your local alcohol/addiction
Alcoholics Anonymous	unit for information on local help
Local alcohol/addiction services	available
Local self-help groups	
Audiocassettes on relaxation and	From alternative health shops and
meditation	alternative health mail order companies

The action stage

The patient modifies his/her behaviour and the detoxification regime takes place. Management should be as positive and comfortable as possible; an unpleasant experience will discourage future attempts to detoxify should relapse occur. Appropriate drug therapy and management of withdrawal is needed — see withdrawal options (Tables 1.3.6 and 1.3.7). The treatment plan should be discussed and agreed with the patient, using problem-solving skills to help the patient resolve problems that threaten the achievement of change. Drink/cigarette refusal skills, social skills, assertiveness and relaxation skills can be taught in order to help the patient cope (Kennedy & Faugier, 1989). Relatives should also be educated to help. It is a common misconception in alcohol-related problems that total abstinence should be the goal of change; in fact, many problem drinkers are able to return to harm-free, acceptable drinking patterns (Heather & Robinson, 1983).

Table 1.3.6: Withdrawal options — alcohol

Withdrawal may be for an agreed short-term period of abstinence or the patient may wish to try to stop using alcohol permanently.
Management should be as positive and comfortable as possible.

- < 10 units per day: sober up with support and information about expected side effects.
- > 10 units per day: reducing regimen 5–10 days — phone addiction unit for prescribing advice.
  — Chlordiazepoxide: is most effective in large doses; range of 100–400 mg on first day (some individuals need higher doses). Dose should be tapered at a rate of 25% of initial dose.
  — Heminevrin is highly addictive and is dangerous if taken with alcohol. It is no longer recommended for use in detoxification.
  — Hallucinations can also be managed by low-dose haloperidol (0.5–2.0 mg 1–2 hourly).
- History of seizures or delirium needs admission for detoxification.
- Support and educate relatives — they may find patient easier to handle when using alcohol than when going through withdrawal.

The nurse should be aware that nicotine reduces blood flow to the skin, so diabetics administering insulin may need to decrease their insulin dose once they have stopped smoking (Clark, 1995).

The maintenance stage

Lifestyle changes and motivation levels are maintained and developed. Nurses can provide continuing encouragement and support aimed at sustaining change. Self-help groups such as Alcoholics Anonymous may be helpful for patients with alcohol-related problems.

Relapses

It is rare to succeed in the first attempt to change — most people relapse at some point. This may happen several times. However, the

Table 1.3.7: Withdrawal options — smoking

1. Behavioural therapy alone — for patients with no physical symptoms of nicotine addiction.
2. Behavioural therapy plus use of nicotine replacement therapy; this can be in
   the form of transdermal, oral gum, nasal spray or inhalator. Transdermal nicotine (see Table 1.3.8) is the preferred method for people with head and neck
   cancer as it has the least effect on the mucous membrane, which may become
   very sensitive during treatment. Nicotine replacement therapy has been shown
   to increase the success of smoking cessation, with concomitant behavioural
   therapy, but the sustained rate is 10% at best (Benowitz, 1997).
3. Behavioural therapy plus use of antidepressant drugs — antidepressants have
   been shown to give a success rate of 44.2 % at the end of 7 weeks treatment,
   and 23.1% at 1-year follow-up (Hurt et al, 1997), and to double the success of
   cessation in another study (Humfleet et al, 1997). All these drugs were given
   with concomitant behavioural therapy. It would be wise to assess the need for
   antidepressants by using a tool such as the Hospital Anxiety and Depression
   Scale.
4. For those who use tobacco/alcohol to cope with stress, their discontinuation
   results in anxiety and the recurrence of the distress previously controlled by
   smoking. Tobacco withdrawal should therefore be managed with the use of
   anti-anxiety drugs and relaxation techniques to minimize discomfort (Breitbart
   & Holland, 1988).
4. An anti-smoking quitline was shown to be associated with successful smoking
   cessation and a campaign resulted in a decline in smoking prevalence (Platt et
   al, 1997). Giving the patient a telephone helpline number should therefore also
   be considered.
5. Intensive telephone contact follow up (four calls in 90 days) after a 30-minute
   behavioural session given by nurses improved cessation rates by 7% at 1-year
   follow up compared to patients given behavioural therapy alone (Miller et al,
   1997). This intervention should therefore also be considered.

process of moving through the change cycle allows people to learn
from previous relapses and they may get better with each attempt. It
is helpful to explain this process to the patient so that initial relapses
do not lower their feelings of self-efficacy.

Managing alcohol in the ward or clinic

The ward or clinic team should agree on a strategy for managing
alcohol use.

The ward

- Should patients be allowed alcohol at all on the ward? — a period
  of short-term abstinence may be more appropriate.
- How do other patients feel if someone is drinking on the ward?

Table1.3.8: Nicotine patches

Transdermal patches maintain a steady blood concentration of nicotine by absorption through the skin. This helps to prevent withdrawal symptoms.
They can be purchased from pharmacies in three strengths:
    High strength: for those smoking 20 + cigarettes per day
    Medium strength: for those smoking 10–20 cigarettes per day
    Low strength: for those smoking < 10 cigarettes per day.

The patch strengths are reduced over a number of weeks (see individual manufacturers' instructions)

The patch should be applied to clean, dry, hairless skin. Occasionally skin irritation may occur; use a different site each day. Refer to product data sheet for additional information on contraindications and side effects.

- Is the hospital liable for damage caused by an intoxicated patient or visitor?
- Why is the patient drinking? — anxiety?
- Ask relatives to help by not bringing alcohol for the patient.
- A planned strategy with the whole team's cooperation and consistency is essential.

Intoxicated or withdrawing patients and relatives have the potential to become aggressive. Nurses therefore need to have a strategy for managing aggression in the department. If patients or visitors become aggressive strategies should be employed to minimize disruption and increase cooperation:

- avoid being aggressive
- explain the reason behind policies on alcohol, procedures, etc. (e.g. it is dangerous for you/ your relative to drink whilst undergoing surgery/treatment)
- ask simple questions
- avoid the potential for violence by providing a calm environment, listening, sitting down
- personalize communication — use names
- use positive, not negative, responses.

The clinic

- If the patient attends the clinic intoxicated, try to identify and define the problem and the situation in which it occurs — e.g. is

the patient drinking to relieve anxiety about attending the clinic,
or because of poor pain control?
- Discuss with the patient the consequences of the behaviour — e.g.
non-compliance with treatment, unsafe behaviour.

Managing smoking in the ward or clinic

Most hospitals are now smoke-free zones. However, some areas
provide facilities for smokers. The ward or clinic team should agree
on a strategy for smokers:

- notices explaining no-smoking policies
- should patients be allowed to smoke at all on the ward?
- how do other patients feel if someone is smoking on the ward?
- why is the patient smoking? — anxiety, boredom?
- ask relatives to help by not bringing cigarettes for the patient
- a planned strategy with the whole team's cooperation and consistency is essential.

Summary

In summary, there is much nurses can do to facilitate smoking
cessation and manage alcohol-related problems effectively. This is
possibly the most important factor influencing a good outcome for
the patient both in terms of surgery and radiotherapy. Early intervention is vital, and outpatient head and neck oncology clinics
should be geared for nurses to provide these interventions. It is
strongly recommended that resources are allocated to these areas
both in terms of numbers and grades of nursing staff, as well as
education of the whole team. This without doubt would reduce
costs in terms of treatment of postoperative complications, length
of hospital stays, and number of hospital admissions during radiotherapy treatment, as well as increase the long-term survival of
patients.

Strategy for practice

- Organize inservice training on addiction management for all
staff.
- Provide comprehensive assessment of smoking and alcohol use at
the first clinic visit.

- Develop individual care packages according to the Model of Change.
- Provide structured educational packages for all smokers.
- Ensure there is a consistent smoking/alcohol policy clearly stated in the department.
- Establish close links with the local addiction service.

Chapter 1.4
Continuity of care: using all the resources

Introduction

Strategies to improve patients' quality of life and coping skills become ever more important as advances in treatment technology mean that more people survive head and neck cancer but live with physical and psychological disability. The provision of healthcare for today's cancer patients is complicated by a healthcare system that has traditionally been orientated to short-term acute care, not to the ongoing needs of people with chronic and often debilitating life-threatening illness (Conkling, 1989). The complex problems they face include financial security, employment, insurance access, loss of body function, pain management, disruption of family and other relationships, emotional and psychological implications.

This means that patients may need the services of multiple agencies in order to cope with everyday living. The challenge is to ensure continuity of care from the point of diagnosis, through the acute care setting, into the community. Attention to psychosocial and rehabilitation issues should be practised from day 1 as an ongoing process of comprehensive care for the patient and family. The goals should be to achieve as much function, as much physical and emotional comfort, and as normal social and occupational living as possible. This should not be merely a post-treatment 'discharge plan', but an ongoing interaction with the patient and family, extending all available resources in a timely fashion.

The nurse is often the key person in accessing the patient to community, voluntary and social services. This chapter will examine the ways in which the nurse can maximize current resources to provide continuity of care. It will also give an overview of community resources to provide the nurse with the knowledge to put patients in touch with all the services they need. It will also explore the ways in which nurses can help patients benefit from support groups.

Developing a coordinated care approach

What is continuity of care?

No single definition simultaneously captures every facet of the concept 'continuity of care'. Taken together, definitions proposed in the literature suggest that continuity of care is a philosophy and standard of care that involves patient, family and healthcare providers working together to provide a coordinated, comprehensive continuum of care. Such a continuum of care facilitates transitions from setting to setting, results in improved outcomes for the patient, and contributes to cost-effective use of health resources (Beddar & Aikin, 1994). This is vitally important in head and neck oncology, where care is often complex, with multiple disciplines involved over a variety of settings; as many as 20 professionals may be involved at some stage (Van Wersch et al, 1997).

Team collaboration

In head and neck oncology, the quality of patient care depends on the capacity of the many professionals involved to work as a team. Poor communication between staff causes dislocated care, failure to communicate with patients and inaccurate recording of clinical treatment. Early identification of problems through comprehensive assessment can do much to prevent crisis and alleviate difficulty for patients. Conkling (1989) suggests that a continuing care programme should include:

- Comprehensive assessment of all factors that will enhance or undermine the patient and family's ability to cope with the treatment and the disease, and to return to as high a level of functioning as possible.
- High risk screening; identification of those at high risk for psychosocial breakdown.
- Plan development; formulation of intervention strategies to identified needs and a treatment programme.

Much of this assessment information is gathered by various professionals in the head and neck team as they evaluate the patient for their specific services. Better methods are required for gathering and documenting this information in a consistent, organized fashion, which is easily accessible to all those involved in the patient's care. It is not realistic to expect that any one individual or care setting should be responsible to oversee a continuing care plan for a patient; these issues should be consistently addressed by the whole team.

Nurses can play a key role in initiating collaborative care; Scott and Cowen (1997) describe how multidisciplinary collaborative care planning was developed in a stroke rehabilitation unit. The benefits were many:

- broke down professional barriers, promoting awareness of each others' roles
- multidisciplinary ownership of patient records improved efficiency of recording information and communication between professionals
- allowed care to be monitored daily and omissions spotted quicker
- care was more individualized
- patient satisfaction increased
- better communication within the team allowing problems to be addressed more promptly
- increased professional satisfaction leading to higher staff morale
- clearer explanations of proposed treatment.

Care coordinators

Evidence shows that healthcare personnel who help to coordinate patient treatment and follow-up have a positive effect on overall patient care. Benninger (1992) compared a group of head and neck cancer patients who were managed by a liaison team, to a group with no access to help. The group managed by the liaison team were more likely to have reliable follow up ($P = 0.001$). Nurses are ideally placed to take on this role and case management by clinical nurse specialists has been very successful (Ethridge & Lamb, 1989; Cronin & Maklebust, 1989). In recognition of the important contribution nurses make, the Calman Hine Recommendations on cancer services (1994) propose that nursing care for all patients must be planned and led by specialist cancer nurses.

Documentation

Good documentation is essential for effective discharge planning and continuity of care. The UKCC (1993) found 'substantial evidence that inadequate and inappropriate record-keeping neglects the interests of clients by impairing the continuity of care'. Poor record-keeping leads to communication breakdown and an increase in the incidence of complaints (Swanson, 1995). The Clinical Systems Group (CSG) (Department of Health) report on clinical record-keeping found that: few records are made of decisions regarding planned care, and who is responsible for carrying tasks out; where care is shared between professionals there is rarely a full record of all events; specific advice or information given to the patient is rarely recorded; some of the recorded information is inaccurate; there is widespread duplication of data collection and transmission. The report reveals a catalogue of communication failures and makes a number of recommendations on record-keeping, one of which states that patient-held records have potential which is not being realized (CSG, 1998).

Client-held records

Client-held records have been explored in many settings to improve continuity of care and are particularly well established in maternity services. I have heard medical professionals question the ability of people with head and neck cancer to keep records safely and bring them to consultations. It is therefore interesting to read reviews in the literature about client-held records in mental health. A project by Essex et al (1990) showed that a client-held record could be used successfully and was helpful to both service users and providers. Another small study also found client-held records helped coordination of care in the homeless mentally ill (Reuler & Balazs, 1991). Stafford & Hannigan (1997) write about the design and use of a client-held record for mental health clients. They recommend that it is easy to carry, easy to use, flexible and hard wearing. Their booklet was in the form of a small pocket sized plastic ringbinder with four main sections: personal details, including a list of names and telephone numbers of agencies involved; appointments; notes; and medication. This booklet has been well established in the pilot locality and they report it being introduced across the whole borough. Clients are able to make an informed choice about whether or not to have a booklet.

Client-held records in head and neck cancer

Van Wersch et al (1997) provide an excellent example specifically for head and neck cancer. They approached the problem of continuity of care and information for head and neck cancer patients in Holland by developing a 'logbook'. The aim was for patients and families to be more informed about care, and for professionals to achieve better continuity of care. Compared to a control group, patients in the trial logbook group received more comprehensive and structured information, with less contradictory material. They also experienced fewer psychosocial problems and were more independent and better informed. Professionals reported that the logbook had contributed to continuity of care in the trial group and that it had enabled them to gain a more rapid and complete view of the patient's case history, despite the fact that many had not used the logbook optimally due to 'lack of time'. This evaluation concluded that a logbook definitely has a contribution to make in continuity of care for patients with a head and neck tumour. The authors recommended that the form and content be designed carefully by the whole team, with a ringbinder in a smaller format than A4 and separation of the communication and information sections into two folders. They acknowledged that the attitudes of care professionals must change so that they are more willing to read and write in a logbook.

Hospital to community liaison

The community team

Primary care, not hospital care, should be the focus of good cancer care. It is provided by general practitioners, district nurses and specialist nurses (palliative care nurses, health visitors, community psychiatric nurses and practice nurses) within the community. The Calman Hine Report (1994) highlighted the need for good communication between the hospital and the primary healthcare team: 'All sectors are important in cancer care. However the primary care team is a central and continuing element in cancer care for both the patient and his or her family from primary prevention, pre-symptomatic screening, initial diagnosis, through to care and follow-up or, in some cases, death and bereavement. Communication between sectors must be of a high quality if the best possible care is to be achieved'. The GP and the district nurse are key carers for the patient and it is important that they are involved in the patient's care from day 1. The outpatient nurse is the key person to ensure this happens.

Sadly, there is often a lengthy delay between the patient's outpatient visit for a cancer diagnosis and a letter informing the GP about the outcome being dictated, typed and posted. The district nurse may not be informed about the patient at all until a crisis occurs, or the patient is discharged home from hospital after surgery, often with severe communication difficulties and complex care needs. The importance of the nurse initiating good communication cannot be emphasized enough. Mackay (1997) developed a nurse-led approach to this problem with a fast-track communication form to complement, not replace, the more detailed letter which would follow in due course from the hospital doctor. This form is completed during the outpatient consultation by the consultant or clinic nurse and given to the patient, with the request that they or a relative hand it to their GP's surgery within 2 days. Use of the form demonstrably improved communication between the hospital outpatients' department and the primary healthcare team.

Early district nurse referrals

Many cancer units now routinely refer to the district nurse when a cancer diagnosis has been given. The district nurse can then meet and assess the patient prior to the commencement of treatment or surgery. This is particularly important for head and neck oncology patients who may have difficulty communicating after their initial discharge from hospital, making a district nursing assessment at this point extremely difficult. If the patient has particularly complex care needs after surgery or radiotherapy, the district nurse may welcome an invitation to visit the patient on the ward prior to discharge for a handover from the ward primary nurse.

Discharge planning

As a result of technological developments older people are receiving treatment for conditions, such as advanced head and neck cancer, that would once have been considered untreatable. However, financial restraints mean hospital stays for these patients are becoming shorter. Patients are now discharged 'quicker and sicker' than used to be the case (Naylor, 1990). The head and neck cancer patient can be extremely vulnerable on discharge from hospital because of huge changes in body function that often require highly technical nursing skills and care (for example, nasogastric or gastrostomy feeding, tracheostomy care, use of nebulizers and suction). Their baseline health status in both the physical and non-physical domains is likely to be significantly below that of their age-matched contemporaries in the general population (Funk et al, 1997). Added to this, most of this patient group are over 65 years of age, and the elderly are known to have a variety of problems after discharge. Mistiaen et al (1997) list a variety of problems from a review of the literature and their own study on patient problems after discharge from an acute care setting:

- limited ability to carry out personal care activities and house-keeping; decreased mobility; difficulty in following prescriptions; difficulty in using appliances
- diminished general health, reduced physical and emotional functioning; fatigue, unstable posture, pain and not sleeping well were the most common physical complaints
- not receiving enough assistance to carry out everyday activities, not receiving enough support in dealing with physical and emotional problems
- not feeling adequately informed; most frequently about the course and signs of recovery and medication.

The authors conclude that these problems can impede recovery and lead to unplanned readmission. They recommend that discharge plans are designed to take all these needs into account and information strategies are designed and evaluated carefully.

Most patients rely on relatives for support; it is therefore important to involve relatives in the discharge plan to make sure they are able to give the help patients need and to avoid burdening care-givers. Mah & Johnston (1993) showed that the major concern for families of head and neck cancer patients was caring for the patient after discharge. Nazarko (1997) summarizes reports of inadequate discharge procedures for older adults over the last 25 years. These reports identify common themes:

- poor interprofessional cooperation
- poor documentation

- inadequate patient consultation
- communication difficulties.

More specifically, Van Wersch et al (1997) cite a study of 133 head and neck cancer patients following discharge: 23% received poor information about aftercare, 73% received little or no information, and 59% little or no support.

Unless head and neck cancer patients are being cared for in designated head and neck oncology units, they are often nursed on ENT and maxillofacial wards where patient dependency may mostly be low, and turnover high. Thus the wards often are not used to, and do not have discharge policies for, patients with complex needs. Discharge planning for the head and neck patient can be very time-consuming and labour-intensive, with the primary nurse working with many members of the team. For example, a discharge plan for one patient may involve the dietitian, speech and language therapist, medical social worker, occupational therapist, district nurse and palliative care team. This takes place in an atmosphere of stress due to the ever-increasing pressure on NHS beds (O'Donnell, 1996).

Even patients whom nurses consider to be of low dependency still need post-discharge support. Van Harteveld et al (1997) looked at 337 cancer patients for whom hospital nurses would normally not have made a community nursing referral. Each patient was offered a community nursing 'continuity' visit. Evaluation demonstrated that 93% of the patients experienced one or more physical, psychological or social problem that had not been identified by the hospital nursing team. Both patients and community nurses found the visit beneficial.

Resources in the community

The key role of the district nursing service and the GP has been emphasized. However, head and neck cancer patients have complex and demanding requirements after discharge. The nurse must therefore have a good knowledge of all the resources available in the community. Nurses will often work alongside social workers to access patients to these services. Outpatient nurses may not always have the luxury of access to a social worker, so it is even more important that they are aware of services.

Social services

All patients have the right to be assessed by the social services department for support in their home. The nurse can help the patients gain access to these services by telephoning the Social Services Department covering the area in which the patient lives. Services provided include:

Emergency alarm systems

Vulnerable patients who live alone and are not in a position to deal with an emergency or contact help can have a 24-hour alarm system installed. This is connected to the telephone system and is activated by the press of a button (usually on a pendant or bracelet). The control centre will contact nominated friends or relatives when the alarm is activated.

The home care service

The home care service helps people to live independently in their own homes by helping with tasks which have become difficult to manage. This may be temporary help for a short-term illness, help for carers to avoid a breakdown in care arrangements, or help for people with a physical disability, mental health problem, learning disability or long-term illness in order for them to live safely at home. The home care service can help in a variety of ways, for example assisting with personal care, shopping, housekeeping, making meals, budgeting. Frozen meals and meals on wheels are available. The service is usually initiated by a referral to the local social services office, and is arranged by a home care manager. Charges are calculated on the patient's financial situation.

Daycare

Many older people have poor social networks which compound the isolation often caused by head and neck cancer. Day centres are a good way of easing loneliness, as are luncheon clubs. Many hospices provide day care services which incorporate creative rehabilitation activities and give the patient access to specialist palliative care.

Services for the hearing impaired

Patients who develop hearing problems should first be referred to an audiologist for a hearing assessment. Most social services departments provide specialist help for people with hearing problems, sometimes through voluntary organizations. Help available will include: someone to talk to and give support, advice and information; equipment to help with everyday life — for example loud doorbells, special telephones; help for the patient and family to adjust to hearing loss; information about lip-reading classes; information about help for tinnitus sufferers.

Services for the visually impaired

People who have sight loss which is affecting their daily life may find it an advantage to be registered as visually impaired; this is done after a visual assessment by a consultant ophthalmologist. Registration leads to a visit by a rehabilitation officer specially trained to help people with sight loss. This includes help with adjustment to sight loss, learning new skills such as Braille, moon, typing, and using writing/signature guides; mobility training (getting about safely inside and outside); advice on special equipment such as clocks, watches, games, talking books; information about voluntary organizations; advice about re-training for employment.

Services for carers

Caring for an ill relative or friend can be very tiring, stressful and complicated. Carers are often completely tied to the house, unable to take a break and cut off from their friends and everyday life. Often, it is not even acknowledged that they are acting as a 'carer'. Carers should not be expected to cope alone and 'stumble across information along the way'. Under the Carers Act, since 1 April 1996 Social Services have had a legal duty to carry out a separate assessment for carers if the carer asks for this, and if the person they care for is being assessed or reviewed. An assessment is a meeting between someone who needs services and people from the agencies who provide or organize the services. Assessments include community care assessments and discharge planning meetings. When such an assessment is being organized, any carer who is regularly providing a substantial amount of care, or is intending to do so, has a right to talk to someone about their own situation and have this recorded as a Carer's Assessment. Services which may be useful to carers include: benefits, home care, daycare centres, family placement (breaks for carers by arranging stays away from home), respite sitting services, residential care and holidays, practical help, equipment and adaptations. Hospices provide daycare and respite care to help carers. The private sector also provides home nursing and home care services. There are also many voluntary organizations to help carers, as well as carers' support groups.

Local voluntary schemes

There are a large number of voluntary schemes, including the Good Neighbour, Helping Hands and Community Care schemes, usually run by local churches. What they provide usually depends on the numbers and talents of local volunteers; for example, befriending, sitting, shopping, gardening, dog walking.

Ethnic minority services

People from ethnic minorities are also able to seek help from a wide range of local groups run by the communities themselves. Advocacy and interpreting services are usually available from social services for people from ethnic minorities. A patient advocate can often attend important hospital appointments with the patient as well as provide advice and help.

Financial benefits

People with cancer often find they need to spend more money because of their illness, or they may find their ability to earn money is affected. A patient currently in employment when diagnosed should be encouraged to speak to their employer to find out how long they can have paid sick leave, what occupational sickness benefits are available and what sickness notes are needed.

Grants from charities

Patient grants from charities can help to deal with financial crises. Macmillan Cancer Relief grants are available for a wide range of goods and services including:

- heating, fuel, bedding, clothing, furniture
- treatment and fares
- domestic appliances
- convalescence

- domestic help, childminding
- telephone installations
- general debts, mortgage and rent arrears.

A patient who has been in the armed forces may obtain a grant from the Soldiers', Sailors' and Airmen's Families Association, the Earl Haig Fund or the RAF Benevolent Fund. The Independent Living Fund helps with the costs of help at home and is accessible via social services. *The Charities Digest* (available at public libraries) contains extensive information about organizations that provide special financial help for respite stays, holidays, etc.

The benefits system

People with cancer may be entitled to several benefits: Disability Living Allowance (DLA) (under 65s) or Attendance Allowance (AA) (over 65s); Disability Working Allowance; Incapacity Benefit; Severe Disablement Allowance; Invalid Care Allowance; Disability Premium and Severe Disability Premium; Income Support; help from the Social Fund. People on a low income can get help with the costs of travelling to hospital and prescriptions. People with a permanent tracheostomy and people taking thyroid hormone replacement are entitled to free prescriptions. People with a terminal illness, who have a prognosis of 6 months or less, are entitled to DLA or AA immediately under Special Rules. The doctor fills in a DS1500 (Special Rules) form which is sent with the DLA or AA application. The Citizens Advice Bureaux offer extra help, advice and support in dealing with benefits and employment issues. Most cancer centres have specialist social workers and welfare benefits advisors to help.

National voluntary organizations

Macmillan Cancer Relief (MCR)

MCR is a national charity working to improve the treatment and care of cancer patients and their families. The organization's aim is to develop and promote new ideas to improve their lives and reduce unnecessary levels of fear. MCR funds doctors, buildings and education for cancer specialists but is perhaps best known for its Macmillan nurses. Macmillan nurses are all clinical nurse specialists. They are highly skilled in pain and symptom control and offer emotional support and practical advice to cancer patients and their families from the moment of diagnosis onwards. Based in either a hospital or the community, Macmillan nurses work in a team with other health-care professionals, ensuring that patient care is continuous. Many Macmillan nurses specialize in certain types of cancer, for example head and neck, helping patients cope with the particular problems associated with each illness. MCR also has a patient grants service that provides one-off grants to help patients in financial difficulty; these can help with items such as fuel bills, clothing and convalescent breaks. An application can be made by nurses, social workers and local voluntary organizations.

Marie Curie Cancer Care

As well as funding specialist cancer care centres and research, Marie Curie Cancer Care nurses can provide care at home through the day or night, giving a carer the chance to have a break or sleep. This service is organized by the district nurse.

CancerBACUP

This organization provides trained nurse counsellors to give support on the telephone, in London and Glasgow, and will help individuals find counselling elsewhere. The organization produces a wide range of patient information booklets on different cancers and treatments, available free to patients.

Cancerlink

Cancerlink provides information about all aspects of cancer by telephone or letter. Information is provided in Bengali, Hindi, Punjabi, Urdu and English. Cancerlink's self-help and support service acts as a resource to cancer support groups and individuals throughout Britain. This service helps people to set up new groups and offer one-to-one support. It promotes continued development of these services through information exchange, training and support. Cancerlink also produces a range of publications on the emotional and practical aspects of cancer.

Age Concern and Help the Aged

These organizations provide information and help on a wide range of services and support, including daycare, visiting and specialist services.

Equipment for people with head and neck cancer

Patients often require equipment at home; feeding pumps (usually arranged by the local dietetic department), nebulizers and suction pumps are often needed. To help with telephone communication, the TalkType system and machines such as the Claudius 2 are available from British Telecom. Liquidizers and magnetic writing boards are very useful. Portable suction pumps and nebulizers can help individuals to get out of the house. However, except for feeding pumps, nurses may find it very difficult if not impossible to get these items in the community.

Nursing teams should therefore investigate establishing their own equipment pool. Funding can be obtained from various sources: MCR provide grants for equipment to help Macmillan teams as well as individual grants to patients; the Hospital League of Friends is also usually willing to help, as are local organizations such as Rotary or Round Table. Cancer centres and units often have money donated in memory of patients, which can be used specifically for patient care. Nurses can use all these sources together to establish a comprehensive equipment pool. Those nurses with plenty of energy may also wish to organize their own fund-raising events!

Self-help and support groups

What are self-help and support groups?

BACUP (1995) and the King's Fund Report on head and neck cancer care (Edwards, 1997) recommend that patients should have the opportunity to meet former patients and that local self-help groups should be formed. There are approximately 500 such self-help groups in the UK, providing advice and support to people with cancer and their families. Some groups are general cancer support groups, open to anybody with a diagnosis of cancer, whilst some are specific to head and neck cancer.

Cancerlink defines a self-help group as a group run for its members by its members; professionals do not normally get involved. Members feel that by helping others they are helping themselves, and they control decisions made by the group. A support group is often more formal; it may be more clearly divided into those being supported and those doing the supporting. The supporters often have some training. Professionals tend to be more involved, as advisors or as part of the committee. Support groups may help a series of patients, who pass through the group as they adapt to the disease with information and support (Cancerlink, 1988).

Speigel et al (1989) noted that 'the provision of psychosocial support for isolated individuals under stress can improve health outcome and self-help groups can counter the social alienation that often divides cancer patients from their family and friends'. Support groups for cancer patients can vary in several ways but can be defined as a voluntary, small group structure for mutual aid and accomplishment of a special purpose. Groups exist for individuals to help each other. Core elements include sharing and distributing information, support, advocating, socializing and affirmation. Sharing of experiences is a key element and groups are reported to provide social support, decrease isolation and facilitate improved adaptation to the disease (Bottomley, 1997). Bottomley's review of the literature on the efficacy of support groups is inconclusive because of the methodological difficulties in studying the effects of such groups. However, the review demonstrates overall that cancer support groups offer the potential for cost-effective help to cancer patients.

A self-help group can help to transform feelings of helplessness, with members regaining a sense of control and independence (Cancerlink, 1988). Members can find their own strengths and use these to help others. As well as providing peer support, groups can offer professionals information about their own experiences and how to handle their problems — they are specialists deeply concerned with their own problems (Brimelow & Wilson, 1982). They can be a consumer watchdog body, educating professionals about their needs. There is also an important role in raising awareness in the local community of their disability and needs.

Support groups in head and neck cancer

A review of the literature on head and neck cancer and support groups shows that peer support is very important in rehabilitation after laryngectomy. No literature on support groups in other head and neck cancers was found, but it seems reasonable to assume that these findings can be generalized to all individuals with head and neck cancer. Patients in the King's Fund study reported that speaking to other patients was helpful; 'they described the relief when they met someone who understood what they had being going through' (Edwards, 1997). Goffman (1963) notes that people with disabilities tend to derive comfort and support from those who share the same stigma and can provide the individual with instruction in 'tricks of the trade' and with a 'circle of lament'. Jay et al (1991) found that 78% of 65 laryngectomees questioned found the laryngectomy club useful as they had the opportunity to share and discuss their problems. Richardson et al (1989) interviewed 60 laryngectomees and found that peer support provides an opportunity for social comparison as other laryngectomees model skills and provide feedback for improvement. Speech adjustment was significantly associated with support from peers and professionals — more support from these sources indicated better communication outcomes and less dysfunction. Stam et al (1991) completed a structured interview with 51 laryngectomees; the need for preoperative counselling proved to be a crucial factor in postoperative adjustment. They found that preoperative counselling, including speech therapist appointments and visits by fellow laryngectomees, strongly predicted later quality of life. Support from peers with the same cancer plays a crucial role in the major adjustment that takes place after surgery, a factor which is independent of family and professional support. The support group also plays an important role for spouses and significant others, as Blood et al (1994) found in their study of 75 laryngectomee spouses.

National support agencies for people with head and neck cancer

• **The National Association of Laryngectomy Clubs** aims to promote the rehabilitation of laryngectomy patients within the British Isles. See Table 1.2.1 for contact details. It encourages the formation of local clubs, coordinates and disseminates all information relevant to the rehabilitation of the laryngectomee, advises on the availability of speech aids and medical supplies, arranges for lectures on mouth to neck resuscitation, and arranges for laryngectomees to visit pre- and post-operative patients. A wide range of leaflets on laryngectomy are available free of charge.

- **Changing Faces** provides help for people with facial disfigurement. See Table 1.2.1 for contact details.
  They emphasize communication skills and developing a positive outlook in people with altered faces. This service is available in person, by telephone or by letter. Regular workshops are organized for individuals to meet in a safe atmosphere and learn positive coping strategies and self-confidence. They also produce a range of booklets, including When Cancer Changes The Way You Look. The organization is constantly developing new rehabilitative ideas. At the time of writing, Changing Faces is exploring an exciting new way of training nurses to lead patient groups with the aim of rehabilitating them socially. Contact the organization for more information.

- **Let's Face It** provides a friendship service for people suffering from all forms of facial disfigurement from others who have experienced similar problems. Regional group meetings are available as well as telephone contacts, letters, social meetings and outings for patients and carers. See Table 1.2.1 for contact details.

Setting up a self-help or support group

The nurse's role in a support group

It is important that nurses consider their role carefully in relation to a self-help group. While professionals can assist in starting a group, there can be difficulties if they take too active a role initially, preventing the group from becoming independent; even with the best will in the world, they are likely to take 'control'. Brimelow and Wilson (1982) found that those professionals who were most effective in maintaining the sensitive balance between offering constructive support and taking over believed in the intrinsic value of self-help and the capacity of members to organize their own affairs. They saw their role as complementary to group members, and described the relationship as one of partnership. Even if they played a significant role in establishing a group, they saw their role as facilitators, bringing people together to provide backup support. It is therefore important that nurses establish limits to their involvement in the starting and running of a self-help group.

Establishing a group

Cancerlink is an organization concerned with the support of self-help groups, and they are an excellent source of advice for anyone thinking about establishing a group. Firstly, it is important to establish whether the clients definitely want a self-help group, and to identify a core group of people who have the time, energy and commitment to run such a group (Cancerlink, 1988). If a few people volunteer, they first need to meet together to get to know each other; it is important that the group members can work together. There is a danger that some of those who have volunteered want to help but are actually more in need of help which the group is not yet ready to give. Each person must be honest about the amount of time and commitment they feel they can give. To help this process, Cancerlink has a team of experts who will offer the volunteers training and supervision in setting up and running a self-help group. They also offer a small start-up grant to cover initial expenses (Cancerlink, 1988).

Establishing a visiting scheme

It is common practice for ex-patients to be asked to see new patients in order to provide encouragement and support. Unfortunately this often happens in a very ad hoc way. An inappropriate visitor can do more harm than good, and visitors, like professionals, need to receive support and ongoing training and development. A common problem is that of the ex-patient who has had a bad experience and 'unloads' this on to the new patient being visited. A visiting panel of patients who are good role models and willing to help other patients going through treatment can be invaluable. It helps to have a range of individuals so that patients and visitors can be matched as closely as possible. Breast Cancer Care provides a good model for practice with their Buddy Scheme, which provides trained ex-patients as buddies for women currently undergoing treatment.

Volunteers should be carefully selected and receive training in basic listening skills and issues such as confidentiality. This should be followed up by ongoing support. It is therefore recommended that senior nurses (e.g. the clinical nurse specialist) should take a key role in the selection and training of visitors. Cancerlink will help in the training of visitors if requested.

The establishment of a Laryngectomy Friendship Scheme with ex-patients trained and selected by the speech therapist and clinical nurse specialist demonstrated a marked improvement in patients' access to, and satisfaction with, a laryngectomee visitor (Feber, 1998).

Summary

In summary, nurses are often the gatekeepers to many other services for the patient, so it is important that they are up to date with the wide range of services available in their area, and that they put the patient and family in touch with colleagues who have the specific knowledge and expertise to help. Nurses may also need to reflect on working practices in order to improve continuity of care and provide a patient-focused service.

Impressive diagnostic and treatment technologies in head and neck oncology, coupled with the medically driven model of care, often mean that the team does not address the other, equally important, disease management considerations. People fear cancer not only for the treatments used against it but because of its physical, psychological, social and economic sequelae. Patients are often discharged with multiple continuing care needs which they and their families are unprepared to handle. A well-informed healthcare team, functioning in a non-hierarchical, non-medically-dominated environment, can be much more sensitive to the biopsychosocial implications of head and neck cancer and is more able to help the patient and family create a personal environment that makes surviving cancer worthwhile.

Strategy for practice

You can improve continuity of care by:

- Performing a comprehensive assessment of the patient at diagnosis.
- Developing a protocol to ensure the right information and support are given at the right time.
- Developing patient-held documentation.
- Developing fast-track information to the primary healthcare team.
- Involving the primary healthcare team from the point of diagnosis onward.
- Developing a discharge protocol for your area — ensure that you invite the whole multidisciplinary team to take part in the design and development.
- Appointing a designated coordinator to take charge of and be accountable for discharge arrangements for each patient.
- Developing effective discharge documentation. This should include a discharge checklist and written information about discharge and aftercare that will be given to the patient and community staff.
- Consulting and preparing patients and family for discharge.
- Informing the district nursing service about all patients.
- Being familiar with all services and equipment available to help patients.
- Being familiar with all local sources of funding.
- Forming good working relationships with national and local voluntary organizations.
- Training and supporting your ex-patient volunteers.

Section Two
Acute nursing management in head and neck cancer

Chapter 2.1
Airway management

This chapter will look at airway management in the head and neck cancer patient, focusing on the care of the patient with a tracheostomy in both the surgical and oncology setting. It is not intended to give information about caring for the tracheostomy patient in intensive care, as this falls within the domain of intensive critical care nursing.

Anatomy and physiology of the airway
Martini, 1992

The respiratory tract consists of the conducting passageways that carry air to and from the alveoli in the lungs. The passageways delivering air to the lungs constitute the upper respiratory tract. These passageways filter, warm and humidify the air, protecting the more delicate conduction and exchange surfaces of the lower respiratory tract, or lungs, from debris, pathogens and environmental extremes. Filtering, warming and humidification of inspired air begins at the entrance to the respiratory tract and continues throughout the rest of the passageways. By the time the air reaches the alveoli, it is at 100% humidity and 37°C and most foreign particles and pathogens have been removed.

Air enters the respiratory tract via the nares, through the nasal cavity. The vestibule is the first portion of the nasal cavity, contained within the fleshy tissues of the external nose. Its epithelium contains hairs that extend across the nares, trapping any large airborne particles such as sand, sawdust, or insects, preventing them from entering the nasal cavity. Air passes from the vestibule to the internal nares, flowing around the conchae; the conchae cause the air to swirl around the nasal cavity, ensuring that it comes into contact with the mucous membrane. The mucous membrane of the nose contains an abundance of arteries, veins, and capillaries bringing nutrients and water to the secretory cells. This extensive vascularization provides a mechanism for warming and humidifying incoming air. As cool dry air passes over the exposed surfaces of the nasal cavity, the warm epithelium radiates heat and the mucus evaporates. Air leaving the nasal cavity has been heated to body temperature and is nearly saturated with water vapour. This mechanism protects the delicate respiratory surfaces from chilling or drying out — potentially disastrous events.

The respiratory epithelium consists of a pseudostratified, ciliated, columnar epithelium with numerous goblet cells. The goblet cells and mucous glands beneath the epithelium produce the mucus that bathes the exposed surfaces of the nasal cavity. Smaller particles may be trapped by the mucus of the nasopharynx or secretions of the pharynx before proceeding farther along the conducting system. Cilia sweep that mucus and any trapped debris or microorganisms toward the pharynx, where they are swallowed. This filtering mechanism removes virtually all particles larger than around 10μm from the inspired air. Particles as small as 5μm are trapped by the mucus lining the larynx, trachea and bronchi. The cilia in these regions beat upwards towards the pharynx, forming a mucociliary escalator. Particles 1–5μm collect in the terminal bronchioles, where they are engulfed by alveolar macrophages that also remove smaller particles stuck into the alveolar surfactant. Exposure to unpleasant stimuli such as cold air, large quantities of dust and debris, allergens, or pathogens results in a rapid increase of mucus production.

The altered airway

Airway obstruction

One of the most frightening and life-threatening acute oncological emergencies in the head and neck patient is airway obstruction. This occurs when the flow of air into the lungs via the airway is impaired by tumour or the effects of treatment. Situations when this emergency may often arise are:

- initial presentation of an advanced laryngeal cancer with acute stridor
- acute laryngeal oedema caused by radiotherapy.

Rapid recognition and treatment are vital to prevent respiratory arrest. An intravenous line should be established and corticosteroids should be administered to reduce inflammation and oedema. Oxygen should also be administered (Chernecky & Berger, 1998). Heliox can be very helpful in this situation as helium has a low density and therefore an increased flow rate, which results in less airway resistance and decreases the work of breathing (Milner et al, 1997). An emergency tracheostomy may be performed to bypass the obstruction.

Tracheostomy

The airway is often altered in the head and neck patient by the formation of a tracheostomy. This may be a temporary tracheostomy to preserve the airway from the massive postoperative oedema associated with oropharyngeal surgical procedures and partial laryngectomy, or a permanent tracheostomy formed after removal of the larynx. Temporary tracheostomy may also be required for non-surgical patients for: obstruction of the upper airway by inoperable tumour; acute laryngeal oedema caused by radiotherapy; and chronic fibrosis of the larynx caused by irradiation. Figure 2.1.1 shows the normal airway, the airway altered by a temporary tracheostomy, and the airway after laryngectomy.

There are two basic techniques for creating a temporary tracheostomy:

- The standard surgical technique involves the dissection and transfixtion of the thyroid isthmus and formation of an opening in the trachea, often by the formation of a flap (Bjork technique) which ensures a large window-like opening which facilitates easy tube insertion (Martin, 1989).
- Percutaneous dilational tracheostomy does not involve a formal incision into the trachea or transection of the thyroid isthmus. The procedure is performed by the introduction of a wire guide percutaneously into the trachea, followed by dilation of the tract formed to enable the insertion of a tracheostomy tube (Carrillo et

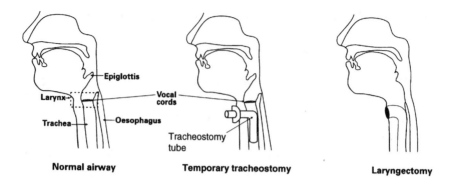

Figure 2.1.1: The altered airway.

al, 1997). It is becoming more popular, as evaluation shows it to have less morbidity and a lower cost than standard surgical tracheostomy (McHenry et al, 1997). Insertion of a tracheostomy tube is much more difficult after this procedure.

After these procedures, a tract forms between the trachea and the skin over a period of around 4 days (Harkin, 1998).

Laryngectomy creates a permanent stoma (see Chapter 4.2 for details of the surgical procedure). Laryngectomy results in a less acute tracheal angle, therefore a tracheostomy tube is unsuitable to accommodate this difference. A laryngectomy tube should be used instead (Martin, 1989).

Management and care of the tracheostomy depends on the type of procedure; the tracheostomy formed after laryngectomy requires different management to that of a temporary tracheostomy.

Temporary tracheostomy care

Tracheostomy care is an extremely ritualized area of practice; each unit has its own particular rituals. There are numerous articles in the literature recommending various approaches to tracheostomy care. Unfortunately, many of these are not evidence-based. This section will examine the evidence available and, from this, attempt to determine optimal tracheostomy care. The aim of tracheostomy care is the maintenance of a patent airway, alongside the prevention of the complications cited below.

Complications of tracheostomy

El Kilany (1980) and Waldron et al (1990) have performed comprehensive reviews of the complications of tracheostomy. El Kilany reviewed 1,982 cases, Waldron et al 150 cases. This information, alongside other reports of complications, provide a useful background on which to plan nursing interventions aimed to prevent, reduce and manage complications.

Haemorrhage
El Kilany, 1980; Regan, 1988; Waldron et al, 1990; Billy et al, 1994; Gelman et al, 1994; Grillo et al, 1995; Holdgaard et al, 1998; Yoshida et al, 1998

Surgical: a vessel may be transected at the time of surgery and result in bleeding when the blood pressure begins to rise postoperatively.

Delayed: erosion of tracheal wall and vessel by excessive tube or cuff pressure. The innominate and right common carotid arteries, which cross the trachea at the level of the clavicle, are particularly at risk from the tip of the tracheostomy tube on the anterior tracheal wall. When a tracheostomy tube is dangerously near a large vessel, it can be seen to pulsate synchronously with the patient's pulse. Later, aspiration of blood may be noted. This should alert the nurse to a serious problem; the tube should be replaced immediately with one of a different size and length (Regan, 1988; Wright, 1996; Yoshida et al, 1998).

Yokoyama et al (1995) report an adjustable flange tube causing fatal haemorrhage of the innominate artery. They recommend great care in the use of such tubes; the correct fit should be verified by radiography. Fibre-optic examination should be performed a few days after insertion to determine whether mucosal damage is present.

El Kilany recommends that treatment of massive haemorrhage should be to suction the airway, insert an endotracheal tube and inflate the cuff. Selecky (1974) recommends over-inflating the cuff already in place to temporarily reduce bleeding. Waldron et al (1990) recommend applying local pressure but do not describe how. Wright (1996) recommends bedside control of haemorrhage by cuff over-inflation, or digital arterial compression. An additional intervention would be to place the patient in head-down position to minimize blood flow into the respiratory tract. The patient will require surgical repair of the damaged vessels.

Tracheoesophageal fistula

El Kilany, 1980; Waldron et al, 1990; Berrouschot et al, 1997; Letheren et al, 1997

This may result from a poor surgical technique, wound breakdown caused by infection, or erosion of the posterior tracheal wall by excessive tube or cuff pressure. Wood and Mathiesen (1991) also cite the concomitant use of a stiff nasogastric tube. Treatment is to insert a longer cuffed tube beyond the level of the fistula, and to minimize leakage from the oesophagus into the trachea by keeping the patient nil by mouth with enteral feeding. The fistula may be allowed to heal spontaneously, or may require surgical repair. Recent trials using fibrin glue to repair fistulas have been successful (Benko et al, 1997).

Infection

El Kilany, 1980; Waldron et al, 1990; Teoh et al, 1997; Crosher et al, 1997; Mazzon et al, 1998; Holdgaard et al, 1998; Harkin, 1998

Peristomal infection: the tracheal stoma is a surgical wound that is difficult to protect with a dressing. It is therefore very vulnerable to infection from the respiratory tract or surrounding skin. Mazzon et al (1998) report peristomal infection after translaryngeal tracheostomy to be linked to oropharyngeal colonization. The stoma needs frequent cleaning using an aseptic technique in the first post-operative days (see Stoma care, p. 107). Any dressings should be changed regularly as they quickly become soaked in secretions, providing an ideal environment for bacterial growth. The tracheostomy mask should also be washed in warm soapy water and dried with paper towels after each use (Ronchetti, 1998) as it tends to become dirty and damp, and thus represents a potential risk for wound infection. Dampened or soiled Buchanan laryngectomy protectors may also present an infection hazard (it is not necessary to dampen these products).

Chest infection: chest infections are also a problem as a tracheostomy bypasses the normal immune protection system of the upper airway. This can be minimized by prevention of stomal infection, use of an effective heat/moisture exchanger, and scrupulous cleaning of tracheostomy mask, nebulizer chambers and humidifier system (see Humidification, p. 116). Suction should be strictly aseptic and only performed when necessary (see Suctioning, p. 113).

Tracheitis
El Kilany, 1980
This can be caused by infection (bacterial or fungal) or chemical irritation. Signs of fungal infection can be seen by a fungal growth on the tube itself. A swab should be taken to confirm the cause. Tubes should not be soaked in disinfectants as they absorb the chemicals, which then irritate the trachea.

Obstruction of tracheostomy tube
El Kilany, 1980; Waldron et al, 1990; Clarke, 1995; Rowe et al, 1996; Forbes, 1997
El Kilany cites obstruction of the tube as being the third most common cause of death in 1,928 cases studied (0.21% mortality rate). Waldron et al report five of their 150 cases experiencing obstruction. The most common cause is the tube gradually being obstructed by secretions. Forbes reports five of 20 tracheostomy patients receiving hospice care experiencing recurrent episodes of blockage. Two patients died as a result of this. Humidification can help to prevent this, but the best method of prevention is the use of tubes with an inner cannula which can be changed easily and frequently. The nurse should be alert to the signs of gradual tube occlusion:

- increased respiratory rate
- decreased oxygen saturation
- difficulty passing suction catheters
- little or no airflow to be felt through the tube.

Tubes may also be occluded by the end of the tube settling against the tracheal wall, decreasing the airway, and herniation of the cuff over the tube end (Sakabu et al, 1997; Rosenberg & Katz, 1997).

Prompt removal of the tube in cases of subtotal and total obstruction will prevent rapid deterioration and cardiopulmonary arrest (Rowe et al, 1996). Forbes concludes, in her review of head and neck cancer care in the hospice setting, that information and training are needed and hospice staff should visit the patient in hospital prior to transfer in order to gain the knowledge and confidence to care for the patient's airway.

Tube displacement/malposition of the tube
El Kilany, 1980; Waldron et al, 1990
The tube can become displaced by the patient coughing if it has not been secured adequately (see Securing the tracheostomy tube, p. 107). The tube position should be checked regularly by a visual check and feeling for the airflow out of the tube with one's hand.

If a tracheal stoma is new and therefore not well formed, if the surgical procedure has not been performed well, or if a percutaneous tracheostomy has been perfomed, it is possible to push the tube into the tissues alongside the trachea instead of into the trachea itself when changing the tube. This can also happen if the patient has a thick neck and the tube is not long enough.

Unscheduled replacement of dislodged tubes can be difficult. Forceful attempts at replacement are painful and may disrupt the soft tissues adjacent to the tracheal tract, creating a false passage. Young et al (1996) describe the use of a nasogastric tube as a 'guidewire' to facilitate replacement of the tube. Harkin (1998) describes the use of a suction catheter (see Changing the tracheostomy tube, p. 105).

It is important to check the airflow after changing the tube. If a good airflow is not present, remove the tube and start again. A pair of tracheal dilators should be kept at the bedside, along with two spare tubes; one of the same size, and one a size down to be inserted in case of difficulty replacing the same size.

Excess granulation tissue
El Kilany, 1980; Prescott, 1992
Granulation tissue forms in the raw tissue of the stoma and subsequent fibrosis requires removal. Prescott recommends that this is avoided by formal skin to trachea stoma formation at the time of tracheostomy. El Kilany recommends treatment by application of silver nitrate (weekly as necessary), or by applying a steroid-based cream.

Tracheal mucosal injury
Regan, 1988; Waldron et al, 1990; Wood & Mathiesen, 1991; Prescott,1992; Partridge & Flood-Page, 1997
This can be due to trauma or ischaemia caused by poor suctioning technique (see Suctioning, p. 113), insertion of a tube without an

obdurator, using the wrong type or size of tracheostomy tube, dragging on the tube by attachments, and the style or pressure of the cuff used. This injury can lead to tracheoesophageal fistula as reported above, tracheal stenosis, trachemalacia and granuloma formation. Tracheal ischaemia occurs when the tube or cuff exceeds the mucosal capillary perfusion pressure (25 mmHg). Flexible tubes with low pressure cuffs are therefore the tubes of choice.

The features of tracheal stenosis include airway narrowing, cough, wheeze and exertional dyspnoea. Management includes insertion of a long tracheostomy tube, and surgical repair if possible (Levine et al, 1978).

Aspiration and swallowing problems
Selecky, 1974; Oermann et al, 1983; Logemann et al, 1998
The tracheostomy tube anchors the trachea to the skin and prevents the laryngeal elevation and relaxation of the upper oesophageal sphincter phase of the swallow. This is worse when a cuff is present and can cause aspiration. Logemann et al (1998) discuss whether the presence of a cuffed tube to protect against aspiration actually makes the situation worse for some patients. To reduce the risk of aspiration of regurgitated enteral feeds, the patient should be in a semi-recumbent or upright position. Oermann et al (1983) reported that 58.8% of patients with tracheostomy (both permanent and temporary) reported discomfort during swallowing, especially patients with plastic cuffed tubes. Chapter 2.3 gives a detailed discussion of swallowing problems caused by tracheostomy.

Foreign body aspiration
Gupta & Ahluwalia, 1996; Partridge & Flood-Page, 1997; Kumar et al, 1997
This includes parts of fractured tracheostomy tubes, insertion devices, and tracheoesophageal valves. Management involves the bronchoscopic removal of the foreign body. Tube and insertion devices should therefore be inspected carefully for any defects before placement is carried out.

Excessive coughing and mucus production
Martin, 1989; Hooper, 1996; Harkin 1998
This is due to initial irritation of the trachea by the tube, and also excessive mucus production due to the response of the lungs to

unhumidified, cold air. The initial irritation will settle, but the patient should be warned about it. This will also occur at tube changes, particularly if a new tube of different size or length is inserted. Use of an effective heat/moisture exchanger will minimize mucus production in the long term (see Humidification, p. 116).

Pressure sore caused by the tube flange

This can particularly be a problem if the neck is oedematous. It can be prevented or relieved by using a swivel flange tube, and by placing a dressing (e.g. Trachi-dress) between the flange and the skin. The only skin complication noted in the literature is contact dermatitis caused by a rubber tracheostomy disc (Mitxelena et al, 1998).

Cuffed tracheostomy tubes

A cuffed tracheostomy tube is the tube of choice in the following circumstances:

- immediately after surgery to prevent aspiration of blood and serous fluid from the wound
- to prevent aspiration of leakage from a tracheoesophageal fistula, or pharyngocutaneous fistula near the stoma
- to prevent aspiration due to laryngeal incompetence
- to seal the trachea when the patient is being mechanically ventilated
- to seal the trachea when the patient is swimming.

Cuffed tracheostomy tubes can cause serious damage to the trachea, as discussed above. Care of the patient with a cuffed tube must therefore be meticulous.

- Keep the cuff pressure below 25 mmHg. Various authors recommend between 15 and 22 mmHg (Selecky, 1974; Mapp, 1988; Regan, 1988).
- Although cuffs are labelled 'low pressure', they are only low pressure if inflated correctly. It should not be assumed that they are the panacea to tracheal mucosal damage. Guyton et al (1991) showed that the pressure in these types of cuffs can often exceed 25 mmHg even when used very carefully. Selecting the correct

size tube is vital; too small a diameter tube will result in over-inflation of the cuff with pressure greater than 25 mmHg to achieve a seal; too large a tube will result in inadequate inflation of the cuff and possible excessive pressure on the mucosa by malposition of the tube itself or the folds of the cuff (Mackenzie, 1983; Hollis et al, 1996). The cuff should be carefully inflated to minimal occluding volume, that is no more air than the exact amount necessary to seal the trachea (Mulvaney, 1976). The only cuff that automatically deflates and inflates to conform to the trachea is the Fome cuff (however, this tube does not have an inner cannula system).

- It is recommended by some authors that the cuff pressure be checked with a cuff manometer every 8 hours (Crosby & Parsons, 1974; Regan, 1988). However, Crimlisk et al (1996) question this practice and recommend 8–12 hourly or daily checks.
- One of the great nursing rituals of the past was the hourly 5-minute deflation of the cuff, but this has been shown to be ineffective (Powaser et al, 1976) and unnecessary if a low-pressure cuff is used correctly (Bryant et al, 1971).
- The amount of air used to inflate the cuff should be recorded and any variation at a later date noted. This could indicate a leaking cuff, tracheal dilatation, or a tracheoeophageal fistula (Regan, 1988; Prinsley, 1992).
- Removal of the cuffed tube will be perfomed on medical instructions. Higgins et al (1997) recommend that patients have a swallowing assessment prior to removal as aspiration may occur due to alterations to motor and sensory functions caused by the tracheostomy tube.

Fenestrated tracheostomy tubes

A fenestrated tube is a tube with a hole in the shaft to allow air to flow through the larynx into the upper airway. They are useful in patients who need a tracheostomy to ease stridor, but still have enough capacity to use the larynx and upper airway to speak by finger occlusion of the tube end, or using a speaking valve such as the Passy Muir. They are also used to wean patients off their tracheostomy as the airway improves after radiotherapy or surgery. A non-fenestrated inner tube should always be inserted before suctioning (see below).

Tracheostomy speaking valves

If the patient can exhale efficiently through the nose and mouth and around the tracheostomy tube, a speaking valve can be fitted to facilitate vocalization (Kaut et al, 1996). This is much more hygienic than fingertip occlusion. It also restores olfaction, and secretion management is improved as patients can cough up secretions as well as blow their noses. Swallowing may also be improved (Dettelbach et al, 1995; Stachler et al, 1996). The tracheostomy tube may need downsizing or changing to a fenestrated tube to allow exhalation around the tube. Valves are available as separate units which fit onto the end of the tracheostomy tube (e.g. Passy Muir), or as an integral part of an inner cannula (e.g. Negus tube, Tracoe Flex, Tracoe Comfort).

Choosing a tube

There are many different types of tracheostomy tube for temporary tracheostomy on the market. These are outlined in Table 2.1.1. Tracheostomy tubes should be selected with safety and comfort in mind. Swivel flange tubes will move to the shape of the patient's neck, reducing the risk of causing a pressure sore. Rigid tubes carry more of a risk of causing tracheal necrosis, fistula and haemorrhage. Patients with thick necks or, for example, large thyroid tumours or large stomal recurrences, making access to the trachea difficult, will require specialist tubes such as the extra long, adjustable flange tubes. Fortunately, all tracheostomy tubes now have low-pressure cuffs, but unfortunately they do not all have inner cannula systems. The routine use of a tube without an inner cannula system is not recommended due to the risk of obstruction.

Sizing a tube

Just to make life complicated, manufacturers of tracheostomy tubes all seem to have their own grading system for sizes. To select the optimum size, the diameter of the patient's tracheal stoma is measured in millimetres and then the tube whose overall diameter (OD) is the same or nearest size down from this measurement is selected. The OD is written on the side of the box and on the tube flange; it should not be confused with the internal diameter (ID) measurement of the tube. See Table 2.1.2 for a guide to sizes.

Table 2.1.1: Tracheostomy tube types (LP = low pressure)

Tracheostomy tube type	Inner cannula system	Flexibility	Swivel flange	Comments
Silver (Negus, Chevalier Jackson) • must not be worn during radiotherapy — causes the beam to scatter	Yes	Rigid	No	For long-term tracheostomy — many patients prefer the appearance Inner cannula with speaking valve
Tracoe Twist (Polyurethane)	Yes Spares available	Flexible at body temperature	Yes — horizontal and vertical	LP cuffed and uncuffed, with and without fenestration Fits Passy Muir valve, has inner cannula with speaking valve on selected tubes
Tracoe Comfort (PVC)	Yes	Yes	No, but light and soft	For long-term tracheostomy — transparent, so discreet appearance Inner cannula with speaking valve. Can be custom made
Shiley (PVC)	Yes Disposables available	Rigid	Yes — vertical	LP cuffed and uncuffed, with and without fenestration Fits Passy Muir speaking valve

(contd)

Table 2.1.1: (contd)

Tracheostomy tube type	Inner cannula system	Flexibility	Swivel flange	Comments
Portex (PVC)	Only in selected tubes	Flexible at body temperature	No	LP cuffed and uncuffed, with and without fenestration No speaking attachment Adjustable neck flange (extra long) model available
Bivona Adjustable Neck Flange — extra long (Silicone)	No	Very	No, but very soft and flexible	Has tight-to-shaft LP cuff for ease of insertion Ideal for patients with thick necks, problems due to recurrence around tracheal stoma, etc
Bivona Fome Cuff (Silicone)	No	Yes	No	Expands to conform to trachea with lowest possible pressure

Table 2.1.2: Tracheostomy and laryngectomy tube sizes

Bivona Soft Laryngectomy Tubes	Portex Tracheostomy Tubes	Tracoe Twist Tracheostomy & Laryngectomy Tubes	Shiley Tracheostomy & Laryngectomy Tubes	Silver Negus & Chevalier Jackson Tracheostomy Tubes	Silver Colledge Laryngectomy Tube	Medasil Button	Kapitex Button
—	size 5 (OD 8 mm) uncuffed tube only; size 6 (OD 9 mm) all other tubes	size 4 (OD 7.2 mm)	size 4 (OD 8.5 mm)	28 French	28 French	—	—
—	size 7 (OD 10 mm)	size 6 (OD 9.2 mm)	size 6 (OD 10 mm)	32 French	32 French	size 10	size 8
size 8 (OD 12.0 mm)	size 9 (OD 12 mm)	size 8 (OD 11.5 mm)	size 8 (OD 12 mm)	36 French	36 French	size 12	size 10
size 9 (OD 13.5 mm)	—	size 10 (OD 13.5 mm)	size 10 (OD 13 mm)	40 French	40 French	size 14	size 12
size 10 (OD 15.0 mm)	—	size 12 (OD 15.9 mm)	—	—	—	—	size 14

(contd)

Table 2.1.2: (contd)

Bivona Soft Laryngectomy Tubes	Portex Tracheostomy Tubes	Tracoe Twist Tracheostomy & Laryngectomy Tubes	Shiley Tracheostomy & Laryngectomy Tubes	Silver Negus & Chevalier Jackson Tracheostomy Tubes	Silver Colledge Laryngectomy Tube	Medasil Button	Kapitex Button
size 12 (OD 17.0 mm)	–	–	–	–	–	–	–
size 14 (OD 20.0 mm)	–	–	–	–	–	–	–
size 16 (OD 24.0 mm)	–	–	–	–	–	–	–

Changing the tracheostomy tube

The frequency of tube changes depends on the type of tube and also the individual patient. If a tracheostomy tube with an inner cannula system is being used, the inner cannulas can be changed as often as necessary with the tube itself being left in place for up to 4 weeks (EEC Directive, 1993). Saah et al (1996) report a case of a patient who had worn the same tube for 2 years without removing it for cleaning. A foreign body was found in his bronchus after investigations for chest infection. It was a fragment of the outer cannula. The authors recommend regular examination of tracheostomy tubes for signs of wear and tear.

Tubes without an inner cannula system need to be changed on a daily basis, or more often, to avoid occlusion occurring. Different units and clinicians have different policies, and there is no evidence in the literature to give clear guidelines.

The first tube change should be performed by an experienced practitioner. Tracheostomy tube changes tend to cause anxiety in both patients and nurses as many people believe that the tube has to be in position for the patient to breathe, and also that the stoma will close as soon as the tube is removed, which is not the case. It is important that the procedure is performed in a calm and confident manner.

Surgical and well-established tracheostomies

- Prepare for the procedure by giving both procedural and sensory information to the patient. Reinforce information that he/she will still be able to breathe whilst the tube is out.
- Until the stoma is formed properly, tracheal dilators and a tube one size smaller should be at the bedside in case the stoma tightens up when a tube is removed.
- Prepare the new replacement tube for insertion; inspect for any defects, insert introducer, attach tapes/tracheostomy holder, apply a small amount of lubricating gel. If tube is cuffed, inflate cuff and observe for any defects, deflate fully, folding the cuff away from the tube tip to form a smooth surface for insertion.
- If a cuffed tube is in situ, fully deflate the cuff, suctioning any secretions retained above the cuff.
- Remove old tube.
- It may be helpful at this point to let the patient breathe without

the tube in situ just so that they know the tube is not vital to breathing to avoid panic at tube changes or if the tube falls out at any time.

- Clean and inspect the stoma using a torch (as described in Stoma care, p. 107).
- Insert the new tube, following the curve of the trachea.
- Remove introducer immediately and insert inner cannula.
- Check the airway patency to ensure the tube is positioned correctly in the trachea.
- Secure with tapes or Velcro holder.
- Inflate cuff if appropriate.

Percutaneous dilational and very new tracheostomies

As replacement of a tube via a percutaneous or newly formed (< 4 days old) tract is difficult, it is recommended that this procedure is carried out only by experienced practitioners (Harkin, 1998).

- Prepare for the procedure by giving both procedural and sensory information to the patient. Reinforce information that he/she will still be able to breathe whilst the tube is out.
- Until the stoma is formed properly, tracheal dilators and a tube one size smaller should be at the bedside in case the stoma tightens up when the tube is removed.
- Prepare the new replacement tube for insertion as described above, but do not insert the introducer.
- Insert a size 14 suction catheter (Harkin, 1998) (with the connector end cut off) into the tracheostomy tube which is to be removed. Remove tube over the catheter. Alternatively, Young et al (1996) describe the use of a nasogastric tube.
- Feed the new tube over the catheter into the trachea. There may be a small amount of trauma as the introducer cannot be used with this technique.
- Use of a size 14 catheter ensures that the airway will be maintained as it has a similar gauge to a mini-tracheostomy (Harkin, 1998).
- Check the airway patency to ensure the tube is positioned correctly in the trachea.
- Secure with tapes or Velcro holder.

Stoma care

- The stoma will need frequent cleaning during the initial postoperative period. The aim is to reduce the risk of peristomal infection and secondary chest infection, and to promote wound healing and the formation of a stoma tract. The stoma should be managed in the same way as any surgical wound until healing has occurred and sutures are removed, around days 7 to 10. It should be cleaned using normal saline and an aseptic technique.
- The stoma should be inspected carefully with a torch at tube changes; watch for signs of necrosis, infection, tracheitis, over-granulation tissue or fistulae. The suture line and peristomal area should be cleaned with normal saline. Dressings can pose an infection risk as they quickly become wet and provide an ideal environment for bacteria. They should be changed regularly.
- The skin around the stoma may become excoriated by mucus secretions and salivary fistulae; it should be cleaned regularly. A skin barrier (e.g. Clinishield Wipes, Cavilon) should be applied if necessary. Tracheostomy dressings should be used with care, as they quickly become soggy and exacerbate the problem. Specifically designed dressings such as Trachi-dress (Kapitex Healthcare) are designed to absorb and retain mucus in a middle layer whilst protecting the skin with a non-adherent layer.
- Dressings with loose fibres (e.g. gauze) should not be used as the fibres can break off and enter the respiratory tract. Pre-cut, specially formulated dressings (e.g. Trachi-dress) should be used.

Securing the tracheostomy tube

The traditional way of securing a tracheostomy tube is with tracheostomy tape. The tape is threaded through the slots in the flange and tied securely in a knot. One finger's breadth should be allowed between the neck and the ties to ensure they are not too tight. If the patient has a flap or graft, care should be taken that the tape does not cause pressure in this area (Martin, 1989). Velcro tracheostomy holders with a soft backing can be more comfortable for the patient, as well as being easy to secure and adjust. They are also much easier for the patient to use at home if a tracheostomy is long-term. They can be obtained from most airway product suppliers but unfortunately are not available on prescription.

Cleaning tubes and inner cannulas

Some tubes and their inner cannulas can be cleaned and reused; for example silver tubes and long-term plastic tubes. There is no specific evidence in the literature on cleaning tracheostomy tubes. Soaking dirty tubes in disinfectant is not recommended because organic matter (e.g. mucus) neutralizes disinfectant (Maurer, 1985). In addition, polyurethane tubes are damaged by agents such as alcohol, hypochlorite and gluteraldehyde (Coates & Death, 1982). Mallinckrodt recommend that Shiley inner cannulae are rinsed, but not soaked, with hydrogen peroxide 0.5% to remove encrusted secretions (Mallinkrodt Medical Inc., 1993). The tube should be cleaned with a tracheostomy brush (available on prescription). Great care should be taken not to damage the tube or cannula with the brush. Tubes should be then be rinsed carefully with sterile normal saline or water as carry-over of the antiseptic causes chemical irritation of the trachea. Tubes should be allowed to air dry. For patients at home, the most sensible advice seems to be to clean the tubes in warm soapy water, then allow both tube and brush to air dry. Tarnished silver tubes should be cleaned with a proprietary silver cleaner, then rinsed thoroughly to remove any residue before use. More research is needed in order to provide evidence for practice.

Patient education

If the tracheostomy is intended for long-term use, a teaching plan should be designed to enable the patient to care for their own tracheostomy. This should be documented in order to ensure consistent information is given, and in order to evaluate progress.

Decannulation

When the upper airway obstruction has resolved, removal of the tracheostomy (decannulation) can be considered. This can be assessed by the patient's tolerance of occlusion of the tube using a decannulation plug. Patients who experience anxiety and difficulty can be weaned off the tube using a tracheostomy valve (e.g. Passy Muir). The patient should be monitored for 48 hours to ensure tolerance to decannulation before removing the tube. It is then removed and the stoma is occluded by an airtight dressing. The patient should be taught to press on the dressing when coughing and speaking to prevent air being forced through the fistula (Harkin, 1998). The stoma should close down and heal completely over a period of approximately 14 days (Heffner, 1995). Surgical closure is only required if a persistent tracheocutaneous fistula occurs (Waldron et al, 1998).

Laryngectomy care

Laryngectomy tubes

After a laryngectomy, the trachea is stitched to the neck to form a permanent tracheostomy. The cartilage rings of the trachea make the stoma very stable and therefore a tube is not normally required (Martin, 1989).

During surgery, a cuffed tube will be in place for ventilation purposes and to protect the airway from any leakage from the wound. This should be removed as early as possible to prevent tracheal mucosal damage and is replaced by a stoma button whose purpose is to prevent the skin around the stoma edge from shrinking as scar tissue forms.

A laryngectomy tube may be required in certain situations:

- extensive reconstructive surgery using flaps which occlude the stoma (e.g. a pectoralis major flap to replace a defect in the neck)
- damage to the cartilage rings in the trachea caused by postoperative wound infection, or tube damage which has caused tracheal stenosis or tracheostomal stenosis (Weissler, 1997; Vlantis et al, 1998)
- severe lymphoedema or obesity which causes occlusion of the stoma
- recurrent tumour in the stoma.

The different types of laryngectomy tube available are shown in Table 2.1.3. The shape of the trachea when a laryngectomy stoma has been formed is much less of an acute angle than a temporary tracheostomy. The laryngectomy tube is therefore shorter with a less acute angle. Long-term use of a tracheostomy tube in a laryngectomy patient may result in internal abrasion of the anterior tracheal wall, with potential haemorrhage from the innominate or right common carotid artery, especially if the stoma is positioned low in the neck (Martin, 1989).

Table 2.1.3: Laryngectomy tube types

Laryngectomy tube type	Description	Comments
Button	Short, soft tube to prevent stoma shrinking. Does not usually prevent tracheoesophageal valve use, but can easily be adapted by cutting a piece out	Most commonly used tube after laryngectomy
Bivona Stomvent Inhealth Laryngectomy Tube	Soft tube available in longer lengths than the button. Can be adapted for tracheoesophageal valve use by fenestrating	For patients with tracheal stenosis, or stomas that tend to collapse or become blocked by skin flaps or submental oedema
Shiley Laryngectomy Tube	Rigid tube with inner cannula. Cannot be adapted for use with tracheoesoephageal valve	For patients with tracheal stenosis, or stomas that tend to collapse or become blocked by skin flaps or submental oedema. Can also be used to maintain a patent airway in stomal recurrence
Tracoe Twist Laryngectomy Tube	Flexible at body temperature tube with inner cannula (spares available). Cannot be adapted for use with tracheoesophageal valve	For patients with tracheal stenosis, or stomas that tend to collapse or become blocked by skin flaps or submental oedema. Can also be used to maintain a patent airway in stomal recurrence
Portex Laryngectomy Tube	Flexible at body temperature tube. No inner cannula. Cannot be adapted for use with tracheoesophageal valve	For patients with tracheal stenosis, or stomas that tend to collapse or become blocked by skin flaps or submental oedema. Can also be used to maintain a patent airway in stomal recurrence
Silver Colledge Tube • must not be worn during radiotherapy – causes the beam to scatter	Rigid tube. No inner cannula. Cannot be adapted for use with tracheoesophageal valve	For patients with tracheal stenosis, or stomas that tend to collapse or become blocked by skin flaps or submental oedema. Can also be used to maintain a patent airway in stomal recurrence

Stoma care

The aim of stoma care is to maintain a patent airway, promote healing and prevent peristomal infection, tracheitis and secondary chest infection.

- The laryngectomy stoma should be managed as a surgical wound until the suture line has healed, and sutures have been removed. It should be cleansed as needed, depending on the quantity of secretions produced, with normal saline using an aseptic technique.
- Stoma buttons can be removed frequently for cleaning. They need to be a good fit to avoid being expelled too easily when the patient coughs. If it is difficult to insert the button, it is helpful to apply lubrication (e.g. yellow paraffin) to the outside of the button and the rim of the stoma — it will then slide in easily.
- During removal of the button and cleansing, the stoma should be inspected with a torch. The nurse should observe for signs of infection, tracheitis, fistulae, necrosis, over-granulation tissue and crusting. Any crusts should be removed with tweezers. If severe crusting is a problem, a pair of curved forceps (e.g. Tilley's) can be used to remove crusts obstructing the airway.
- After healing has taken place, stoma care should become part of the patient's own daily routine. The patient should be taught to clean the stoma with cotton buds and tweezers to remove any mucus and crusting. Sterile saline should be used in hospital, but on discharge the patient can be instructed to use boiled water.
- There is not usually a need for tracheal dilators, as the permanent stoma will not close down
- During postoperative radiotherapy, crusting of secretions in the trachea can be a major problem, and these should be removed using curved forceps or tweezers. Severe radiation reactions in the trachea may necessitate admission to hospital in order to monitor the airway carefully. Extra humidification via steam inhalation will help to manage this problem during radiotherapy. Again, use of an efficient heat/moisture exchanger will minimize the crusting problem.
- If stoma shrinkage has occurred in a laryngectomy stoma, it can be redilated using a rigid laryngectomy tube.
- Care of the tracheoesophageal puncture and valve are discussed in Chapter 2.5, p. 201.

The patient should be taught to care independently for their laryngostomy as early as possible. An individual teaching plan should be designed and documented in order to ensure that consistent information is given and progress is evaluated.

Airway resistance in the laryngectomee

The physiological airflow resistance from the upper nares to the upper trachea is important in preventing alveolar collapse and maintaining optimum lung ventilation : perfusion ratio. This resistance is lost in the laryngectomee, causing a subsequent decline in lung function and oxygen saturation. A product to correct this situation has now been developed. Trachi-naze replaces the normal airway resistance. Laryngectomees wearing it demonstrated a rapid increase in oxygen saturation (McRae et al, 1996). This device also acts as a heat/moisture exchanger and filter (see p. 116). It is available on prescription in the community.

Other problems associated with laryngectomy

- Loss of nasal function. Anosmia will be experienced, due to loss of airflow through the upper airway (see Chapter 2.10, p. 262). Nose blowing can be difficult; Jay et al (1991) found that 65% of a sample of laryngectomees found this a problem. In addition, 62% were troubled by not being able to sniff, and 31% complained of a troublesome running nose.
- Loss of the sphincteric function of the larynx. Fixation of the chest in inspiration by the adduction of the vocal cords facilitates a rise in intra-abdominal pressure for activities such as weight lifting, defecation and micturition. Jay et al (1991) report 6% of laryngectomees experiencing difficulty with micturition, 18% with defecation and 57% with lifting weights.
- Use of bronchodilator and corticosteroid inhalers for laryngectomees with coexisting airways disease is very difficult; it is impossible to achieve an airtight seal with devices made for oral use. Nakhla (1997) describes the use of a spacer device with a homemade adaptation of a plastic soft drink bottle. However, spacer devices made for infants are ideal for use with inhalers for tracheostomy patients and can be easily obtained on prescription.

Suctioning

Complications

- Hypoxia, when a tracheostomy is suctioned, air is removed from the lungs as well as secretions. Therefore suction should not be applied for any longer than 10–15 seconds (Mapp, 1988), and the patient should take deep breaths of oxygen both before and after the procedure (Carroll, 1989).
- Atelectasis, negative pressure during suctioning can cause alveolar or even lung collapse; Demers and Saklad (1976) state that 'as mild to moderate degrees of negative pressure are transmitted to unstable airways during suctioning, even the most meticulous of operators will probably inflict diffuse microatelectasis'. Pressure of suction apparatus should never exceed 80–120 mmHg and catheter diameter should be less than half the diameter of the tracheostomy tube (Regan, 1988). The patient should take deep breaths of oxygen both before and after suctioning (Carroll, 1989).
- Tracheal irritation caused by the suction catheter can result in coughing and excess mucus production (Mapp, 1988). This rather negates the effect of suctioning. Instilling a bolus of saline into the trachea also causes irritation (see Saline lavage, p. 115).
- Tracheal mucosal trauma is caused by the catheter brushing against the mucosa. Every single insertion will cause some degree of trauma. Rough introduction can damage the mucosa and cause bleeding (Regan, 1988); therefore the catheter should be inserted gently. The design of the suction catheter is also important. The catheter should be able to reach at least 10 cm beyond the end of the tracheostomy tube, but not so far that it enters the right main bronchus. The catheter should not have any sharp edges and should be flexible enough to exert minimal pressure against the mucosa yet stiff enough to be easily pushed into the airway. The catheter should have a smooth surface to reduce trauma during insertion and removal. A standard catheter with a plain end hole and a single eye results in the eye 'grabbing' and damaging the mucosa; they are not recommended for airway suction. An aerodynamic design with multiple eyes prevents contact of the tip with the tracheal wall whilst applying suction.

- Excessive suction pressure will also cause damage (from 80–120 mmHg is recommended by various authors). Folding the suction catheter and then releasing it applies a very rapid vacuum to the catheter tip and can be dangerous. A catheter with a fingertip vacuum control gives low residual tip vacuum, reducing the risk of damage and hypoxia (Health Devices, 1977). However, Jung and Gottleib (1976) felt that trauma was more likely to be due to repetition of suctioning, vigour of insertion and amount of suction applied, whatever the type of catheter used. Duration of uninterrupted suction also influences the amount of damage caused (Jung & Gottleib, 1976); again use of a fingertip vacuum control catheter allows intermittent suction to be applied. Authors recommend that suction should be applied for a maximum of between 10 and 15 seconds. However, Czarnik et al (1991) examined the effects of continuous suctioning (for 10 seconds) versus intermittent suctioning (2 seconds with and 1 second without) and found that there was no significant difference as both methods caused trauma. Intermittent suctioning is less effective in secretion clearance. Carroll (1989) states that use of suction pressure over 120 mmHg causes mucosal damage. Using high negative pressure does not mean that more secretions will be removed, but that more damage will be caused. The best intervention for thick tenacious secretions is optimal humidification and hydration.
- If a fenestrated tube is in situ, the suction catheter touches the mucosa and can cause over-granulation. To avoid this risk, a non-fenestrated inner cannula should be inserted during suctioning (Harkin, 1998).
- Infection can easily be introduced into the trachea by poor aseptic technique when suctioning. First, the mucous membranes are more vulnerable to infection than the skin. Second, the upper airway, where antimicrobial defence mechanisms are centred, is bypassed (Demers & Saklad, 1976; Fiorenti, 1992). There are arguments both for and against using a new suction catheter each time the trachea is entered (Crow & Carroll, 1985).
- Dysrhythmias (bradycardia) may be caused by myocardial hypoxia and stimulation of the vagus nerve, whose receptors line the tracheobronchial tree. Inserting the catheter too far results in carinal stimulation, producing syncope.
- Hypotension may result from the above.

- Oermann et al (1983) found that 79% of patients in their study experienced sensations of pain, pressure, coughing and choking during suctioning but that some of this group said they did not have sensations if 'nurses were gentle'. Sawyer describes his experience of tracheal suction as "the closest I have come to hell on earth ... In the hands of a skilled, sensitive practitioner suction need not be more than a very necessary discomfort. On occasions however, it was horrific. The coughing, the gagging and the choking spasms produced by the 'sink plunger' technique were terrifying ... I dreaded the words 'just one more go'." (Sawyer, 1997).

Saline lavage

This is another of the great nursing rituals in tracheostomy care. It has been advocated as a way of loosening secretions and lubricating the suction tube. Dried secretions are often cited as the main reason for instilling saline bolus; Ackermann (1985) dismisses this practice as ineffective because water and mucus do not mix, even after being shaken vigorously together in a test tube. He cites an experiment by Hanley et al, who instilled radio-tagged saline into the tracheas of five dogs and two humans. Subsequent X-rays showed that all of the saline remained in the trachea and main bronchi and suctioning recovered only 10.7% and 18.7% of the saline in the dogs and humans respectively. Thus none of the saline reached the dried secretions and only a small percentage of the saline itself was retrieved. He concludes that saline instillation has no value, and it is much more important to prevent the formation of dried secretions by effective humidification of the airway and ensuring the patient is well hydrated systemically. In another paper, he examined the effect of saline instillation on oxygen saturation and found that saturation levels fell more in patients who had saline instillation than in those without saline. This negative effect increased with time. He concludes from this that saline instillation disadvantages the patient by causing bronchospasm, as well being a barrier to gaseous exchange (Ackerman, 1993).

Implications for practice

- Only suction when absolutely necessary. If the patient can expectorate his/her own secretions this should be encouraged in preference to suctioning. Change the inner tube to remove secretions from the tracheostomy tube, rather than using suction.

- Ensure the patient is well hydrated as this will ensure secretions are not tenacious and dry, and thus are easy to expectorate.
- Ensure the patient is using humidification or a heat/moisture exchanger at all times to prevent drying of secretions.
- Do not instil saline prior to suctioning.
- Ask the patient to take deep breaths of oxygen both before and after suctioning.
- Use a catheter specifically designed for tracheal suctioning, e.g. Gentle-Flo or Aero-Flo, and no greater than half the diameter of the tracheostomy tube. Be very gentle when inserting the catheter. Do not insert any more than 15 cm of the catheter.
- Ensure the suction machine setting is no higher than 120 mmHg.
- Apply suction for no more than 15 seconds whilst withdrawing the tube.
- Use a strict aseptic technique and thorough handwashing; monitor for early signs of infection: raised white cell count, temperature, sputum cultures.

Humidification and heat/moisture exchangers

Tracheostomy can have potentially disastrous effects by bypassing the normal humidification and filtration system of the upper respiratory tract (Shelley et al, 1988). This effect can be aggravated by the administration of dry gases such as air and oxygen. There can also be considerable heat and moisture loss from the body via the tracheostomy (above the normal 250 ml water and 350 kcal heat per day) because the heat and moisture conservation mechanism has been bypassed. Drying of the mucous membrane, which compromises 95% water, causes drying and crusting of the viscous layer, destruction of the cilia, damage to the mucous glands, disorganization and flattening of pesudostratified columnar epithelium and cuboidal epithelium, disorganization of the basement membrane, desquamation of cells, mucosal ulceration, and reactive hyperaemia. This leads to sputum-retention atelectasis and reduced tissue elasticity, with collapse of bronchioles and mucosal swelling. Surfactant activity is reduced, and there is a fall in residual capacity and static compliance. Dehydration of the mucous membrane seriously increases the risk of infection.

Jay et al (1991) found that 35% of laryngectomees were troubled by crusting in their trachea. Fifteen per cent suffered from troublesome bleeding and 54% reported frequent chest infections. Humidification and filtration of air and gases is therefore vital for the tracheostomy patient. Some kind of humidification or heat/moisture exchanger should be used at all times.

Dry gas humidifiers

A humidification system will normally only be used in the initial postoperative period or when administering medical dry gases such as oxygen. Dry oxygen should never be given to a patient with a tracheostomy as it will quickly cause airway dehydration. Distilled water and saline reservoirs in humidification systems have been shown to be important sources of infection. Where these are used, 500 ml bottles should be used in preference to 1,000 or 1,500 ml bottles, and opened bottles should be discarded after 24 hours (Brown et al, 1975). However, evaluation of a closed system sterile prefilled humidifier (Aquapak) showed that it reduced the occurrence of bacterial contamination completely (Castel et al, 1991). Modern humidification systems such as Respiflo provide fine water particles (2–8 μm) that are able to penetrate deep into the smaller alveoli and bronchi alongside a sterile prefilled closed system, which eliminates bacterial contamination. Heated water systems are preferable as cold water humidifiers dry the airway as it gives up a proportion of its moisture content to try to saturate the inspired cold gas (Fell & Boehm, 1998).

Over-humidification

Excessive artificial humidification of inspired gases may produce as much harm as under-humidification (Shelley et al, 1988). Excessive heating may cause mucosal damage, pulmonary oedema and stricture formation. Again the cilia may be damaged and there may be an increased volume of secretions exceeding the capacity of the mucociliary escalator. Condensation of water droplets within the airways may block them and cause atelectasis. These systems must therefore be used with care.

Nebulizers

Nebulizers produce water droplets (not water vapour) at room temperature. Administration of water droplets into the respiratory tract may result in water overload and atelectasis. They can become contaminated and represent a source of infection. Nebulizers can be useful, especially to administer bronchodilators, but should not be used instead of an effective heat/moisture exchanger. The mask and chamber should be washed in hot soapy water and dried thoroughly after each use (Critchley & Roulsten, 1993).

Heat/moisture exchangers

Heat/moisture exchangers conserve heat and moisture during expiration and return them to the inspired gas or air. The Buchanan laryngectomy/tracheostomy protector or the Deltanex consist of a special type of foam (Hydrolox) which acts as both a filter and a heat/moisture exchanger. Laryngofoam acts in a similar way. It is not necessary to wet these products. They are available on prescription in the community. There is no specific data available on their efficiency.

The Swedish nose type heat/moisture exchange is placed on the end of the tracheostomy tube and can be used in conjunction with oxygen therapy. It can be blocked by secretions and therefore needs regular changes; recommended maximum use time is 24 hours. A similar device is available for laryngectomy patients not wearing a tube; this has been shown to reduce coughing, sputum production and frequency of stoma cleaning (Hilgers et al, 1991). More recent technology has produced a heat/moisture exchanger that also contains a bacterial filter. Trachi-naze has been shown to raise air temperature in the trachea by 44%, and humidity by 50% (McRae et al, 1995 & 1996). It is available on prescription in the community.

Water and the neck breather

Patients with tracheostomies must take precautions when bathing and showering. Shower shields are available to allow these activities to be carried out as normal, either as a 'stick on' unit or, more simply, as a plastic apron to tie around the neck. Jay et al (1991) report that 29% of their sample of laryngectomees were swimmers preoperatively and of these 53% were unhappy about not being able to swim. Swimming is still possible, using a swimming aid consisting of a cuffed tracheostomy tube with a snorkel or mouth attachment. Patients need to be trained to use these safely and details of centres that provide this facility are available from the National Association of Laryngectomy Clubs (NALC).

Resuscitation in the neck breather

All nurses should ensure that they are familiar with resuscitation of a tracheostomy or laryngectomy patient. This becomes an issue particularly when they leave the safety of the head and neck unit; many healthcare professionals do not know how to resuscitate a neck breather. Resuscitation lectures do not usually cover the neck breather, and it is not routinely taught on first aid courses. The NALC can supply both a video and poster on resuscitation, as part of their awareness-raising campaign of the problems of neck breathers among first aid organizations and healthcare professionals.

Whether resuscitating a tracheostomy or laryngectomy patient, the nose and mouth should always be occluded as many laryngectomy patients now have tracheoesophageal valves that will allow air to escape via the upper airway.

It is recommended that all neck breathers carry a card or wear a bracelet stating that they have a tracheostomy, in case of accident or illness. Cards and car stickers are available from the NALC.

Summary

Tracheostomy has serious implications for the wellbeing of the patient, with many reports of complications in the literature. It is vital that the nurse is conversant with current management and feels competent and confident to care for the tracheostomized patient.

It is also important that the nurse remains up to date with airway management products in order to ensure that the correct devices are supplied in order to give maximum benefit to the patient, helping to improve quality of life and comfort. Nurses should be knowledgeable about their benefits in order to make a convincing case for the need to purchase such products.

This chapter has attempted to provide as much evidence as possible on which to base tracheostomy care interventions. However, many areas of tracheostomy care are based purely on individual clinical experience, which varies between areas. With clinical governance now a priority for the NHS, it is important that nurses evaluate the care that they are providing, using audit and research to ascertain what exactly are the best interventions for the patient with a tracheostomy.

Strategy for practice

- Develop evidence-based tracheostomy care guidelines for your unit.
- Develop evidence-based suctioning guidelines for your unit.
- Be aware of the potential for harm that a tracheostomy presents and know how to minimize the risks.
- Select tracheostomy tubes with care and ensure your patients have the best available.
- Always measure cuff pressure: your unit should have its own cuff manometer.
- Never leave tubes soaking.
- Always ensure a heat/moisture exchanger is used at all times.
- Ensure the patient receives all the necessary equipment to manage their tracheostomy at home; use a discharge checklist. People with permanent tracheostomies are entitled to free prescriptions.
- Ensure the whole team knows how to resuscitate a neck breather. Have a copy of the NALC poster and video on the ward. Ask your hospital resuscitation trainer to incorporate this into training for all staff. Approach local first aid organizations and offer training in resuscitation of neck breathers.

Chapter 2.2
Mouth care

Anatomy and physiology of the airway
Martini, 1992

The oral cavity

The oral cavity is formed by the cheeks on either side, which are continuous with the lips anteriorly. The area between the teeth and lips is called the vestibule. The gums (gingivae) cover the tooth-bearing surfaces of the upper and lower jaw: the alveolar ridges. The roof of the oral cavity is formed by the hard and soft palates. The floor of the mouth is dominated by the tongue. The free anterior portion of the tongue is connected to the underlying epithelium by a fold of mucous membrane, the linguinal frenulum.

The oral cavity is lined by mucous membrane consisting of three layers. The top layer is stratified squamous epithelium. This covers a layer of loose connective tissue called the lamina propria, which contains blood vessels, sensory nerve endings, lymphatic vessels, smooth muscle fibres and areas of lymphatic tissue. The submucosa is a layer of loose connective tissue containing larger blood vessels and lymphatics, exocrine glands, and a network of nerve fibres. A basement membrane lies between the lamina propria and submucosa. It is here that the epithelial stem cells replicate. These cells have a life span of 7 days and are continuously renewing. The outer epithelial layer is replaced completely every 7 to 14 days. This high cell turnover makes the epithelium very prone to damage by cytotoxic agents such as radiation and chemotherapy. After 12 days of radiotherapy, the epithelium begins to slough off with no new cells to replace it. This leaves a denuded mucous membrane with large areas of bleeding, painful ulceration. These areas are very vulnerable to infection, both bacterial and fungal.

Saliva

There are three pairs of salivary glands. The large parotid glands lie just underneath the zygomatic arch. The parotid duct empties into the vestibule at the level of the second upper molar. The parotids produce a thick serous solution containing large amounts of salivary amylase. The sublingual and submandibular glands are located in the floor of mouth. They have ducts emptying into the mouth on either side of the linguinal frenulum. They produce saliva containing large numbers of glycoproteins and mucins. Mucins are responsible for lubrication properties of saliva. The most important antibacterial enzymes in saliva are lysozyme and lactoperoxidase.

The salivary glands produce 1.5 litres of saliva per day, with a composition of 99.4% water, plus an assortment of ions, buffers, waste products, metabolites, immunoglobulins, lysozymes and enzymes. Saliva is continually produced throughout the day, with extra large amounts at mealtimes. Production falls during the night. Saliva flushes and lubricates the oral surfaces, controls bacteria levels (e.g. plaque-causing mutans streptococci and lactobacilli) and remineralizes the teeth. During eating, salivary amylase (produced by the parotids) begins breaking down complex carbohydrates, and mucin containing saliva from the submandibular and sublingual glands lubricates the mouth and food bolus to facilitate chewing and swallowing. Saliva also dissolves chemicals in the food to stimulate the taste buds; for a substance to be tasted it must be in aqueous solution.

At rest the saliva mixture in the mouth comprises approximately 70% submandibular, 25% parotid and 5% sublingual fluid. At mealtimes flow rate increases to up to 7 ml per minute and the mixture changes to include more parotid secretion (approximately 50%). Saliva is pH 6.7 at rest, shifting to pH 7.5 when eating.

The salivary glands are very sensitive to radiation; a radical course of radiotherapy will cause permanent loss of salivary function. Other factors such as emotional distress and dehydration can also reduce salivary flow. The absence of saliva (xerostomia) has dramatic adverse effects on both a physical and emotional level:

- a rapid increase in oral bacterial levels (often compounded by the need for supplements high in sugars to maintain nutrition)
- recurring oral infections
- progressive erosion of the teeth and gums, dental caries
- loss of lubrication causing mucosal abrasions, difficulty eating and swallowing, difficulty articulating
- discomfort causing distress and sleep disruption.

Enderby and Crow (1995) report that a diet high in dairy foods and calcium makes saliva more viscous (thick and sticky), which can be a cause of discomfort for some patients.

The teeth

Teeth are important for processing food in the mouth. The incisors are responsible for biting off chunks of food, whilst the molars perform mastication, breaking down food and helping to saturate the materials with salivary lubricants and enzymes. The bulk of a tooth consists of dentin, a mineralized matrix similar to that of bone. Under the dentin there is a central pulp cavity containing blood vessels and nerve fibres; cytoplasmic processes extend into the dentin. The blood vessels and nerves enter via the root canal at the base (root) of the tooth. The root sits in a socket of the jawbone (alveolus). The neck of the tooth refers to the boundary between the root and the crown. The crown of the tooth is the visible part, covered by a layer of enamel. Enamel contains calcium phosphate in a crystalline form and is the hardest biologically manufactured substance. Adequate amounts of calcium, phosphates and vitamin D are essential to maintain the enamel. Fluoride increases the density and hardness of the enamel. Erosion of the enamel exposes the dentin, which is very sensitive and gives access to decay-causing bacteria. Epithelial cells of the gingiva form tight attachments to the tooth above the neck to prevent bacterial access to the root. Erosion of and damage to the gingiva allow bacterial access, as well as exposing sensitive dentin.

Dental plaque

Plaque is a film on the teeth surface consisting of bacterial cells in a matrix of extracellular polymers and salivary products. Effective toothbrushing prevents plaque formation, except in inaccessible crevices. Plaque accumulates rapidly between brushings. Plaque bacteria ferment carbohydrates to lactic acid. Lactic acid causes decalcification of the enamel, which allows bacteria to erode into the matrix. *Streptococcus mutans* is one of the main organisms implicated in dental caries; it produces a dextran polysaccharide which is strongly adhesive to the tooth. This can only be produced when sucrose is present (Brock & Madigan, 1991).

The causes of impaired oral integrity

All oncological treatment to the head and neck can cause impaired oral integrity:

- Surgery: impaired mucous membrane due to surgical wound, xerostomia due to removal of one or more salivary glands or nerve damage to salivary function, impaired clearance of debris from the mouth due to restricted tongue movement.
- External beam radiotherapy: oral irradiation surpasses all other treatment for its severe stomatoxic effect, having a profound effect on physical, emotional and psychological well-being. The oral mucosa, tongue and lips become painfully inflamed, oedematous and ulcerated, with white pseudomembranes being formed. The tongue is dry, coated and blistered. Saliva becomes thick and ropey. Nutrition is rapidly affected, and oral infections quickly take hold. Infections are caused by organisms found in the normal oral flora (e.g. *Candida albicans, Staphylococcus aureus*) which take advantage of the impaired mucosal barrier. Unchecked, they spread to cause oesophagitis, gastritis, chest infection and septicaemia. Pain, malnutrition, and difficulty in communicating rapidly cause depression. Due to a combination of these factors, patients may fail to complete the prescribed course of radiotherapy (Madeya, 1996). Long-term xerostomia predisposes to high rates of dental caries and oral infections.
- Brachytherapy: insertion of radioactive wires causes a surgical wound and the radiation causes localized mucositis.
- Chemotherapy: certain cytotoxic drugs have a significant effect on the mucous membrane, 5-fluorouracil and methotrexate are notable drugs often used to treat head and neck cancer. These

drugs are antimetabolites and cause cessation of epithelium replication leading to mucosal atrophy and ulceration. They also
cause bone marrow suppression and the resulting neutropaenia
can have an indirect effect on the mucosa by predisposing to
bleeding and infection (Madeya, 1996).

- Extensive, fungating oral cancers cause significant oral problems
  including infection, halitosis, altered taste.
- Drugs used to control symptoms: for example antidepressant
  drugs and narcotic analgesics, cause dry mouth.
- Eating and drinking have a mechanical cleansing effect on the
  mouth, so patients on enteral feeds often experience dry, dirty
  mouths and coated tongues.
- Oxygen therapy and mouth breathing have a negative effect on
  the mouth.

The psychosocial effects of impaired oral integrity should not be
overlooked. The mouth has a vital role to play in speech, the appreciation of food and drink, and the expression of intimate affection. A
patient with a sore mouth will experience difficulty in speech and
eating, cracked lips will make smiling painful, and halitosis leads to
mutual avoidance of the patient and their nearest and dearest.

Skilled nursing care is essential and aims to prevent or minimize
all these side effects. There are four key components to good nursing
management:

- an evidence-based oral care protocol
- careful assessment and evaluation
- patient education
- intensive emotional support.

Despite the fact that there is now a body of literature on oral care
to guide practice, many centres continue to use unsuitable products.
Because of the extreme problems caused by stomatitis, anecdotal
remedies and mouth rinses abound; they represent large profits for
pharmaceutical companies. The nurse must be very careful to evaluate these products before use, as many of them can actually be
contraindicated. A review of the literature gives a good indication of
which oral rinses and oral cleaning tools to use.

Oral rinses and remedies

Chlorhexidine digluconate (Corsodyl)

Chlorhexidine is an alcohol-based mouthwash that prevents plaque formation and the development of gingivitis. It is an antimicrobial and reduces bacterial and fungal levels in the mouth, being effective against Gram-positive bacilli and yeasts. However, Gram-negative bacilli have a low susceptibility to chlorhexidine (Raybould et al, 1994). Its major action is the control of plaque-forming organisms. Studies also claim that it helps to promote wound healing after oral surgery (Lang & Brecx, 1986). Please note that it does not contain any analgesics or ulcer-healing drugs!

Chlorhexidine is absorbed into the oral mucosa and dental surfaces and then slowly released in active form. Two daily rinses with 10 ml of 0.2% chlorhexidine will assure complete plaque inhibition (Loe & Schiott, 1970). Rinsing with chlorhexidine should last for 35–45 seconds to assure good absorption. It may temporarily affect taste sensations so rinsing should not be done before meals. To assure optimal substantivity, no swishing with water should follow the rinse (Lang & Brecx, 1986). It can stain teeth yellow-brown after a few days of use, and concentrations of 0.2% have been shown to produce mucosal desquamation and ulceration (Flotra et al, 1971). However, chlorhexidine can be diluted with water 50 : 50 to reduce mucosal irritation (Joyston-Bechal et al, 1992). Chlorhexidine combines with nystatin to form a chlorhexidine–nystatin salt compound, rendering the combined drug complex ineffective as an antibiotic agent. The two agents should therefore not be used together (Barkvoll & Attramadal, 1989).

Chlorhexidine can also be applied to the teeth in gel form in customized trays to give chemical plaque control thus reduce caries in patients with high levels of mutans streptococci and lactobacilli, for example those with xerostomia due to oral irradiation (Joyston-Bechal et al, 1992).

The literature is very confusing on the usefulness of chlorhexidine in stomatitis; whilst Ferretti et al (1987) claimed that it reduced mucositis in a selection of 33 bone marrow transplant patients (they compared chlorhexidine to an alcohol-based placebo), Foote et al (1994) found that oral irradiation patients using chlorhexidine experienced significantly more side effects than a placebo (no alcohol) group and concluded that it appeared to be detrimental (52 patients). Samaranayake et al (1988) compared chlorhexidine to benzydamine oral rinse (Difflam) (alcohol plus an anti-inflammatory) and found no difference between the two groups undergoing irradiation for pain, mucositis, coliform or yeast levels (25 patients). Dodd et al (1996), in the most comprehensive study (222 patients), compared chlorhexidine to water and found no significant differences in mucositis for patients receiving chemotherapy. They conclude that, as chlorhexidine was no more effective than water, substantial cost savings can be realized by rinsing with water.

In summary, from the evidence available, the following recommendations are proposed:

- for patients undergoing radiotherapy or chemotherapy; only dentate patients should be prescribed chlorhexidine in order to prevent caries, and they should use it diluted with water. These patients should never be prescribed nystatin concurrently
- patients should be prescribed chlorhexidine after oral surgery to reduce the risk of wound infection.

Benzydamine (Difflam)

Difflam is a mouth rinse marketed for 'the relief of pain and inflammation'. It is a non-steroidal anti-inflammatory drug in a 10% alcohol carrier, reported to possess topical analgesic, anti-inflammatory and antimicrobial properties (Kim et al, 1985; Samaranayake et al, 1988; Epstein et al, 1989). As it has no antimicrobial agent in it, it is difficult to understand how it can be said to possess this property; perhaps it is the alcohol carrier. It did manage to outperform chlorhexidine in reduction of bacteria and yeasts in Samaranyake's study! Paradoxically, in the same study, chlorhexidine (which does not contain an anti-inflammatory drug) was reported to cause much less discomfort than the benzydamine. The studies by Kim et al and Epstein et al are both extremely dubious in quality and findings. The abstracts claim wonderful properties for benzydamine, but a critique of both studies reveals poor design with several flaws. In fact patients in both studies found that benzydamine made their mouths sting. Neither study actually has any statistically significant findings.

Hydrogen peroxide

A review of the literature on the use of hydrogen peroxide (H_2O_2) as an oral rinse shows that although it may have some benefits (Passos & Brand, 1966; Beck, 1979), these are not proven and the evidence in more recent studies shows concerns that it may act as an irritant on the oral mucosa. Daeffler (1980) proposes that H_2O_2 promotes overgrowth of yeasts in the oral cavity and also that it inhibits mucosal tissue granulation. In a more recent study Tombes and Gallucci (1993) compared H_2O_2 to saline rinses in normal volunteers. The H_2O_2 users reported taste alterations, stinging, oral pain, dry mouth and nausea. Highly significant differences in oral assessment scores were found ($P < 0.001$), suggesting mucosal abnormalities. Elongation of the filiform papillae were noted, with colour changes on the dorsal surface of the tongue. The authors conclude that H_2O_2 is an irritant and should not be used for oral care. This correlates with a study comparing saline 0.9% with H_2O_2 in patients undergoing oral irradiation; on average the patients using saline had better outcomes (Feber, 1996).

Selective elimination of Gram-negative bacilli

Spijkervet et al (1990) hypothesized that the inflammatory aspect of radiation stomatitis could be due to the presence of Gram-negative bacilli in the mouth, releasing potent endotoxins. They compared 15 patients using 1 g lozenges containing polymyxin E 2 mg, tobramycin 1.8 mg and amphotericin B 10 mg (PTA lozenges) with patients given chlorhexidine and water rinses, and reported much less severe mucositis with complete absence of pseudomembranes in the PTA group. Their patients also had the benefit of an oral care protocol using a deionized water solution administered by a dental hygienist. This is encouraging data but it was not a randomized or double blind trial and used data for comparison from patients studied in a previous trial. Symonds et al (1996) randomized 275 patients to receive a PTA lozenge or placebo and had less dramatic results; there was no significant difference in patients developing pseudomembranes. They report that a more sensitive mucositis test revealed a significant difference ($P = 0.009$) and that patients in the PTA group lost less weight ($P = 0.009$). However, an examination of the patient characteristics shows that the placebo group contained more patients undergoing hyperfractionated therapy (3%), and more having the oral cavity (5%) and oropharynx (8%) treated. The PTA group had 14% more larynx patients, who would not be having large areas of the oral cavity treated (if any). The patients were all using sodium bicarbonate rinses; no strength is mentioned. No oral care protocol was in use. An important variable, smoking status, has not been allowed for in the analysis.

In summary, more research is needed before introducing PTA lozenges routinely into oral care protocols.

Sucrulfate

Sucrulfate is a non-absorbable, basic aluminium salt of a sulphated disaccharide reported to be effective for the treatment of gastric and duodenal ulcers. Authors propose that it may be useful to relieve stomatitis (Pfeiffer et al, 1990; Epstein & Wong, 1994; Makkonen et al, 1994; Allison et al, 1995), but their studies are inconclusive. Pfeiffer et al noted that when it was used for chemotherapy patients, aggravation of nausea was a major problem. A critique of these studies shows several flaws and they do not provide sufficient evidence to merit the recommendation of sucrulfate.

Sodium bicarbonate

Although sodium bicarbonate is frequently used for mouth care, a literature review reveals no research on its efficacy; it relies rather on anecdotal evidence. It creates an alkaline environment in the mouth which is not recommended as the oral pH is normally slightly acidic, and alterations may have an adverse effect on the oral mucosa (DeWalt & Haines, 1969). If the solution is too strong, it can cause superficial burns (Heal, 1993).

Lemon and glycerin

This is frequently used in the form of swabs. However, it reduces the pH of the mouth from 6.7 to 2.2–3.9 (Wiley, 1969). Lemon stimulates salivary secretion but overuse may lead to exhaustion of the salivary glands as well as erosion of enamel (Griffiths & Boyle, 1993). Glycerin has hygroscopic properties and therefore may dehydrate the mucous membrane (Trenter Roth & Creason, 1986). The use of lemon and glycerin is therefore not recommended.

Glycerin thymol (pink mouthwash tablets)

This solution is useful for refreshing the mouth, but it has no therapeutic effect and is not antimicrobial (Heals, 1993).

Prostaglandin E2 tablets

Prostaglandin E2 tablets have been investigated for potential prophylaxis of mucositis. Matejka et al (1990) report a small study on 15 patients which has major flaws; they ascertain that the prostaglandin E2 has no systemic side effects, but no data at all on major variables such as radiotherapy or chemotherapy dose, mucositis score, pain score, etc., seem to have been collected. Labar et al (1993) report a study on 60 patients undergoing bone marrow transplant which found that patients in the prostaglandin group had a higher incidence of mucositis than patients receiving the placebo tablet. They conclude that prostaglandin is not effective for prophylaxis of mucositis.

Granulocyte macrophage-colony-stimulating factor (GM-CSF) mouthwashes

Rovirosa et al (1998) studied the effects of GM-CSF (Leucomax) mouth rinses on 12 patients undergoing head and neck irradiation. The GM-CSF was used only when ulceration was present. They do not discuss whether an oral care protocol using other oral rinses was in use. However, their results were promising, with eight of the 12 patients experiencing complete healing of ulceration during the course of irradiation, although it is difficult to ascertain the level of pain relief obtained. The authors conclude that larger prospective randomized multi-centre studies are needed in order to effectively evaluate this promising but expensive new therapy.

Other remedies

There are anecdotal reports in the literature suggesting that tea-tree oil (Mennie, 1997) and a rinse based on camomile (Kamillosan) may be helpful in oral mucositis (Carl & Emrich, 1991). Amifostine is reported to selectively protect mucosal cells from the effects of chemotherapy (Bukowski, 1996), and clinical trials to examine its effect in head and neck irradiation are underway. It is given as a 15-minute infusion. The use of an adhesive water-soluble film containing topical anaesthetic and antibiotics (AD film) has been reported

(Oguchi et al, 1998). Further randomized controlled studies are required in order to evaluate all these agents properly before recommending them for use in clinical practice. Allopurinol mouthwashes have been examined as a potential preventor of 5-fluorouracil-induced mucositis, but were not effective (Loprinzi et al, 1990).

Oral care tools

The oral care tool to clean the patient's mouth should be chosen on the basis of evidence in the literature, and also on an assessment of the individual's needs. For example, questions the nurse should ask are: is the patient dentate, or do they wear dentures? Are they neutropaenic? What is their manual dexterity like? How wide can they open their mouth? All these variables are important when considering the best tool for the job.

The toothbrush

A vital consideration in the dentate patient is the control of plaque. Addy et al (1992) provide a wide review of the dental literature on effective oral hygiene and conclude that the toothbrush is the most effective and widely used tool in the Western world. Used correctly, it is the only tool that removes plaque effectively. The toothbrush filaments, when placed at the neck of the tooth and moved horizontally in very short strokes, dislodge the sticky water-insoluble plaque from the protected areas at the gum margins and from between the teeth. Toothbrushes should be of soft to medium texture, with small heads for ease of access and densely packed nylon filaments. Too hard a brush can cause gum recession and bleeding, allowing bacterial access to the bloodstream. It is thought that the massaging action of the brush stimulates the mucosa of the gums. The toothbrush requires manual dexterity and adherence to good brushing techniques (Kite & Pearson, 1995).

Dental floss

The toothbrush does not remove plaque from areas between the teeth, and dental floss can be used to do this. It should be used with care to avoid damaging the gums. Flossing requires manual dexterity (Kite & Pearson, 1995). It should not be performed if the patient has platelet levels of less than 40,000 mm^3 (Madeya, 1996).

Toothpaste

Toothpaste is not essential to remove plaque, but as an abrasive agent it helps the mechanical effect of brushing. It provides topical application of fluoride and its pleasant taste refreshes the mouth (Kite & Pearson, 1995). If teeth are sensitive, patients can use a desensitizing toothpaste.

Foam swabs

Foam swabs are not effective in removing plaque (Pearson, 1996). However, if they must be used, they are more effective in preventing plaque if they have been soaked in Corsodyl (Ransier et al, 1995). They are, however, useful for cleaning the cavity of a maxillectomy.

Swabs and forceps

Swabs and forceps do not remove plaque and forceps can damage oral tissue if not used carefully (Howarth, 1977). Swabs and fingers do not remove debris and plaque, but rather compress them between the teeth (Shepherd et al, 1987).

Lip care

Lubricants such as petroleum jelly and yellow paraffin are often recommended for lips. These should be used with care, as several layers can build up and produce a bolus effect if radiotherapy is being directed on to this area. There is also evidence that their hygroscopic qualities dehydrate the tissues. Moisturizing cream is a good alternative.

Pain relief

Oral mucositis is extremely painful; good pain management is essential in order for the patient to be able to tolerate oral care procedures and maintain nutrition. However, patients with severe stomatitis will frequently require enteral feeding as eating and swallowing become impossible however good their oral care and pain control.

Topical local anaesthetics are not optimal treatment for the continuous burning pain of radiation-induced mucositis as they provide relief for only a short period of time (Weissman et al, 1989). They also anaesthetize the pharynx and so put the patient at risk of aspiration. They block taste perception, which may further diminish the sensory quality of eating (Berger et al, 1995). Topical steroids have often been used in stomatitis; although local corticosteroids may be beneficial in reducing inflammation, there is evidence that they enhance the development of candidiasis and promote tissue friability, therefore they cannot be recommended for the patient with stomatitis (Daeffler, 1981). Soluble aspirin rinses and mucaine are a good alternative. Such simple measures can be helpful in the early stages of stomatitis, but are unlikely to be adequate in later severe stages, where systemic analgesics should be titrated to the patient's need. Most patients undergoing oral irradiation will require an opiate such as Oramorph to control pain. This can be converted to a slow-release morphine preparation or transdermal fentanyl according to patient preference. Transdermal fentanyl (Durogesic) is very useful in this situation as swallowing medication may be impossible at this stage. Janjan et al (1992) showed that daily nursing review of pain control with prompt changes in analgesic therapy according to a three-step analgesic protocol significantly improved pain control, reduced weight loss and improved wellbeing in patients undergoing radiotherapy for head and neck cancer.

Berger et al (1995) describe a novel approach to pain relief in stomatitis using sweets containing capsaicin (the active ingredient in chili peppers). This is a very small study and although patients reported significantly less pain after sucking the sweets, pain control was not complete and only temporary. Although all the patients in the study are described as having mucositis, the reasons for this are not given; there are only two head and neck cancers in the sample. The sucrose in the sweets was necessary to reduce the initial burning of the capsaicin, and so they would be contraindicated in dentate patients. The authors conclude that additional research is needed before recommending this particular remedy.

See Chapter 2.11 for more information on pain control.

Xerostomia

A dry mouth has a profound effect on oral health and function. There may be several reasons for dry mouth: the major causes of severe xerostomia are irradiation of the salivary glands, drug therapy (see Table 2.2.1), dehydration, mouth breathing and oxygen therapy. Marunick et al (1991) reported that multimodality therapy for head and neck cancer (surgery and radiotherapy) reduced salivary flow rates by 83% (resting) and 86% (stimulated) in the patients they studied. A major predicting factor of xerostomia is the amount of salivary gland in the radiation field area. This hyposalivation is a long-term problem as the salivary glands do not recover from radiation damage.

Table 2.2.1: Drugs associated with xerostomia

Anticonvulsants
Antidepressants
Antihistamines
Antineoplastics
Antiparkinsonian agents
Antipsychotics
Atropine
Diuretics
Hypotensives
Tranquillizers
Muscle relaxants
Narcotics
Sympathomimetics

Xerostomia is intensely distressing for patients, who complain that it affects speech, eating and sleep. It becomes impossible to eat starchy food such as potato or bread as it tends to stick in the mouth and refuses to form a food bolus because of the lack of salivary amylase and mucin. Meals become an ordeal, with large amounts of water required to wash food down. Speech is impossible without frequent sips of water. A bottle of water is a constant companion. Sleep is frequently disturbed by the discomfort of a dry mouth.

Symptomatic treatment

Pilocarpine

Pilocarpine hydrochloride can be used to stimulate residual salivary function. It is a direct-acting cholinergic parasympathetic agent. It acts through direct stimulation of muscarinic receptors and can have broad, widely distributed effects on smooth muscle and exocrine tissues. Pilocarpine produces increased smooth muscle tone of the gastrointestinal and genitourinary systems, eye and respiratory tract. Exocrine glands of the lacrimal, gastric, intestinal, respiratory and salivary systems are stimulated. Adverse reactions include nausea, vomiting, abdominal cramp, indigestion, diarrhoea, urinary frequency, headache, syncope, tremors, flushing, hypotension, hypertension and arrythmias. Contraindications are cardiac failure, asthma, urinary tract obstruction, peptic ulcer, hyperthyroidism and Parkinson's disease (Hamlar et al, 1996).

Studies report that pilocarpine 5 to 10 mg three times per day (Salagen) improves saliva production with minimum side effects and therefore represents significant therapeutic benefits for the symptomatic relief of xerostomia. Patients should be advised to titrate the exact dose needed to balance benefits against side effects. However, some patients will not tolerate pilocarpine due to side effects which may range from mild to moderate (LeVeque et al, 1993; Johnson et al, 1993). Patients should also be selected carefully with the contraindications above in mind. The effectiveness of pilocarpine depends on the amount of residual functioning salivary tissue.

Artificial saliva

The four main saliva substitutes currently available on the UK market are Glandosane, Luborant, Saliva Orthana and Oral Balance Saliva Replacement Gel. The first three products are sprays; Glandosane relies on sodium carboxymethylcellulose (CMC) to provide viscosity and does not contain fluoride. It has a pH of 5.06 and uses carbon dioxide as a propellant. Luborant also contains CMC for viscosity but its pH is higher at 6.0 and it contains 2 ppm fluoride. Saliva Orthana contains mucin manufactured from the gastric mucosa of the pig instead of CMC. Like Luborant it contains 2 ppm fluoride and has a pH of 6.69. An in-vitro trial of all three sprays on tooth enamel showed that Saliva Orthana and Luborant were potentially good remineralizing agents. In contrast Glandosane produced subsurface demineralization; the low pH and absence of fluoride in this product means it should not be recommended for dentate patients (Joyston-Bechal & Kidd, 1987). Artificial saliva has been shown to offer greater symptomatic relief than water (Duxbury et al, 1989). In a comparison of CMC saliva and mucin saliva, it was found that patients preferred the mucin saliva. They complained that the CMC saliva felt sticky. Both types of saliva improved denture retention. Mucin saliva tended to last longer and therefore less was required per day (Vissink et al, 1983). Saliva sprays are not effective unless used correctly; the whole of the oral mucosa should be coated by several sprays of the product.

The Oral Balance Dry Mouth System comprises Oral Balance Dry Mouth Saliva Replacement Gel, Biotene Dry Mouth Antibacterial Toothpaste and Biotene Mouthwash. This system contains lactoperoxidase, glucose oxidase and lysozyme to mimic the salivary peroxidase system and thus improve oral health. The manufacturers recommend that Biotene toothpaste and mouthwash are used with the gel as the presence of detergents and foaming agents in other products can destroy the enzymes in the gel. There is evidence that these products are potentially beneficial, but none of the studies is conclusive (Lenander-Lumikari et al, 1993; Toljanic et al, 1996). It has not been compared to other saliva substitutes to date.

Oil

Kusler & Rambur (1992) give a case report demonstrating that a small amount of butter, margarine or vegetable oil can be used to coat the oral mucosa and relieve dryness. Walizer & Ephraim (1996) conducted a small controlled trial comparing vegetable oil to an artificial saliva used in the United States (Xerolube) and found vegetable oil to be at least as effective. The oil did not impair oral health.

Preventing caries

Xerostomia carries a high risk of caries. Dentate patients should be monitored closely every 3 months after radiotherapy; oral hygiene instruction should be reinforced during these checkups and scaling carried out when necessary. Regimes using fluoride and chlorhexidine gel applied daily in custom-made carriers have been shown to reduce radiation caries. For patients not able to use carriers, fluoride and chlorhexidine rinses should be used. Sweet drinks and snacks should be avoided. Patients should not choose sugary sweets, gum or drinks to relieve xerostomia; a sugar-free gum should be used instead (Joyston-Bechal, 1992). Simons et al (1997) demonstrated that a xylitol gum produced significant reductions in mutans streptococci, whilst a chlorhexidine/xylitol gum significantly reduced mutans streptococci, lactobacilli and yeasts.

Dentures

Dentures frequently present a problem in the head and neck cancer patient. Alteration to the mouth caused by surgery, radiotherapy and weight loss means that dentures may no longer fit. Ill-fitting dentures can cause trauma and irritation. Great care must be taken as ulcers caused by denture irritation may precipitate osteoradionecrosis (Jansma et al, 1992).

During radiotherapy, dentures may aggravate mucositis and wearing should be discouraged (Jansma et al, 1992). An exception must be made for patients wearing resection prostheses and obdurators, which are needed for closure of the surgical defect. Dentures and obdurators become coated with plaque and food debris just as teeth do, and they can harbour infection (e.g. *Candida*). They must therefore be cleaned meticulously using a soft brush and unperfumed soap and water after meals and every time oral care is performed; rinsing and soaking alone will not remove plaque and debris effectively. Patients should be instructed to remove dentures at night and soak them in a hypochlorite denture cleansing agent two or three nights per week (e.g. Dentural or Steradent), after removing all debris with a brush. Hypochlorites can damage the fabric of the dentures and therefore should not be used too often (Griffiths & Boyle, 1993).

Timing of fabrication of new or replacement dentures after radiotherapy is controversial. Patients will be understandably impatient for a dental prosthesis but care must be taken to allow the mucosa to heal and oedema to settle to avoid irritation or trauma. Jansma et al (1992) recommend waiting for 3 months, and extending this to 6 months for patients who have extractions performed immediately before radiotherapy. The fit of dentures should be checked regularly; if any irritation develops they should be removed immediately and the mouth examined by the dental team.

Self-applied commercial soft linings and denture fixatives should not be used as they may mask problems that need professional dental attention, and they act as a medium for the rapid proliferation of micro-organisms, particularly yeasts (Griffiths & Boyle, 1993).

Trismus

Trismus is difficulty in opening the mouth caused by scarring and fibrosis of the masticatory muscles (the temporalis, masseter, medial pterygoid and lateral pterygoid), causing restricted mobility of the temporomandibular joint (TMJ). This may be due to surgery and radiotherapy, or tumour invasion. Prevention of trismus, rather than its treatment, should be the goal of care. Patients at risk are those whose treatment involves the TMJ:

- those having oropharyngeal, retromolar trigone and maxillary sinus resections
- those having oropharyngeal, retromolar trigone, maxillary sinus, and nasopharyngeal irradiation.

All patients who fall into these groups should have their maximum mouth opening recorded before treatment and perform daily preventative exercises to maintain maximum opening and jaw mobility. Normal opening of the dentate jaw will accommodate the first three fingers on the nondominant hand placed vertically between the central incisors. Edentulous jaws will normally accommodate four fingers between the anterior alveolar ridges (Giuliano & Rudy, 1995). Trismus is present when the maximum interincisal opening is 35 mm or less. However, there are a number of variables that must be considered (height, weight, age, sex, dental status) when making a clinical judgement. Where there is unilateral trismus, the jaw will deviate towards the affected side (Giuliano & Rudy, 1995).

Preventative exercises

There are several mechanical devices for jaw stretching, but the most widely used and least expensive is the use of a stack of wooden tongue depressors. This device can be helpful and stimulating because it acts as a measurement against which the patient and professional can assess deterioration/progress. The patient should be instructed to practice exercises at least three or four times per day for 15 minutes per session, holding their stack of blades in place for a count of 10, removing them, then replacing them. At no time should the patient attempt to use the device as a 'lever' as this will loosen the incisors. Trismus may develop as late as 3–6 months after treatment and therefore exercises must continue, with regular monitoring of the jaw mobility (Jansma et al, 1992). Trismus can severely inhibit eating, speech, prosthesis wearing and oral hygiene and may even require surgical management if it is not prevented.

Treatment of trismus

For patients who unfortunately develop trismus (usually as a result of lack of preventative exercises), treatment consists of gradually stretching the TMJs. A stack of wooden tongue blades is again used. Enough tongue blades to fill the current maximum opening distance are inserted between the teeth/alveolar ridges, then an extra blade is inserted into the middle of the stack to force the jaws open a little further. A rubber band around the stack helps to make handling easier. Over a period of weeks, additional blades are added to increase jaw opening. Administration of non-steroidal anti-inflammatory drugs prior to exercises can be beneficial. Additional measures are the application of warm, moist heat over the TMJs for 15 to 20 minutes prior to exercising, massage and ultrasound (which a physiotherapist will provide).

The patient with trismus will require coping strategies to deal with eating problems; liquidized foods can be given through large diameter plastic straws, or syringes with a short piece of tubing attached (Giuliano & Rudy, 1995). Oral hygiene can be facilitated by use of a small toothbrush, irrigation via a syringe, and by being performed immediately after jaw stretching exercises (Giuliano & Rudy, 1995). The dental hygienist should be consulted for help with techniques and equipment. Communication will also be a problem, and the assistance of the speech therapist should be sought.

Candida

Oral candidiasis is a frequent complication in head and neck cancer. Superimposed on therapy-induced stomatitis, it can significantly increase pain and inflammation. It can also spread from the oral cavity in the immunocompromised patient, to cause oesophagitis and even septicaemia. The most common type is pseudo-membranous candidiasis (thrush), which appears as white patches of various sizes on the oral mucosal surface. These can be wiped off to reveal a red, bleeding surface. Atrophic candidiasis appears as smooth red patches on the palate, buccal mucosa or back of tongue. *Candida* can sometimes cause hyperkeratosis, which presents as white lesions that cannot be wiped off. Angular cheilitis, cracks and sores at the corners of the mouth can be due to *Candida* infection (Pettifer, 1992). Table 2.2.2 shows common *Candida* species.

Table 2.2.2: Common *Candida* species

Candida species	Sensitivity to antifungals
C. albicans (commonest)	Usually sensitive to all antifungals
C. glabrata	Resistant to nystatin, ketoconazole, fluconazole; about 20% are also itraconazole resistant
C. tropicalis	Resistant to nystatin and ketoconazole
C. krusei (rare)	Resistant to nystatin and fluconazole
C. parapsilosis (rare)	Resistant to nystatin

Finlay, 1995.

Confirmation of *Candida* by culture is unnecessary if the patient is apyrexial and has not yet been treated with an antifungal agent. Culture of different *Candida* species requires specialized techniques; testing for different species and resistance to antifungal agents is not a routine, therefore liaison with the microbiology department is necessary if these procedures are required (Finlay, 1995). Nystatin is probably the best-known topical antifungal agent. It should be swished around the mouth for 2 to 3 minutes before swallowing, or sucked as a pastille four times per day. It should be continued for 48 hours after the lesions have resolved. The mouth should not be rinsed, and no food or drink should be taken for 1 hour after treatment. It should not be used in conjunction with Corsodyl (see above). Amphotericin lozenges (100–200 mg every 6 hours) can also be used as a topical agent. There must be enough saliva production to dissolve pastilles or lozenges, therefore they are often unhelpful in head and neck cancer. As these agents are only topical they must be used fastidiously, so their effectiveness is limited if the patient is unable to perform effective oral 'swishing' or sucking due to functional impairment from surgery or tumour. Topical agents are not helpful if *Candida* extends into the oropharyngeal and hypopharyngeal area.

Systemic antifungal therapy should be used if the *Candida* extends into the oropharynx and hypopharynx, if the patient cannot apply topical agents effectively, and if topical agents have been ineffective. Systemic agents include fluconazole (50 mg daily for 7–14 days), ketoconazole (200 mg daily for 7–10 days) and itraconazole(100 mg daily for 7 days). The efficacy of ketoconazole and fluconazole appears to be similar in cancer patients, but fluconazole would appear to have a lower incidence of side effects compared with keto-conazole, which can cause hepatotoxicity after prolonged treatment (Finlay 1995). It is contraindicated in liver disease. Itraconazole is effective against most *Candida* species, and is particularly useful for immunocompromised and AIDS patients. It should be used with care in cases of liver and renal impairment.

Oral hygiene protocols

Studies show that implementation of a systematic oral care protocol alongside patient education significantly reduces mucositis, improves oral comfort, and promotes patient wellbeing (Beck, 1979; Daeffler, 1981; Dudjak, 1987; Graham et al, 1993; Feber, 1995; Dodd, 1996). Consequently, it also makes a significant positive difference to nutrition. There is now so much evidence to support the use of an oral care protocol that it would seem to border on the negligent for nurses not to use one; nurses would not dream of practising without policies for pressure area care and infection control policies, so why not oral care?

The literature shows that the most important factor in oral care is the frequency of care (Ginsberg, 1961; DeWalt, 1975). Ginsberg found that the omission of oral hygiene over an extended period of time (2 to 6 hours) nullified the past benefits of care. She also noted that the frequency required depended on the condition of the individual patient, and so the oral cavity must be observed frequently for signs and symptoms. The literature on oral rinses seems to show that the important factor in oral care is frequent mechanical cleansing, rather than any particular agent used (see section on oral rinses and remedies, above).

Involvement of a dental hygienist and dental team in an oral care protocol is very important (Jansma et al, 1992) to identify risk factors and perform necessary treatment and prophylaxis, particularly before treatment begins. This is especially important if the mandible or maxilla are to be irradiated, as this will lead to long-term impaired blood supply to the bone, resulting in osteoradionecrosis if dental caries occur, or if dental extractions are performed at a later date. A dental assessment and any necessary extractions should be carried out 2 to 3 weeks prior to radiotherapy to allow the mucosa to heal. Doerr & Marunick (1997) report that patients who underwent extractions at the same time as tumour resection had better outcomes in terms of infection and fistula rates. It is therefore recommended that patients undergoing surgery with postoperative radiotherapy have a dental assessment preoperatively so that extractions can then be performed with surgery. It also saves the patient from undergoing a second operative procedure to perform extractions.

A dental hygienist is an important team member to initiate a comprehensive preventative care programme. Fluoride carriers may be made for patients to apply topical fluorides, needed to prevent radiation caries. If the patient is unable to tolerate these, fluoride rinses may be used instead (Madeya, 1996).

An oral care protocol should incorporate written patient education (Beck, 1979; Dudjak, 1987; Feber, 1995) as the majority of patients will perform oral care themselves; radiotherapy is generally performed on an outpatient basis and therefore the patient must be well prepared to manage oral care and side effects at home (Ganley, 1996). Patient education should also include advice and help with smoking cessation, as smoking can increase the severity and duration of mucositis (Rugg et al, 1990).

An example of an oral care protocol for patients undergoing head and neck irradiation is shown in Table 2.2.3.

Oral assessment

Comprehensive oral assessment does not usually form part of nursing documentation; again this can be compared with skin care, where a pressure sore risk assessment is always done. Eilers et al (1988) developed, tested and applied an Oral Assessment Guide, which seems to be the most valid tool in the literature for patients

Table 2.2.3: Oral care protocol for head and neck irradiation

Pre-radiotherapy
- All dentate patients except T1 and T2 larynx should be referred for a dental assessment. Extractions should be performed a minimum of 10 days prior to commencement of radiotherapy to allow healing to occur
- Measure maximum mouth opening if TMJ is in the radiotherapy field; teach patient to maintain jaw mobility
- Advice and help should be given on smoking cessation and excessive alcohol consumption.

Basic oral care
To commence on first day of radiotherapy; initiate documentation and perform baseline Oral Assessment Score. Provide an oral care education session and give patient education booklet.

Table 2.2.3: (contd)

Dentate patients:
- Referral to dental hygienist
- Brush teeth with fluoride toothpaste after every meal or 4-hourly, then
- Rinse mouth 4-hourly with sodium chloride 0.9%
- Rinse twice daily with Corsodyl diluted 50 : 50 with water
- Apply moisturizing cream to lips

Edentulous patients:
- Dentures must be meticulously cleaned after every meal or 4-hourly, with a brush, unperfumed soap and water
- Soak dentures overnight two or three nights per week in a hypochlorite cleaner (Dentural or Steradent)
- Clean around mouth 4-hourly with foam sticks soaked in sodium chloride 0.9%, then rinse
- Apply moisturising cream to lips

Advanced oral care
In addition to above:
- Hourly oral rinses with sodium chloride 0.9%
- Dentures should not be worn
- Provide Saliva Orthana Spray and lozenges to relieve dryness
- Topical antifungals *
- Regular analgesia **

Post-radiotherapy care
- Continue oral rinses until mouth has completely healed. Dentate patients should use 0.4% stannous fluoride gel applied in a custom-made splint for 5 minutes daily. Every 3–4 months the fluoride should be replaced with 1% chlorhexidine gel for 14 days. Patients should be reviewed by a dentist every 3 months
- Dentures can be made for edentulous patients after 6 months if a smooth, well contoured denture-bearing surface is present
- Monitor jaw mobility

*Antifungals
- Mild *Candida* confined to the oral cavity: nystatin suspension 1 ml QDS until mucosa healed post-radiotherapy
- Using Corsodyl; *Candida* not responding to nystatin: fluconazole 50 mg daily for 7–14 days
- *Candida* in oropharynx, hypopharynx, larynx: fluconazole 50 mg daily for 7–14 days

**Analgesia
1. Soluble aspirin: two tablets to rinse, gargle and swallow 4-hourly plus mucaine 10 ml 20 minutes before meals
2. Tylex or Solpadol two tablets four times daily plus mucaine plus NSAID
3. Oramorph: start at 10 mg 4-hourly — titrate to control pain; consider conversion to transdermal fentanyl or slow-release morphine
- Codanthramer 10 ml BD or senokot syrup 10 ml BD should always be prescribed with 2 and 3
- Monitor bowel function and titrate aperients as required

with stomatitis. It has been adapted for use by several authors and has readily identifiable categories with easily differentiated descriptive ratings for use in both clinical and research settings. The Western Consortium for Cancer Nursing Research (1991) tested several oral assessment tools and found that self-report by patients was unreliable as they frequently reported no perceived changes, whilst examination of their mouths revealed definite oral changes. Heals (1993) demonstrated that an oral assessment tool used on admission improved the oral awareness of nurses and thus improved oral status in patients. The unit subsequently went on to use the oral assessment on a daily basis. Thus, for patients with actual or potential impaired oral integrity, daily assessment of oral status is imperative; this should be systematic and documented to allow daily evaluation of care needs. An oral assessment guide is also a helpful teaching tool for inexperienced staff and can be adapted so that the score indicates the level of intervention required (Feber, 1995). Schweiger et al (1980) describe a detailed assessment and found that nurses were able to do a thorough oral assessment in 10 minutes when they had been taught the basic techniques. No specific oral assessment tools were found in the literature for surgical head and neck oncology patients, but a tool could easily be adapted from those reported.

An example of an oral assessment guide is shown in Table 2.2.4 (based on the tool developed by Eilers et al, 1988).

Table 2.2.4: Oral assessment guide

Name
Date

Voice
1 = Normal
2 = Deeper/raspy
3 = Difficult/painful speech

Swallow
1 = Normal
2 = Painful
3 = Unable to swallow

Lips
1 = Smooth, pink, moist
2 = Dry/cracked
3 = Ulcerated/bleeding

Table 2.2.4: (contd)

Tongue
1 = Pink, moist, papillae present
2 = Dry/cracked
3 = Ulcerated/bleeding

Saliva
1 = Watery
2 = Thick or ropey
3 = Absent

Mucous membranes
1 = Pink and moist
2 = Reddened/coated
3 = Ulcerations/bleeding

Gums
1 = Pink and firm
2 = Oedematous/red
3 = Spontaneous bleeding

Teeth/dentures
1 = Clean, no debris
2 = Localized plaque/debris
3 = Generalized plaque/debris

Candida
0 = No
2 = Yes

Oral Cavity Total Score:

Maximum jaw opening: number of tongue depressors

Oral Cavity Total Score	Interventions
8	Perform basic mouth care as defined in Oral Care Protocol
8–10	Perform basic mouth care. Add Step 1 analgesics as defined in Oral Care Protocol
10 or more	Perform advanced mouth care. Add Step 2 and 3 analgesics and antifungal therapy as defined in Oral Care Protocol

Summary

Good oral hygiene is essential for people with head and neck cancer as both the disease itself and the treatment modalities cause significant oral problems. Nurses must ensure that their practice in this area is evidence-based, and this may often lead to reviewing of out-of-date, ritualistic practices. All patients should receive regular, comprehensive, documented oral assessments and care should be guided by evidence-based oral care protocols. A dentist and dental hygienist are essential members of the head and neck cancer team.

Strategy for practice

- Ensure that an evidence-based oral care protocol is in use in your ward.
- Ensure that an oral assessment guide is used daily for all patients.
- Do not use rinses that have not been proven to be effective; they may be harmful, and you may be wasting money.
- Avoid the use of alcohol-based rinses during radiotherapy. If the patient is dentate, Corsodyl should be used, but diluted 50 : 50 with water.
- Never use Corsodyl and nystatin together.
- Do ensure your patients are receiving appropriate pain relief during radiotherapy; topical analgesics are not adequate.
- Always assess the risk of trismus and take preventative action.
- Ensure that a dental team is involved in the patient's care.

Chapter 2.3
Eating and swallowing problems

Maria Harvey

Many patients will experience feeding and swallowing problems during treatment for head and neck cancer, and it is vital that nurses are able to help people in difficulty from both a physical and psychological point of view. This chapter attempts to explain the normal process of feeding and swallowing, the disruptions that occur following resection for cancer, and appropriate management.

Anatomy and physiology of normal feeding and swallowing

Anatomical structures

The oral cavity, pharynx, larynx and oesophagus have important anatomical structures necessary for the physiological coordination required for normal feeding and swallowing.

Structures within the oral cavity include the lips, teeth, the hard and soft palates, the tongue, the floor of the mouth, the mandible and the faucal arches. The most important structures of the pharynx are the three constrictor muscles (superior, medial and inferior), which attach to the structures of the larynx anteriorly (i.e. the cricoid and thyroid cartilage and hyoid bone), and to the base of the tongue, the mandible and soft palate above.

The oesophagus consists of a flaccid muscular tube approximately 23 to 25 cm long with a sphincter at each end. It has two layers of muscle, the inner circular and the outer longitudinal. Each layer is made up of striated muscle in the upper third, a combination of striated and smooth muscle in the middle third, and smooth muscle in the lower third (Ponzoli, 1968; Hansky, 1973).

147

Nerve supply

A total of 26 muscles of the oral cavity, pharynx, larynx and oesophagus are involved, with innervation from six cranial nerves:

Vth Trigeminal
VIIth Facial
IXth Glossopharyngeal
Xth Vagus
XIth Accessory
XIIth Hypoglossal

The Olfactory nerve I also provides sensory input during feeding and swallowing.

Saliva production

Up to 1 litre of saliva is produced by four glands, i.e. the parotid, parotid accessory, submandibular and sublingual glands.

Saliva serves as an emollient to soften the bolus, and as a demulcant to reduce irritation and protect oral mucosa and teeth (Zemlin, 1981). It augments the sensation of taste and must be present to keep the oral cavity moist.

Studies have shown that an average adult swallows 35 times per hour while awake, and six times per hour while asleep, for a total of approximately 600 swallows per day (Lear, 1965).

The three stages of deglutition

Deglutition is a complex process that is dependent on the coordinated actions of the oral cavity, pharynx, larynx and oesophagus. It is often described in three sequential stages, the oral, pharyngeal and oesophageal. The *oral* stage is typically referred to as feeding. The pharyngeal and oesophageal stages constitute the physiological process of *swallowing*.

The oral stage (Figure 2.3.1)

This stage is under voluntary control, such that the timing and movement patterns vary depending on the size of the bolus, the texture, and how enjoyable the food is. It begins with the entry of food or liquid into the oral cavity and ends with the initiation of the pharyngeal swallow. This stage can be further divided into oral preparation and oral transit.

During *oral preparation*, food or fluid is placed in the mouth and the lips seal to prevent drooling. Liquids are cupped with the tongue against the hard palate. Thick liquids and smooth pastes are similarly contained, though they may be manipulated in the mouth by the tongue if the taste is pleasurable. Solid food requires a rotary lateral movement of the mandible and tongue to distribute it between the teeth for mastication, whilst mixing it with saliva. Premature entry of the bolus into the pharynx is prevented by the soft palate resting on the base of the tongue sealing off the nasal cavity, whilst buccal tone increases to prevent escape of food into the cheeks. Peripheral feedback of the position of the bolus on the tongue and the location of the tongue between the teeth is given to prevent injury during chewing. The oral stage is complete when the food is adequately mixed with saliva, and of an appropriate consistency for swallowing. The tongue collects the food from around the mouth to form a cohesive bolus ready for easy passage into the pharynx.

During *oral transit* the food bolus is pushed posteriorly by a squeezing and rolling motion of the tongue on the hard palate from front to back. The base of the tongue retracts towards the posterior pharyngeal wall, and propels the bolus further towards the pharynx.

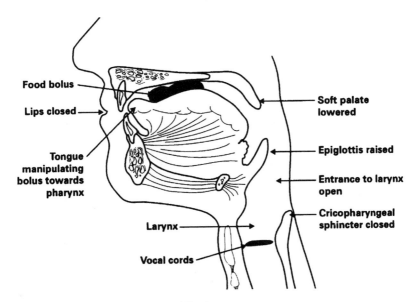

Figure 2.3.1: The oral stage of swallowing.

Pharyngeal stage (Figure 2.3.2)

This stage is triggered as the bolus passes the pillars of fauces. It is involuntary, takes less than a second, and necessitates a temporary pause in breathing. Four key physiological events occur simultaneously.

1. The soft palate elevates and retracts to contact the posterior nasopharyngeal wall, thus preventing nasal reflux.
2. The tongue base retracts and the pharyngeal constrictors contract in a peristaltic wave to push the bolus downwards and clear residue.
3. The larynx elevates by approximately 2 cm, the epiglottis is displaced downward, and the whole of the glottis closes, from the aryepiglottic folds to the true and false vocal folds, in order to prevent aspiration of food into the airway.
4. The cricopharyngeal muscle, which is normally closed to prevent the entry of air into the stomach and the reflux of material from the oesophagus, now opens to allow passage of the bolus into the oesophagus.

The oesophageal stage (Figure 2.3.3)

This stage is also involuntary. It is characterized by a peristaltic wave that travels the length of the oesophagus, lasting between 8 and 20

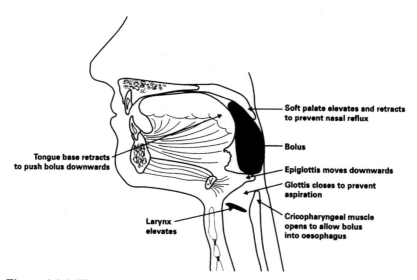

Figure 2.3.2: The pharyngeal stage of swallowing.

seconds (Kronenberger & Meyers, 1994). At any given time, only one peristaltic wave can occur in the oesophagus, moving the bolus downwards towards the stomach. The contents of several rapid swallows may be carried together in the oesophagus by one peristaltic wave.

Alterations to the eating and swallowing mechanism

The term dysphagia is used to describe disorders in feeding and swallowing, and they may be oral or pharyngeal. The type and severity of dysphagia is based largely on the number of structures resected, as well as the reconstructive procedure. In head and neck cancer patients, the dysphagia may be caused by impaired neurological control following surgery, necessitating resection of the nerves involved in deglutition, or due to mechanical dysfunction related to impaired control of the food in the mouth or pharynx.

Neurological disorders

Compression on, or injury to the Xth (vagus) or IXth (glossopharyngeal) nerve caused either by skull base tumours such as chordomas

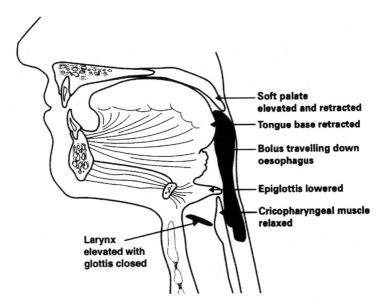

Figure 2.3.3: The oesophageal stage of swallowing.

and nasopharyngeal tumours or surgery employed to treat them
may result in dysphagic symptoms. The dysphagia may be mild and
largely unnoticed or may be so severe as to be life-threatening when
patients are not able to eat or manage their own secretions (Perlman
& Schulze-Delrieu, 1997).

The vagus nerve innervates the muscles of the palate, pharynx
and larynx, such that injury to this nerve can impair closure of the
soft palate, clearance of the pharynx and vocal cord closure during
the pharyngeal stage of the swallow (Netterville & Civantos, 1993).
The glossopharyngeal nerve provides sensation to the base of the
tongue and lateral wall of the pharynx, and is essential to initiate the
pharyngeal swallow. It also provides the motor innervation which is
needed to elevate the larynx.

Paralysis of the VIIth (facial) nerve can also result from parotid
and skull base tumours. Feeding and swallowing are affected by
impaired oral closure and bolus control (Perlman & Schulze-
Delrieu, 1997).

Lower cranial nerve involvement at the base of the skull can cause
unilateral pharyngeal, laryngeal or lingual dysfunction (Groher,
1977).

Mechanical disorders

Oral lesions

Lip seal may be diminished following surgical intervention, resulting in drooling of food and fluid anteriorly with each swallow
attempt. It may also affect ability to generate enough intraoral
pressure to propel the bolus into the pharynx (Appleton & Machin,
1995a). Buccal tone can be reduced because of scar tissue or facial
palsy, leaving the patient with pocketing of food in the lateral
sulcus.

Resections of the tongue and floor of the mouth result in difficulty
with bolus formation and transit of the bolus posteriorly, particularly
for thicker consistencies. When tongue movement is damaged, a
delay in triggering the pharyngeal swallow is often observed and the
patient is vulnerable to aspiration. Reduced range of tongue movement can result in difficulty retrieving food and fluid from around
the oral cavity and there is risk of premature entry of the bolus into
the pharynx and consequent penetration of fluid into the laryngeal
vestibule, or aspiration deeper into the airway.

As a general rule, it is stated that in patients who have had less than 50% of their tongue resected in the surgical procedure, it is the nature of the reconstruction that determines the pattern of function, whereas if more than 50% of the tongue is resected, the extent of resection, as well as the nature of reconstruction, determines functional swallowing abilities (Logemann, 1983). It has been said that the ultimate goal of the reconstruction of the anatomic region is to duplicate the form and function of the normal part (Urken et al, 1994).

Reconstruction using primary closure is an option, but mobility of the tongue secondary to scar contracture may result (Urken et al, 1994). Skin grafts are needed for larger resections, but not only is it important to preserve the mobility of the tongue as far as possible, it is also necessary to maintain sensation. Patients with large amounts of nonsensate tissue have more difficulty eating and swallowing owing to their inability to recognize the presence of food in their mouth, and to manipulate it for an effective swallow. Reconstruction using a radial forearm free flap is a technique used to provide sensation to parts of the reconstructed mouth (Urken & Biller, 1994). The effects are more favourable than reconstructions using myocutaneous flaps (McConnel & Logemann, 1990). Often, if some residual movement is maintained, a prosthetic appliance may be fabricated to utilize the existing function better (Davis, 1989).

Frequently, resections for cancer of the tongue include surgery to the mandible. The patient may be left particularly incapacitated during mastication and swallowing. Associated problems may be exacerbated by dental extraction, loss of bony supporting structure, disturbed alignment of the jaw and trismus (reduced range and flexibility of jaw movement).

If hard palate defects are present, it is not possible to seal the bolus between the tongue and the palate in order to squeeze the bolus backwards. Food and fluid is consequently ejected into the nasal cavity instead.

Oropharyngeal lesions

These include resections of the soft palate, tonsil, base of tongue and superior and lateral wall of the pharynx. Typically the problems experienced following resections of the above structures are nasal regurgitation, decreased bolus transit and aspiration, either before, during, or after the pharyngeal swallow is initiated.

Palatal insufficiency is defined as inadequate length of the soft palate for closure in spite of normal physiological movement, and may occur after ablative surgery. It is distinct from *palatal incompetence*, in which the neuromuscular mechanism is unable to affect closure in spite of normal anatomy, due to cranial nerve damage. The patient remains unable to seal the nasopharynx, thus experiencing problems with nasal regurgitation of food or fluid and premature entry of the bolus into the pharynx whilst attempting to chew. The patient is at risk of aspiration prior to initiating the pharyngeal swallow.

Poor velo-pharyngeal seal may additionally affect the patient's ability to generate sufficient intraoral pressure to drive the bolus into the pharynx (Appleton & Machin, 1995a).

Tumours arising in the tonsillar region often spread quickly to adjacent structures, including the soft palate, the faucal arches, the lateral pharyngeal walls and the tongue base because there is no bone to inhibit the spread. Composite resections of the tonsil and adjacent areas may give rise to a combination of palatal insufficiency or palatal incompetence, difficulty initiating a pharyngeal swallow, reduced tongue base retraction, and impaired pharyngeal peristalsis. The degree of swallowing difficulty increases as the size of the base of tongue resection increases.

Extensive tumours involving the base of tongue may necessitate a total glossectomy. Patients lose the ability to move the bolus from the mouth into the pharynx, resulting in premature leakage into the pharynx and aspiration or nasal regurgitation (McConnel & Mendelsohn, 1987). It is possible for patients to learn to compensate, particularly when provided with a modified diet of pureed food and thin liquids, and tilting the head backwards to facilitate oral transit. However, the point at which aspiration becomes intolerable, and the larynx a liability instead of an asset, is not well defined. Adequate deglutition can still be achieved when up to 80% of the tongue is resected and reconstructed. When deciding if a patient can tolerate total glossectomy with laryngeal preservation, the patient's age, medical condition, attitude, tumour location and whether radiation is to be given, are factors to be considered.

Pharyngeal tumours can be removed without laryngectomy (McNeill, 1981), but constrictor contraction can be so compromised that the remaining larynx again becomes a liability due to aspiration. If pharyngeal contractions do not fully clear the bolus from the pharynx while the larynx is closed, then the residue will be aspirated when the patient inhales after the swallow.

Partial laryngectomy

Partial laryngectomy is a surgical option performed for less extensive tumours of the pharynx or larynx, to control the malignancy whilst preserving voice and swallowing functions. Each resection may vary slightly, but they generally fall into either the category of hemilaryngectomy or supraglottic laryngectomy.

Vertical hemilaryngectomy is indicated for localized tumours on the free margin of one vocal fold. The resection may involve complete removal of the vocal cord, laryngeal ventricle, false vocal cord, and a portion of the thyroid cartilage on the side of the cancer. A pseudocord of muscle taken from the strap muscle is reconstructed at the same level and opposite the remaining vocal cord so that normal laryngeal closure can still be achieved. The hyoid bone and epiglottis are preserved, for laryngeal elevation and deflection of the bolus away from the laryngeal vestibule, thus maintaining airway protection. Studies demonstrate that these patients will experience a temporary dysphagia (Jenkins et al, 1981), but as described later in this chapter, postural changes to the head will help to alleviate these immediate postoperative functions.

Frontolateral hemilaryngectomy is indicated if the tumour is located anteriorly on both vocal cords. In this instance approximately one-third of the front of the larynx, the anterior commissure, is excised on both sides, and replaced with some bulk usually taken from the strap muscles. Both arytenoid cartilages remain so that full laryngeal closure can be achieved, and as with the vertical laryngectomy, the hyoid bone and epiglottis continue to provide airway protection. Any postoperative dysphagic symptoms are temporary and alleviated by modifying the head position. This surgical resection may be more extensive if the tumour extends from the anterior commissure along half the length of one of the vocal cords. The procedure becomes a *three-quarter laryngectomy*. Aspiration can be prevented postoperatively by advising the patient regarding the best head posture, the most appropriate textures of food to eat, and by giving a programme of adduction exercises to follow to improve sphincteric action for airway protection (Logemann, 1983).

A *supraglottic* or *horizontal* laryngectomy may be performed to resect a small supraglottic tumour, whereby the hyoid bone, epiglottis, aryepiglottic folds, false vocal cords, and at least one of the superior laryngeal nerves is excised. The remaining larynx is elevated and sutured to the tongue base.

Aspiration in this client group is common in the immediate post-operative period for a number of reasons. Since the glottis is tucked just below the tongue base, the swallowed bolus falls within close proximity to the airway, and the only remaining airway protection is provided by the true vocal cords. Sensation to the whole of the pharynx is also often markedly reduced, so that the patient fails to close the glottis sufficiently during the swallow, and they may exhibit residual food in the pharynx particularly on top of the airway, with aspiration after the swallow.

It has been found that in these surgical patients, there are two critical factors in recovery of swallowing: airway closure at the laryngeal entrance, and the movement of the tongue base to make complete contact with the posterior pharyngeal wall. Patients who are able to achieve both of these components of the oropharyngeal swallow at 2 weeks postoperatively are able to swallow normally from that point forward (Logemann et al, 1994).

Additionally, a safer *supraglottic swallow* technique can be taught whereby the patient is instructed to voluntarily close the airway or hold their breath prior to the swallow, in order to voluntarily close the true vocal folds. After the swallow, the patient breathes out forcibly to clear any residue of food away from the top of the airway, and then swallows again (Jones & Donner, 1991).

Near-total laryngectomy (shunt)

This is a conservation operation done in cases of extensive but unilateral transglottic, glottic and advanced supraglottic tumours (Casper & Colton, 1993a). It requires interruption of the airway and a tracheostoma.

The entire larynx is removed, with the exception of a narrow strip of tissue which is preserved and fashioned into a shunt connecting the trachea with the pharynx above the uninvolved arytenoid. A form of voicing can be achieved when the patient obstructs the stoma and forces air up the shunt into the pharynx. Though the shunt remains innervated, aspiration may become a problem due to removal of the structures that normally protect the airway.

Total laryngectomy/pharyngolaryngectomy

This procedure involves excision of all laryngeal structures including the cricoid and thyroid cartilages, true and false vocal cords, the epiglottis and the hyoid bone. A permanent tracheostomy is required. The alimentary and respiratory tracts are separated so that pulmonary air cannot be directed into the pharynx. Aspiration of food and fluid from the pharynx into the trachea is not possible. A portion of the tongue base may need to be removed in the resection if the tumour has breached the supraglottic area and extended to the vallecula.

A partial pharyngectomy is required for tumours invading the pyriform sinus. It is these changes to the pharynx and tongue base that can result in a dysphagia (Kronenberger & Meyers, 1994), particularly if tissue grafts are necessary to replace excised tissue.

Jejunum grafts occasionally result in oesophageal dysphagic problems. The jejunum is made of similar striated muscle to that of the oesophagus, but the peristaltic wave can go in both directions. A patient with a jejunum graft may experience retrograde peristalsis causing reflux of food and fluid into the pharynx for up to 6 months after surgery. A second problem occasionally encountered is caused by a stricture at the upper or lower anastomosis which blocks the passage of food through the graft. Such patients may need periodic stretching of this stricture in order to continue with oral foods.

Other causes of dysphagia are fistula formation in the acute stages of recovery, a weakened cricopharyngeal muscle (Hanks et al, 1981), benign strictures in the hypopharynx (Balfe et al, 1982), and increased pharyngeal resistance (McConnel et al, 1986). The reported incidence of dysphagia after total laryngectomy ranges from 10% (Balfe et al, 1982) to 58% (Kirchner et al, 1963). However, the mere presence of an abnormality does not indicate dysfunction, and despite seemingly large amounts of oral and pharyngeal residue, patients may not complain of dysphagia (Pauloski et al, 1995).

Tracheoesophageal puncture

This involves the creation of a tracheoesophageal fistula into which a prosthetic valve is placed to facilitate voice whilst preventing aspiration (as described in Chapter 2.5). Numerous studies report the complications that may affect swallowing, such as aspiration or leakage of saliva and food; aspiration of the voice prosthesis; stenosis of the hypopharynx, tracheostoma, or oesophagus; stoma and fistula infection; development of a secondary fistula; pharyngoesophageal spasm; migration of the fistula; and progressive fistula enlargement (Groher, 1997).

Radiotherapy

Most patients undergo combined treatment for head and neck cancer and have radiation therapy either before or after surgery. If patients have already undergone radiation therapy prior to surgery of the larynx or pharynx, it is important to prepare them for potential disruption to their swallowing ability. Studies using cineradiography have shown that patients who receive radiotherapy prior to resection of the tumour demonstrate paresis, dysfunction of the laryngeal vestibule, and cricopharyngeal incoordination (Ekberg & Nylander, 1983). Stricturing occurs 6 to 8 months post-therapy or earlier with combined radiation and surgery (Lepke & Lipshitz, 1983).

It is equally important to prepare those patients undergoing radiotherapy after surgery to the head and neck for further dysphagic complications to those already incurred through the surgery. Common problems are mucositis, or inflammation of the mucous membranes of the oral cavity and pharynx, which results in pain on swallowing; and xerostomia, following radiation to the salivary glands. When the normal mixture of serous and mucous saliva is no longer produced, the patient may accumulate thick, stringy mucus in the pharynx which is difficult to clear and does not lubricate the oropharynx. As a consequence of xerostomia, dental caries may develop and if left untreated the patient will experience further discomfort whilst eating. Those patients with dentures or a prosthesis may need to discontinue wearing them, since further irritation to the painful mucositis may lead to open sores that will have difficulty healing. Candidiasis is also associated with a dry mouth.

Osteoradionecrosis occurs at the primary site of radiation where fibrosis and a reduction in blood supply can cause necrotic ulcers to form. If left untreated, they can infect bony structures and cause such pain that the patient is no longer able to eat orally.

Trismus develops after irradiation to the nasopharynx, tonsil, retromolar trigone, or paranasal space and is believed to occur secondary to fibrosis of the muscles of mastication (Parsons, 1984). Jaw excursions may be painful and limited, and dental extraction may be necessary for feeding. See Chapter 2.2 for more information on trismus.

The patient may experience a loss of taste and smell, with aversions to certain foods. This can lead to loss of appetite, lack of interest in food and a nutritional deficiency.

Chemotherapy

Chemotherapy may be used if the tumour is large and there is a risk of metastasis, or to reduce the chance of any residual tumour cells re-establishing themselves. It may be administered before or after surgery. Generally chemotherapy alone does not give rise to dysphagia, but some drugs can exacerbate oral mucositis (Raufman, 1988) and changes in taste (Huldij et al, 1986).

Tracheostomy

Most patients undergoing oral or pharyngeal resection or partial laryngectomy will have a tracheostomy performed, to maintain the airway at the time of surgery and to avoid aspiration of blood and saliva in the immediate postoperative period. Initially the cuff is inflated, but it must be deflated as the patient commences with oral feeding.

Many studies have shown that the presence of a tracheostomy tube may worsen a swallowing problem rather than solve it, particularly in patients who have undergone surgery or radiotherapy for head and neck cancer and whose swallowing is already compromised. As previously described, swallowing is a complex process necessitating precise coordination of anatomic structures and sequencing of physiologic events occurring within a closed aerodigestive tract. Tracheostomy interferes in this process, causing a mechanical or physiologic disruption at a number of levels.

1. Tracheostomy causes fixation of the larynx anteriorly, thus limiting laryngeal elevation and reducing airway protection. The degree of laryngeal fixation can be exacerbated by a horizontal incision since it restricts the amount of movement in a vertical direction. Patients who have been intubated over a long period of time may also have decreased base of tongue movement, with a consequent reduction in associated laryngeal elevation. Furthermore the weight of equipment such as a T-piece may impede the upward movement, and fully inflated cuffs — even lower pressure cuffs — may drag along the tracheal walls during each attempt at swallowing (Dikeman & Kazandjian, 1995).

2. Cricopharyngeal opening may become a problem secondary to reduced laryngeal elevation, leaving a residue of secretions in the

pharynx (Bonanno, 1971), and a risk of aspiration after the swallow (Logemann, 1985).

3. A fully inflated tracheostomy tube cuff can distend the walls of the trachea, causing oesophageal compression and consequently a partial blockage to the passage of food and fluid in the oesophagus. Pooling may occur above the level of the cuff, eventually reaching the pharynx and posing a risk of spillage into the larynx. Stagnation of food and secretions can lead to chondritis of the tracheal cartilages, eventually causing tracheomalacia, so that there is no longer a tight cuff-to-trachea seal (Feldman et al, 1966).

4. During the normal pharyngeal stage of the swallow, expiration momentarily ceases and then resumes immediately, clearing any residue away from the larynx. However, in the presence of a tracheostomy tube, air is diverted from its usual route through the larynx and does not reach the vocal folds. Consequently, expiration cannot function to clear the pharynx (Dikeman & Kazandjian, 1995).

5. The diversion of normal airflow through a long-term tracheostomy may cause a desensitization of the larynx so that the patient is unaware of aspiration (Feldman et al, 1966).

6. The protective cough mechanism that would ordinarily clear the airway may also become blunted since, whilst the patient is intubated, the laryngeal reflexes related to normal airflow, such as coughing and clearing the throat, will be eliminated (Tippetts & Siebens, 1991). This eventually results in a decrease in the glottic closure response, the reaction of the larynx to aspirated material (Dikeman & Kazandjian, 1995).

7. It has been postulated that the presence of an unoccluded tracheostomy tube does not allow for sufficient subglottic air pressure to enable the patient to firmly close the vocal folds during the pharyngeal stage of the swallow, thus reducing airway protection (Nash, 1988). A study conducted on head and neck cancer patients with a tracheostomy tube in situ found that aspiration increased when the tracheostomy tube was unoccluded (Muz et al, 1989). A subsequent study reported that aspiration occurred in all patients with an unoccluded tube but in only half of the same patients with an occluded tube (Muz et al, 1994). Other reports indicate that although tracheostomy causes neurophysiologic changes in vocal cord closure, after decannulation for 3 minutes,

some motor function returns (Sasaki et al, 1977; Buchwalter & Sasaki, 1984). There has been much debate whether aspiration is caused by the unoccluded tracheostomy tube or whether it merely exacerbates an already existing dysphagia resulting from treatment for head and neck cancer. A recent study conducted on patients with normal anatomy and physiology of the upper airway, other than the presence of a tracheostomy tube found that the prevalence of aspiration is not affected by the occlusion status of the tube in these patients, leading us to conclude that the patient's oral and pharyngeal physiology is most likely to be the cause of the aspiration (Leder et al, 1996).

NB. It is recommended that patients should not be fed by mouth with the cuff inflated. Therefore, the initial swallowing trials should be deferred until the cuff can be deflated and the patient can tolerate occlusion of the tracheostomy tube at least during each trial swallow. In the case of a fenestrated tube the inner cannula should be removed. In cases of doubt, the speech and language therapist will perform the Blue Dye Test to assess for aspiration.

The role of the speech and language therapist

Speech and language therapists have a thorough knowledge of the anatomy of the vocal tract and the physiology of swallowing. They are skilled in the assessment and management of clients with dysphagia caused by structural or neurological impairment. Any patient with a dysphagia, or at risk of developing a dysphagia following treatment for a head and neck cancer, should be referred to a speech and language therapist.

It has been demonstrated that the intervention of a trained and experienced speech and language therapist leads to more appropriate management of feeding, and a reduction in aspiration (Neufmann et al, 1995). Similarly, the carers of patients with dysphagia are less anxious and learn improved methods of coping with feeding problems (Bryn & Younger, 1988).

Preoperative role

The timing of the initial consultation depends on when the referral is made. Ideally, it is after the physician has given the patient a clear diagnosis and explanation of the recommended treatment, but prior to their admission to hospital. Patients are often admitted to hospital on the eve of their surgery and can easily be overloaded with information from other sources. They have a limited time to absorb this information, and they may be anxious and unable to concentrate or be able to retain information given to them at this stage.

If such an early consultation is not a possibility, the therapist should still meet the patient and if possible his or her carers during the preoperative stage. The preoperative consultation is important for a number of reasons:

1. To review what the patient knows and to correct any misunderstandings about the diagnosis and treatment.
2. To provide information about what to expect in the postoperative period and any difficulties anticipated with feeding and swallowing.
3. To discuss postoperative therapy and the responsibility that the patient has toward his or her own feeding and swallowing rehabilitation. It is most difficult to initiate treatment postoperatively with a patient who has been unprepared for any problems with swallowing. Many patients will assume that their swallowing will recover normally without any effort on their part, and can become quite depressed if after several weeks it has not improved spontaneously.

Postoperative role

The patient's nursing requirements are paramount in the immediate postoperative period, so the speech and language therapist may not visit for the first few days. The nature of this first visit depends on the patient's progress, and whether any postoperative problems have been experienced. The speech and language therapist may take the opportunity to repeat and clarify information and to make general observations. However, no form of swallowing intervention, either for assessment or rehabilitation purposes, is performed until sufficient healing has taken place and the physician signifies that the patient is ready.

Assessment of dysphagia

A number of factors may compromise the patient's ability to swallow and should alert the health professional to the presence of a dysphagia:

1. The patient's cognitive state would not normally change post-operatively, but any confusion or learning disability may predispose the patient to difficulties with swallowing rehabilitation, and such patients may need more support postoperatively.
2. The presence of a facial palsy, sialorrhea (drooling), dysarthria (slurring of words), or nasal emission of air indicates a weakness from neurological impairment that will also affect eating.
3. A wet or gurgly voice is suggestive of pooling in the pharynx and a risk of aspiration.
4. Coughing and choking on secretions, food or fluid signifies a problem with the pharyngeal stage of the swallow.
5. A weak and ineffective cough, or weak and breathy voice.
6. A history of chest infection or aspiration pneumonia is grossly related to the presence of dysphagia.
7. Evidence of aspiration of food and fluid on suctioning patients with a tracheostomy tube.
8. Unexplained weight loss, slow eating and lack of interest in food would all be indicative of a problem. It is important to listen to the patient's account of his or her difficulty in swallowing. However, it has been found that when a patient does complain of a swallowing difficulty, the severity of the problem may be grossly understated (Baker et al, 1991).

Any patient manifesting any of the above warning signs should be seen by the speech and language therapist as soon as possible, in order that a comprehensive dysphagia assessment can be performed.

Evaluation of dysphagia depends on two major factors: meticulous attention to the examination itself and an in-depth knowledge of normal and abnormal anatomy of swallowing (Jones & Donner, 1989). In patients with head and neck cancer it can take a variety of approaches.

Bedside evaluation

Firstly, the clinician can perform a bedside assessment of oral preparatory and oral stages of swallowing. Labial, lingual and palatal range of movement can be observed during a variety of tasks, including speech and manipulation of material in the mouth. However, this method of evaluation gives limited information about the pharyngeal stage of the swallow, in particular whether the patient aspirates.

It does not always follow that patients who aspirate will cough. In the absence of a cough reflex it cannot be assumed that it is safe for the patient to swallow, since sensitivity may be reduced and the patient may be aspirating silently (Logemann, 1989).

Cervical auscultation

This is increasingly being used as an additional tool at the bedside to listen for an abnormal swallow. A stethoscope is placed on either side of the neck and the pattern of sounds created during the swallow can be helpful in identifying spillage of the bolus into the pharynx prior to initiation of the swallow, a delayed pharyngeal swallow and presence of residue in the pharynx after the swallow.

Modified barium swallow

The most widely used objective and physiological approach to the assessment of dysphagia in the head and neck cancer patient is *video-fluoroscopy*. This is a radiological study of structure and function during the three stages of the swallow. The patient sits upright in his or her usual eating position, and the oral cavity and pharynx are viewed in the lateral, and then anterior plane. The patient is given a number of different food consistencies, usually liquid, paste and solid, in different quantities, to assess for problems at any stage, and to rule out silent aspiration. The speech and language therapist can recommend a variety of compensatory strategies to be tried during the study, and their effect on the patient's swallow observed accordingly (as described below).

Other diagnostic techniques include the use of fibre-optic endoscopy to observe the pharynx before and after the swallow, ultrasound to visualize tongue and hyoid movement, scintigraphy to measure speed of bolus transit and the presence and amount of aspiration, and manometry which can provide information on the pharyngeal pressures generated during the swallow (Logemann, 1989).

Management decisions

The management of the dysphagic patient is of course multidisciplinary, but depending on the outcome of the comprehensive swallowing assessment, a number of recommendations may be made by the speech and language therapist, as described.

Patient safety

Patient safety is a priority in those undergoing treatment for head and neck cancer and not only must we ensure that their nutritional needs are met (see Chapter 2.4), but it is vital to ensure that it is safe for them to feed orally. Some patients may be able to tolerate small amounts of aspiration, particularly if generally fit and mobile, but it must be kept to a minimum to prevent the development of aspiration pneumonia.

If the patient is deemed unsafe to continue with oral feeds, a non-oral method of feeding should be considered (as discussed in Chapter 2.4). A non-oral method of feeding may also be considered in cases where patients have some swallow function, but are not yet able to eat enough orally to meet their nutritional needs. At this time the speech and language therapist will be able to suggest some compensatory strategies and embark upon a programme of swallowing therapy.

Compensatory strategies

Compensatory strategies involve providing the patient with techniques that reduce the risk of aspiration and increase the efficiency of the swallow. The following list is not comprehensive and should only be recommended after a full assessment by the speech and language therapist.

The first technique involves manipulating the textures of foods given to the patient, depending on the outcome of the assessment. For example, a patient with limited tongue control during the oral stage may have difficulty manipulating solid foods and will benefit from a soft or pureed diet instead. A patient with a delayed pharyngeal swallow or poor airway protection during the pharyngeal swallow will benefit from eliminating thin liquids from their diet and using a thickening agent in all drinks. Patients presenting with an oesophageal stricture may manage liquids and soft sloppy foods, but not fibrous or cohesive food consistencies. Patients with a very dry mouth after radiotherapy will also benefit from a very soft and sloppy diet and may need to drink plenty of fluid during a meal in order to aid oral and pharyngeal stages of the swallow.

Secondly, postural changes can change the way food flows through the oral cavity and pharynx, and when matched with the patient's individual swallowing physiology, can make significant improvements in both swallow efficiency and safety (Logemann, 1989). Again the following list is not comprehensive and should only be recommended after a full assessment by the speech and language therapist.

Examples would include tipping the head backwards to facilitate transit of a bolus posteriorly in a patient with an anterior resection of the tongue. Alternatively, the head can be tipped forwards to increase the overhang of the epiglottis in a patient exhibiting poor airway protection during the pharyngeal stage of the swallow. (All possibilities are not given in this text.)

When used in combination, the elimination of food consistencies that a patient finds difficult, and suggesting changes to their posture, may enable the patient to tolerate oral feeds. At the same time, swallowing therapy may be administered to improve the patient's residual function.

Swallowing therapy

Swallowing therapy may be indirect or direct. Indirect therapy is a term given to exercises that are aimed at improving strength and range of movement of the muscles involved in eating and swallowing, but do not act on the swallow itself. For example, jaw range of motion exercises may be given to a patient presenting with trismus, or tongue range of motion may be necessary following a hemiglossectomy. Vocal cord adduction exercises may be beneficial after a partial laryngectomy.

Direct therapy involves the provision of exercises designed to change the coordination of the swallow itself. Frequently a safer supraglottic swallow is recommended to patients with reduced airway protection. The patient is instructed to hold his/her breath, swallow hard whilst keeping the vocal cords closed and then to cough on the exhalation after the swallow. Other manoeuvres are also available to improve lingual control during posterior propulsion of the bolus, muscle effort and cricopharyngeal opening.

It is rare for patients to experience a delayed swallow reflex following head and neck surgery. In such cases a technique known as *thermal stimulation* can be used, whereby a cold stimulus is used to contact the base of the patient's faucal arches in an attempt to trigger the swallow (Logemann, 1983).

Once the bolus has entered the oesophagus it is beyond volitional control and does not respond to exercise programmes.

Feeding tools

A further recommendation by the speech and language therapist might be to provide the patient with alternative feeding utensils. Examples include providing a flatter utensil to a patient with trismus, or a plastic feeding utensil to those complaining of a metallic taste after radiotherapy. Glossectomy feeding spoons are available with a plunger to deposit the food in the oropharynx, and patients with less than 50% of their tongue resected may benefit from using a syringe to place a pureed bolus into the position in their mouth where they have greatest sensation and ability to move the bolus with the remaining tongue (Groher, 1997).

Prosthodontic management

The speech and language therapist and maxillofacial prosthodontist may continue to see the patient for some time after discharge from hospital if an intraoral prosthesis is necessary to assist the patient's swallowing.

Case examples

Case one: Alfred

Alfred presented with a T3 N1 squamous cell carcinoma within the right pyriform fossa. He therefore underwent a partial pharyngolaryngectomy which was repaired with a radial forearm flap, a right functional neck dissection, and some dental extractions. He had a temporary tracheostomy during the operation and for a few days afterwards. Immediately postoperatively Alfred was kept nil by mouth (NBM).

Five days after his surgery, the tracheostomy tube was removed and Alfred was commenced on thin fluids.

After another 2 days Alfred developed a chest infection related to aspiration and was recommended to be NBM again. A swallowing assessment was requested from the speech and language therapist.

A bedside assessment demonstrated a difficulty with thin fluids, with evidence of aspiration into the airway. He also had a difficulty chewing solid foods, because of pain and discomfort.

Compensatory strategies were found to help, and the following were recommended:

1. All thin liquids, including drinks and soups, were to be thickened to a custard-thick consistency.
2. Only very soft foods requiring very gentle chewing were to be attempted.

3. He was to turn his head towards the right side during the pharyngeal swallow to encourage transit of the bolus down the intact, left side of his pharynx.
4. Alfred was encouraged to use a Safe-Supraglottic Swallow technique at all times.

Two weeks later Alfred`s eating and swallowing had improved to such an extent that he chose to stop using thickeners in his drinks, and did not persevere with the other compensatory strategies. He was discharged from hospital on oral feeds.

Two months later, Alfred was receiving his radiotherapy treatment and his swallowing was reported to be deteriorating once again. By April he had lost 7 lb and was unable to maintain his weight on oral feeds alone. He was given nasogastric feeds to maintain nutrition until his swallowing ability improved.

After another 5 months he was still having great difficulty feeding orally. His dysphagia was exacerbated by a severely dry mouth as a consequence of the radiotherapy.

Alfred was given a gastrostomy feeding tube through which he would receive the bulk of his nutrition. He was encouraged to persevere with 6 teaspoons of thickened liquids or smooth purees in an attempt to continue to rehabilitate his swallow.

A year after his initial surgery, and after little improvement to his eating and swallowing ability, a formal assessment of his swallow was requested and a videofluoroscopy arranged. The results of this were as follows:

Thin liquids
No difficulties during the oral stage.
During the pharyngeal stage, a small amount of liquid was aspirated due to reduced laryngeal elevation and poor airway protection. Alfred was able to clear the aspirate with a strong cough.

Thick liquids/purees
No difficulties demonstrated with the contrast during the oral stage.
During the pharyngeal stage the contrast passed freely through the pharynx. Airway protection for this consistency was adequate and there was no aspiration.

Solids
This consistency was not tried during the assessment. Commonly bread or biscuit is used, which Alfred reported that he would not manage due to his dry mouth.

As a consequence of the videofluoroscopy, Alfred was encouraged to persevere with his thickened drinks and soft sloppy diet. He continues to struggle to eat and remains with a gastrostomy tube to this day.

Case two: Alan

Alan underwent a total pharyngolaryngectomy repaired with a jejunum graft, and bilateral functional neck dissection.

He healed quickly and generally recovered from the surgery very well. Six days after his surgery, a gastrografin swallow demonstrated that the jejunal anastomosis had healed and he was therefore commenced on liquids and soft foods.

He was discharged from hospital on his eleventh postoperative day. Some concern was expressed by the speech and language therapist, because whilst Alan appeared to be eating and swallowing well, he had been observed to be experiencing regurgitation of food and fluid during a meal, thus slowing his eating considerably and reducing his overall intake.

He was monitored by the speech and language therapist over the next 6 weeks during his appointments at the combined head and neck oncology clinic. He reported that he could manage liquids only.

Alan persevered with his liquid diet and supplements provided to him by the dietitian throughout his radiotherapy, and by sheer determination avoided having to have a nasogastric tube passed.

Four months later, little progress had been made and a videofluoroscopy was requested to assess the reason for Alan's dysphagia to solids. It demonstrated very clearly that the difficulty arose during the oesophageal stage of the swallow, within the jejunum graft.

Liquids
A liquid bolus passed freely through the jejunum. There was minimal pooling of the contrast below the upper anastomosis, where the tail-end of the graft lay in the side of his neck. This caused no discomfort and could very easily be cleared by Alan tilting his head slightly towards the right.

Thick liquid/puree
The flow of a thicker bolus was slowed considerably through the jejunum graft, until it stopped halfway along, and then was refluxed back forcibly by retrograde peristalsis. There was no evidence of a stricture at either upper or lower anastomosis.

Since this was found to be an oesophageal stage dysphagia, the speech and language therapist had no further recommendations or therapeutic techniques that would alleviate his symptoms. The nature of the dysphagia was explained to Alan and his wife, and he was encouraged to take a trial-and-error approach with food textures, in the hope that the reflux would diminish with time.

Summary

Often the ultimate functional outcome of swallowing cannot be determined until several months after treatment when healing is complete, any facial swelling has reduced, and the effects of radio-therapy diminished. Therapy continues until a patient reaches a point that both therapist and patient agree is their maximum swallowing potential. However, it is important to continue to offer support to the dysphagic patient on an outpatient basis for as long as required.

The speech and language therapist has a vital role in the rehabilitation of the head and neck cancer patient. Throughout the rehabilitation process it is important for the entire multidisciplinary team to cooperate and continually reinforce the patient's practice. Difficulties arise if different professionals give different advice to the patient. The best outcome is achieved when a single set of instructions is given to the patient and reinforced by all concerned in the patient's care. It is the speech and language therapist's role to educate the team about the needs of a particular patient and ensure cooperation amongst staff.

Chapter 2.4
Nutrition

Julie Batty

Introduction

Nutrition plays a vital role in the care of the individual with head and neck cancer from the point of diagnosis onwards. Individuals may present at diagnosis with nutritional problems, or these may develop during their course of treatment or beyond.

The consequences of progressive malnutrition are well documented. Malnutrition and weight loss can have a marked effect on the morbidity and mortality of cancer patients (Smale et al, 1981; Daly et al, 1990). The clinical and psychological status of the cancer patient can be significantly aided by providing adequate nutritional support (Shils, 1979).

Malnutrition will undoubtedly lead to depletion of subcutaneous fat stores, progressive muscle wasting and lethargy. Impairment of the immune system, risk of infection and increased risk of pressure sore development are also possible consequences (Haydock, 1986; Higgs, 1987). An adequate source of nutrients is essential to meet the metabolic demands of the immune system. Protein energy malnutrition is known to provoke a decreased immune response, which often worsens the malnutrition when infection follows as a consequence.

Optimizing nutritional intake and status is paramount both in the prevention and treatment of delayed wound healing and pressure sores. Weight loss and muscle atrophy can predispose an individual to pressure sore development by reducing subcutaneous padding between skin and bone. Adequate protein intake is also essential as protein depletion can affect protein synthesis and the maturation of connective tissue.

171

The psychological effects of malnutrition are significant and can include apathy and depression. It has been reported that patients suffering from malnutrition often have a lower morale and reduced will to recover (Theologies, 1978).

Patients with head and neck cancer are particularly at risk of developing nutritional problems and malnutrition. Many patients with head and neck cancer have chronic histories of excessive alcohol intake, heavy tobacco abuse (Department of Health, 1998) and poor dietary habits. These factors alone often place the individual 'nutritionally at risk'. Malnutrition can often arise when alcohol contributes a significant percentage of the individual's daily energy intake at the expense of their diet. This can often result in an inadequate nutrient intake.

Tumours of the head and neck can lead to nutrition-related problems even before the cancer is diagnosed. Pain on eating, ulcerated mouth, dysphagia and poor-fitting dentures are all examples of factors that may interfere with an individual's ability to chew and swallow. The head and neck patient can then go on to be treated with a single therapy or combination of therapies: surgery, radiation therapy or chemotherapy. Each treatment approach has the potential for precipitating further nutritional problems, which will be explored in greater detail in this chapter.

Assessment and dietetic intervention

Early identification of patients who are malnourished, at risk of becoming malnourished or at risk of developing nutrition-related problems is essential.

A number of different protocols for the assessment of nutritional status are currently in use throughout hospital and community settings. Although not all protocols currently used have been validated, their routine use raises awareness for early nutritional intervention and referral to a state registered dietitian.

All protocols should include assessment of the following (British Association of Parenteral and Enteral Feeding [BAPEN], 1996):

- weight and weight change (percentage of weight loss over a stated period of time)
- height
- appetite

- ability to eat, i.e. chewing/swallowing difficulties
- psychological state, i.e. confused/depressed
- risk factors associated with the disease or potential treatment, i.e. obstruction secondary to the tumour, surgery, radiotherapy or chemotherapy.

It is important that any protocol developed is quick and simple to use and appropriate to this patient client group. Many nutritional assessment screening tools available have limited value because they were developed for use with specific patient groups and cannot therefore be applied to other categories of patients.

If it is highlighted that diet-related problems exist, then early referral to a state registered dietitian is advisable. The dietitian will assess fully the individual's nutritional intake and status, and take appropriate action. Individual plans and goals of dietary care will be devised after consultation with the patient, family, carers and other team members. Consideration of disease state, proposed or current treatment and prognosis is essential to ensure the appropriate level of nutritional support is given.

Nutritional effects of treatment

Specific problems occur during the course of treatment that will have a direct effect on nutritional intake and therefore nutritional status. It has been estimated that more than 80% of head and neck cancer patients lose a significant amount of weight during multi-modal treatment (Chencharick & Mossman, 1983). The head and neck team need to incorporate nutritional assessment and monitoring into each stage of the cancer treatment process to ensure that dietetic intervention is optimized.

Surgery

Surgical-related nutritional problems can be both complex and extensive. Early nutritional assessment is required to ensure that preoperative nutritional support is provided if required. Van Bokhorst-de van der Schueren et al (1997) studied 64 patients undergoing major surgery for advanced cancer and found that patients with a weight loss of more than 10% which occurred during a period of six months prior to their surgery, had a greater risk of postoperative complications. These included wound infections, anastomotic leakage and septicaemia. In some cases aggressive preoperative nutritional support will need to be initiated. Post-surgical risk of malnutrition is increased in this patient group, and prolonged enteral feeding is often needed (Gardine, 1988). Surgical resection of tumours of the head and neck area have the potential to severely restrict or eliminate oral intake. Additionally, postoperative complications, such as infection and development of fistulas and sepsis, will increase the individual's nutritional requirements (Elia, 1990).

Treatment approaches may weigh heavily in the decision to initiate artificial feeding. If it is anticipated that short-term artificial support is required, enteral feeding via a nasogastric tube is often the most appropriate choice. Gastrostomy feeding may be a preferred method if it is indicated that long-term enteral feeding is required. In order to anticipate length of feeding period it is important to consider preoperative oral intake and nutritional status alongside potential post-surgical rehabilitation problems in feeding.

Chemotherapy

Chemotherapy can compromise the individual's nutritional status and intake in the following ways:

- Nausea and vomiting, if not well controlled with anti-emetics, can lead to dehydration, weight loss and lethargy. Anticipatory nausea and vomiting can also be a problem. Factors found to be involved in this response include taste, smell and anxiety (Nerenz et al, 1986).
- The rapidly dividing cells of the gastrointestinal tract are often affected by chemotherapy. The mucosal lining of the mouth can become damaged, leading to pain and ulceration. These factors can, in turn, further limit nutritional intake and the enjoyment of eating.

Radiotherapy

Radiotherapy of the head and neck compromises the nutritional status of the patient by affecting the normal tissues in and around the oral cavity. As a result of normal tissue damage to this area, patients commonly experience reduced or abnormal taste sensations, dry mouth, mucositis, loss of appetite and dysphagia. Chencharick et al (1983) reported that head and neck cancer patients are subjectively aware of nutritional problems before radiotherapy and that radiotherapy exacerbates these problems.

Xerostomia can be temporary or permanent. Alongside good oral hygiene, adjusting the patient's food texture and consistency and increasing fluid intake can help. The use of artificial saliva immediately prior to meals may benefit some patients, as may utilizing extra sauces or gravies with meals or using sugar-free chewing gum. The reduction of salivary function during radiotherapy can cause loss of palatal seal in denture patients and general difficulty in chewing. It may also cause alterations in taste sensitivity (Palmer, 1984).

Chencharick et al (1983) found that taste problems were a common consequence of radiotherapy. In their study, aversion to meat was common, as was increased 'sweet tasting threshold'. An increase in sugar consumption was evident as a result of the latter. Salt was avoided because it irritated the oral cavity and because patients reported that their saliva already tasted salty. Further subjective studies of this kind need to be conducted.

The sore oral mucosa may also be irritated by alcohol, smoking, extremes of temperature and spicy food. Patients often discover their own individual food sensitivities by trial and error.

Dysphagia, a difficulty in swallowing, can occur during radiotherapy treatment. Changes in food texture and/or utilization of nutritional supplementation may be the first line of intervention to facilitate eating whilst maintaining adequate nutritional intake.

Artificial feeding needs to be considered, either alone or as an adjunct to the individual's oral intake if it becomes obvious that oral intake alone is failing to meet nutritional requirements. If, in the planning stage of radiotherapy, an individual is identified as being at high risk of nutritional compromise, instigation of early artificial feeding needs to be considered.

Oral nutritional support

Nutritional goals

The main goal for providing nutritional support in the patient with head and neck cancer is to achieve and maintain a desirable weight and to correct or prevent nutritional deficiencies (Kouba, 1988). A variety of feeding choices exist to achieve this goal, but it is important to ensure that any feeding approach is both individualized and realistic.

Ideally, adequate oral feeding should be encouraged where possible. Maintenance of normal eating patterns is important to both patients and their carers (Mattes et al, 1992). Patients often feel that they are in control of their food intake, whereas they often have little control over other aspects of their care. The carers too, may feel that they are able to contribute to the patient's care through food. It is paramount that health professionals empathize with patients' eating problems and help them to find alternative eating strategies.

Initial nutritional intervention should be an evaluation of the patient's present dietary intake and advice on how nutritional requirements can be maintained.

Maintaining nutrition via oral intake

Poor appetite — early satiety

Cancer can produce profound changes in an individual's appetite. As previously discussed, reasons for this can be multifactorial. Various relatively controllable symptoms, such as pain, nausea or constipation, can also precipitate a loss of appetite for the individual. Often the first step in improving the individual's appetite and nutritional intake is improvement of symptom control.

Finding practical coping strategies for the patient can be helpful at this time. Suggestions may include:

- Small, frequent meals and snacks to maximize intake.
- Using smaller plates/dishes so the patient doesn't feel daunted by the size of the portions.
- Making food look attractive.
- Ensuring that the individual is relaxed when eating.
- Eating at times of the day when compromising symptoms are reduced.
- Taking part in family meals.
- Consideration of use of alcohol pre-meals as an appetite stimulant.
- Consideration of use of medication as an adjunct to dietary intervention, e.g. low-dose steroids or megestrol acetate may help to improve appetite, and prokinetic agents (e.g. metoclopramide or cisapride) may help if early satiety or chronic nausea are reported by the individual.

- Advice regarding the fortification of the individual's diet, i.e. maximizing the protein and energy content of foods. Items such as dried milk powder, butter, milk and cheese can be used for this purpose, e.g. grated cheese in soup, extra butter on vegetables, dried milk powder added into puddings/custards.

It is important to provide the patient and carer with written practical advice and simple action plans, based on their individual needs.

Dysphagia

Patients will undoubtedly find it difficult to achieve an adequate dietary intake if dysphagia is a problem. It is important that the cause of dysphagia is identified, i.e. mechanical, secondary to surgery or radiotherapy and appropriate food texture chosen. Close liaison with a speech therapist is often a priority to establish what the dysphagic patient can swallow safely in terms of texture and consistency (see case example). Modified consistencies may include soft consistencies, e.g. scrambled egg, fish pie, mince; 'thick pureed' consistencies, e.g. custard, smooth porridge, milk puddings; or the consistency of a thin liquid. Commercial thickeners are available if thin liquids need to be thickened.

Changing food textures

Liquidizing foods may often be necessary to produce a smooth and even texture for the patient. A wide variety of foods can be altered to a suitable consistency, although this can also make foods more filling and dilute nutrients. Liquidized foods may look and taste better if different parts of the meal are liquidized separately rather than altogether. This retains a range of colours and flavours to make eating more appealing for the individual. If additional liquid is needed to texture food, the utilization of milk sauces, gravies or milk, rather than water, will be advised to improve the nutritional content of textured food.

Nutritional supplements

Often, in spite of increased snacks, fortifying foods or changes in food consistency, the patient may still fail to meet his or her nutritional requirements. The next option would be to consider nutritional supplements. A variety of liquid or powdered supplements are now available and most commercial supplements are available on prescription. The majority of sip feeds are not only high in energy and protein but also contain a full range of vitamins and minerals. For this reason they can be an important adjunct to an individual's inadequate oral intake, or can be the individual's sole source of nutrition. A major problem with the use of nutritional supplements can be their palatability, which may affect the individual's tolerance and compliance. On a long-term basis tastes and flavours can become monotonous, leading to taste fatigue. Practical advice such as incorporating certain sip feeds into jellies or mousses, and utilizing neutral flavours, can be essential to aid compliance to the dietetic plan.

Artificial feeding

Enteral feeding refers to nutritional support administered into the stomach or intestine. For reasons already discussed, adequate oral nutritional intake may not be achievable for all patients during their course of treatment. If this is the case, artificial feeding must be considered. As the majority of head and neck patients have a functional gastrointestinal tract, they are ideal candidates for enteral feeding. Unlike parenteral feeding, which bypasses the gastrointestinal tract, enteral feeding maintains gut mucosal integrity and prevents gut mucosal atrophy. Gut mucosal atrophy can initiate translocation of bacteria and endotoxin into the portal circulation (Herndon et al, 1993). There is an extensive variety of enteral nutrition sites, tubes and mechanical delivery devices.

Nasogastric feeding

Each of the many methods of enteral feeding has their own advantages and disadvantages. The simplest and cheapest method in the short term is via a nasogastric tube. This method has improved significantly with the replacement of wide-bore plastic tubes (Ryles) with fine-bore enteral feeding tubes. The use of wider-bore plastic tubes has been associated with complications including pharyngitis, oesophagitis and rhinitis (Payne, 1995). The introduction of fine-bore tubes has improved patient comfort and reduced tube-associated complications.

Most fine-bore tubes have an internal diameter of 1–2 mm and an external diameter of 2–3 mm (6–9 French Gauge [FG]). Obviously the smaller the external diameter the more comfortable it will be for the patient. Tubes intended for short-term use (approximately 7–10 days) can be made from polyvinyl chloride (PVC), whereas longer-term tubes should be made of either polyurethane or silicone. The latter two materials will remain resistant to gastric acid erosion over prolonged periods of time.

Nasogastric tube placement should be carried out by a qualified nurse or dietitian. BAPEN (1996) stated in their standards for the placement of enteral feeding tubes that medical staff have a responsibility for the insertion of fine-bore feeding tubes in patients who have maxillofacial disorders or surgery, laryngectomy or any disorder of the oesophagus. They state, however, that if medical staff feel that it is appropriate and safe for a nurse to pass the tube, this should be documented in the patient's medical notes.

Placement of nasogastric feeding tubes can be confirmed by aspiration of stomach contents and litmus testing. Radiographic confirmation of placement is required if positive aspirate cannot be obtained (BAPEN, 1996). It is important to consider that treatment with H_2-receptor antagonists or antacids may affect pH measurements (Nakao et al, 1983).

Complications of nasogastric feeding

Risk of aspiration

The potential for aspiration needs to be considered with nasogastric feeding. The risk can be reduced by elevating the patient's head during and after feeding, and ensuring the adequacy of gastric emptying of the patient (Bastow, 1986).

Once nasogastric feeding has commenced, the position of the tube should be checked at least daily. This should be carried out before starting or restarting a feed. If the patient is confined to bed, or needs to be fed overnight, he or she should be fed in an upright position or at least have the head and shoulders raised 30–40 degrees to avoid aspiration of the feed (Taylor & Goodinson-McLaren, 1992).

Tube blockage

Maintaining the tube's patency will prevent occlusion and therefore the need for tube replacement. Fine-bore tubes should be flushed according to the manufacturer's guidelines. In the author's experience, flushing the fine-bore nasogastric tube every 4 to 6 hours before and after the feeding interval, and after the administration of medication, has proved effective. Blockage may sometimes be resolved by the instillation of cola or fresh pure pineapple juice into the tube. Check local policies before proceeding because some Trusts only allow sterile water to be instilled down the tube.

Risk of infection

Often the patient requiring artificial feeding may have some degree of malnutrition which, as already stated, can affect immune status thereby increasing the individual's susceptibility to infection.

Potential bacterial contamination of enteral feeds and feeding equipment must always be considered. Commercially prepared liquid feeds should be sterile until opened and sterile procedures are required when decanting feeds (Anderton & Aidoo, 1990).

The re-use of feed containers and administration sets can also be a significant source of contamination (Grunow et al, 1989; Anderton & Nwoguh, 1991). Therefore both feed containers and administration sets should be changed every 24 hours.

Psychosocial problems

The psychosocial aspect of nasogastric feeding is another issue to consider. The presence of a nasogastric tube can markedly affect the individual's body image. If it becomes obvious that enteral feeding will be required on a long-term basis, gastrostomy tube placement will need to be considered.

Comfort

Nasogastric tube feeding should also be limited to short-term use because of potential mucosal erosion and nasopharyngeal irritation (Taylor & Goodinson-McLaren, 1992). Another limitation of nasogastric tube feeding is frequent tube displacement and the trauma the patient experiences with repeated tube placement.

Gastrostomy feeding

Gastrostomy is the placement of a tube in the stomach for feeding, and it involves the creation of a tract between the stomach and the abdominal surface. The advantages of this technique include easy access to the stomach and the bypassing of proximal mechanical, surgical or functional obstructions (Taylor & Goodinson-McLaren, 1992). Gastrostomy feeding is considered more aesthetic than naso-gastric feeding, and there is a reduced risk of tube misplacement or blockage (Shike et al, 1989).

Percutaneous endoscopic gastrostomy

Since its introduction in 1980, the percutaneous endoscopic gastrostomy (PEG) technique, unlike the surgically placed gastros-tomy, has made it possible to place a feeding tube directly into the stomach without either a general anaesthetic or laparotomy. The PEG technique allows the placement of a gastrostomy feeding tube under simple intravenous sedation with the assistance of an endoscope. It can be performed in either an endoscopy unit or at the bedside and takes about 15 minutes (Matthewson, 1995).

Radiological gastrostomy

For the head and neck cancer patient the development of the radio-logically placed gastrostomy has proved most valuable. The radio-logical procedure does not require an endoscope for placement, which can be troublesome for this patient group. This technique requires the stomach to be inflated with air through a nasogastric tube to aid radiological visualization, and then external puncture of the stomach.

Complications of gastrostomy feeding

Despite reports that complication rates of percutaneous gastrostomy techniques are low (Gutt et al, 1996), it is important to be aware of some of the associated complications.

Wound infection: Wound complications include cellulitis at the tube site, abscess in the abdominal wall, and leakage around the gastros-tomy tube (Deveney, 1990). A small study by Shike et al (1989) reported that three out of 39 patients developed localized skin infections after the placement of PEGs. All three infections cleared with appropriate antibiotic therapy. By comparison, Ghosh & East-wood (1994) reported that 31% of patients studied with long-term gastrostomy tubes had stomal infections.

Separation of the stomach from the abdominal wall: This complication can occur following inadvertent tube removal and early re-insertion of the gastrostomy tube before firm adhesion between the stomach and anterior parietal peritoneum. During the attempt to replace the tube, the stomach may be pushed away from the abdominal wall and allow leakage of gastric contents into the peritoneal cavity. If recognition of this is delayed, severe peritonitis may result (Rombeau & Palacio, 1990).

Bleeding: Major bleeding following gastrostomy placement can occur. This problem can be minimized by preoperative assessment of the individual's coagulation status. The patient should be monitored for signs of haemorrhage post-procedure.

Gastrostomy tube replacements

If either tube, i.e. the PEG tube or radiological tube, becomes displaced or irreparably damaged, various replacement gastrostomy tubes exist. Insertion of replacement gastrostomy tubes is a relatively simple procedure as long as the tract of the gastrostomy is well established.

Most replacement tubes are secured in the stomach by a balloon containing water. The water in the balloon should be checked weekly as some may be lost by osmosis. Patients, carers and/or other health professionals can be trained to replace balloon-retained tubes. Confirmation of tube position is paramount before any feeding is commenced via the enteral tube.

Another development in replacement gastrostomy tubes has been the 'gastrostomy button', which is a low-profile replacement device fitted to the size of the gastrostomy tract. This can be an ideal choice for certain patients, especially where body image or interference with sexual activity had formerly been a problem. Unfortunately, the external fixation device will not move on the 'button' and therefore if weight changes are expected the lifespan of the tube will be limited.

Home enteral feeding

A small qualitative study undertaken to explore the psychological effects of percutaneous gastrostomy feeding on both patients and carers revealed a wide spectrum of difficulties (Rickman, 1998). These problems included the physical and mental ability of the patient to set up feeds, changes in body image and the loss of enjoyment of food and drink. Artificial feeding is often a familiar, straightforward procedure for dietitians and nursing staff, but for patients it can be very frightening and the cause of much anxiety. Preparation for home should ideally involve close liaison with the patient and/or their carer, in addition to both hospital- and community-based multidisciplinary teams.

Developing structured teaching programmes and setting learning goals can help to reassure the patient and the team of a safe transition to the community. Often the use of discharge checklists can aid communication between the team.

Psychosocial aspects

The psychosocial aspects of artificial feeding must always be considered and, if issues are identified, appropriate intervention must be taken.

An individual's social life can be markedly affected if he or she is on continuous or restricted feeding regimes. It is important to consider changing feeding regimes or using ambulatory feeding pumps to ensure the patient does not come to resent 'artificial feeding'. The option of bolus feeding may also be a consideration. For many patients, pump-assisted feeding may be appropriate initially to allow a constant low volume of feed to be instilled into the patient when poor gastric emptying, nausea or vomiting are factors to consider. However, once the patient is stabilized on his or her feeding regime, the option of bolus feeding may be more practical. Bolus feeding can release the patient from long periods attached to a feeding pump, and appears to help the transition to oral feeding and regulate appetite.

The social impact of not being able to eat and drink can be devastating for some patients. Grindel et al (1996) reported that patients receiving home enteral nutrition felt excluded from the daily routine of meals and festive occasions in which food played a part. The impact of this should not be under-estimated or ignored. More information on psychosocial problems and their management can be found in Section Three.

Palliative care

Dilemmas regarding the provision of nutritional support in both the palliative and terminal stages of disease continue and can create much discussion and controversy. Copp & Dunn (1993) reported that palliative care nurses found nutrition to be one of the most difficult problems in palliative care.

Food and drink can hold different meanings for different individuals. For some, it has both social and pleasurable links, while for others it is simply a way to sustain their existence. Nutritional intervention during palliative or terminal care needs to be aimed at helping the individual obtain an optimum quality of life. This will undoubtedly involve the individual taking control over his or her nutritional intake.

Before any nutritional intervention is undertaken, it is paramount to establish what patients, their families or carers and the team expect from their care.

Setting nutritional goals can often help clarify realistic aims of nutritional intervention. Such goals may include:

- improving general health and sense of wellbeing
- preventing clinical malnutrition
- improving body image by preventing further weight loss
- preventing hunger
- improving wound healing/prevention of pressure sores.

Progressive weight loss can often be the cause of anxiety for individuals and their carers. Cancer cachexia in end-stage disease can be the cause of excessive weight loss, changes in body image and increasing weakness. Cancer cachexia is the well known but ill-defined syndrome whereby the severity of weight loss is in excess of that which may be expected from the degree of reduction in nutritional intake. At present, the cause of cancer cachexia is thought to be multifactorial. Research suggests that cytokines and peptides secreted by the host in response to the tumour have a role in the development of cachexia. However, whilst metabolic abnormalities are the main cause of malnutrition, decreased nutrient intake can also contribute to the cancer cachexia (Bruera, 1997).

As previously discussed, the reasons for reduced nutrient intake in the head and neck cancer patient can be multifactorial, and the practical suggestions previously discussed in this chapter can be utilized at this stage. Any nutritional intervention should, however, be patient driven. It is essential to promote quality of life, dignity and self worth.

In some circumstances, such as mechanical obstruction or an impaired swallowing mechanism, artificial feeding may need to be considered for the head and neck patient undergoing palliative treatment. Decision-making with regard to nutritional care needs to include the opinions of not only health professionals, but also of patients and their carers. All possible options available need to be discussed with the patient and the benefits and burdens of each option discussed honestly.

Nutritional care for patients in the terminal stages of disease often poses a considerable challenge for the team. It can often be the cause of much anxiety for the patient and family as food intake deteriorates. Aggressive nutritional support is not appropriate at this stage. It may be more appropriate to assist eating and drinking by improving symptom control. Oral feeding should be advocated whenever possible. Food and control of food intake may give comfort and pleasure. The most important priority is to provide food according to the patient's individual wishes (American Dietetic Association Report, 1987).

Many patients with end-stage cancer feel neither hunger nor thirst (McCann et al, 1994) and others are comforted by only small amounts of food, or oral care and sips of liquid (Dunlop et al, 1995). Difficulties may arise when patients have artificial feeding tubes in situ before they reach this stage. Reducing volumes of feed or discontinuing feeding can be seen as withdrawal of essential treatment. The patient's informed preference for the level of nutritional intervention is paramount at this point. Often feeding volumes need to be reduced to reduce gastric discomfort or nausea — these issues need to be fully explained to the patient and their carers (Boyd & Beeken, 1994).

Feeding may not be desirable if death is expected within hours or days, and the effects of partial dehydration or the withdrawal of nutrition support will not adversely alter patient comfort (American Dietetic Association, 1987).

Case example

Alfred

Alfred was referred to the oncology dietitian at the start of his postoperative radiotherapy outpatient treatment. He had previously undergone a partial pharyngolaryngectomy. He weighed 44.6 kg and reported that he was struggling to maintain his weight, despite being able to manage normal food textures and complete liquid nutritional supplements three times per day.

Alfred was given practical dietary advice — high-protein, high-energy — to improve his nutritional status and intake. Recipe ideas were also given to incorporate nutritional supplements into a variety of puddings, cereals and drinks. Twice-weekly monitoring of weight and nutritional intake was commenced. After 15 fractions of radiotherapy, Alfred was experiencing further problems with eating. His taste had been markedly affected and his mouth was excessively dry, despite use of regular drinks and artificial saliva.

After 17 fractions of radiotherapy Alfred was unable to cope as an outpatient. His weight had decreased by 1.5 kg and he was experiencing severe dysphagia. He was admitted to hospital and a fine-bore nasogastric tube was placed (6 FG). Full blood profile revealed mild dehydration and he was pyrexial secondary to a chest infection.

Nasogastric feeding was initially slow to establish due to nausea and vomiting experienced secondary to morphine administration for pain control. Anti-emetics were prescribed and extra fluid was given via sterile waterflushes through the tube, until full feeding requirements could be met. Once established, Alfred and his wife decided that overnight feeding would be more convenient for home. It was decided that 75% of Alfred's requirements would be met via a complete fibre-combining enteral feed via the nasogastric tube. The remainder of his requirements would be met via a variety of commercial fluids and milk-based drinks.

Alfred was discharged with district nurse support, home enteral feeding equipment and practical information. He had now regained the weight he had lost during radiotherapy.

One week post-discharge Alfred was reviewed by the dietitian, who found he was experiencing poor oral intake, including liquids, secondary to pain on swallowing. He had lost 1 kg in weight and it was decided that his full nutritional requirements would be met via artificial feeding.

Swallowing rehabilitation was very difficult for Alfred in the weeks that followed. He had not only lost his sense of taste but also his confidence to eat. A trial of reduced nasogastric feeding was commenced with the aim of stimulating his appetite. No increase in oral intake was noted and full nasogastric feeding was recommenced. The option of gastrostomy feeding was discussed at this point but Alfred declined. During the following weeks, Alfred found that he was feeling stronger and had started to go on long weekends away. One significant problem experienced was the practicality of getting a nasogastric tube replaced when it accidentally fell out away from home.

Six months later Alfred reported that there had been no changes in his eating. He still had pain on swallowing and coughing episodes with thin fluids. At a joint assessment with the dietitian and speech therapist, he agreed to have a radiological gastrostomy tube placed. A gastrostomy tube was therefore placed and Alfred was successfully discharged home. He was taking full feeding requirements via the tube and weighed 51 kg.

Alfred was pleased with the gastrostomy tube and felt that it would alleviate his anxieties regarding tube displacement. Problems experienced in the weeks that followed included stoma leakage and infection. After-care information was reinforced to the patient and the infection was treated with antibiotics.

Four months later Alfred was fully established on gastrostomy feeding but still struggled with oral diet and fluids. He was seen by the speech therapist and a videofluoroscopy arranged. As a result of the videofluoroscopy, Alfred was encouraged to persevere with oral intake. Soft and semi-solid meal plan ideas were given and practical ideas regarding thickened drinks and commercial sip feeds were suggested.

At the time of writing Alfred has successfully gained weight (56 kg) and is confident with gastrostomy feeding. Unfortunately, his confidence with eating has not improved. He finds that eating is no longer a pleasurable event. He still has limited taste and, despite experimenting with textures, eating is still very time consuming. Eating socially is also a problem for Alfred; choking and coughing episodes cause much distress to both himself, family and friends.

Summary

Nutritional assessment should be an integral part of any treatment for the head and neck cancer patient. Nutritional support is one area in which family and carers make an important contribution to the management of the patient. Nutritional care of the patient with head and neck cancer should be directed towards early intervention to provide optimal nutritional support as soon as it is feasible.

Strategy for practice

- Work with the dietitian to develop a nutritional assessment tool for people in your unit with head and neck cancer.
- Ensure that all patients are assessed in the diagnostic stage.
- Ensure nutritional support by the dietitian is instigated as early as possible to ensure the patient is in the best possible nutritional state preoperatively/pre-radiotherapy.

- Ensure enteral feeding is given safely with minimum complications.
- Consider gastrostomy for long-term feeding problems, but be aware of potential complications.
- Ensure patients discharged on enteral feeds receive all appropriate training and equipment — use a discharge checklist.
- Consider the use of feeding in the palliative setting carefully — it is often beneficial. However, before instituting such feeding, discuss with both the patient and the family the fact that feeding will be withdrawn during the last days or hours of life. It is necessary to explain this so that everyone is prepared for, and understands, this intervention when the time comes.

Chapter 2.5
Altered communication

MARIA HARVEY

The anatomy of voice and speech

It is important for nurses caring for head and neck cancer patients to have some understanding of the normal anatomy of voice and speech so that they can comprehend the impact of surgery on communication. Unlike swallowing, where the anatomy and physiology is described from the oral cavity down through the pharynx, oesophagus and on to the stomach (the route the bolus falls), it is convenient to describe the anatomy of voice and speech in the reverse, as air is expired from the lungs, up the trachea, larynx and into the vocal tract.

Voice production

Firstly it is worthy of note that the larynx serves more than one important role.

1. It serves a respiratory function ensuring the free flow of air into and out of the lungs. Inhalatory stridor would result from obstruction of the airway at the level of the larynx and may be a symptom of a mass within the larynx.
2. The swallowing function of the larynx has already been explained in Chapter 2.3, it protects the lungs from ingestion of food and fluid during the pharyngeal stage of the swallow. Additionally, it enables us to clear any aspirated material from the airway by coughing and throat clearing.
3. The larynx also has an effort closure function allowing us to hold breath in the lungs against which we can bear during effortful

physical work, such as lifting and pushing, and to enable us to compress the abdominal cavity for defecation, micturition, parturition, etc.

4. Finally, it provides a phonatory function, producing voice by regular vibrations of the vocal folds (Aronson, 1990a).

Voice production is normally dependent on a steady flow of expired air from the lungs. As the air travels upwards through the larynx, the vocal folds are brought together by the 'Bernoulli effect', i.e. the velocity of the air increases as it passes from the wider lumen of the trachea to the narrowing at the level of the vocal cords, causing a negative pressure which draws the vocal folds together. As this happens repeatedly, a wavelike motion of the vocal folds is created (phonation). Consequently, the air molecules vibrate creating sound.

Clear voice can only be produced if the vocal folds are in a healthy condition and if they can move freely. A tumour arising anywhere along the vocal folds, or scarred or dry vocal fold mucosa (as can happen following radiotherapy), will impair their three-dimensional waveform and give rise to a hoarse and breathy voice quality.

Speech production

Speech is formed by the active movement of the articulators (soft palate, tongue and lips), which modifies the shape of the vocal tract. The acoustic waveform created by the vocal folds is formed into vowels and consonants as the shape of the vocal tract changes. In order to produce clear articulation and smooth speech, the structure and function of the vocal tract must be intact. Speech impairments result from altered anatomy following resections for oral cancer.

Articulation of consonants

Consonants are produced by creating an obstruction of the airstream through the vocal tract. They are classified according to place of articulation and manner of this obstruction. They may be voiced or voiceless, depending on whether the air causes the vocal folds to vibrate or whether it passes through silently. They may also be oral or nasal, depending on the position of the soft palate and the amount of nasal airflow.

Simplistically, there are six places of articulation in the English language (places of articulation vary from one language to another). Four of these involve contact between the tongue and other structures:

- bilabial (contact between the two lips, e.g. p b m)
- labiodental (contact between the lower lip and the upper front teeth, e.g. f v)
- dental (contact between the tongue tip and upper front teeth, e.g. th)
- alveolar (contact between the tongue tip behind the top teeth on the alveolar ridge, e.g. t d)
- palatal (contact between the front of the tongue and hard palate, e.g. ch j)
- velar (contact between the back of the tongue and the hard palate, e.g. k g).

There are three common manners of articulation:

- plosives (complete closure of the articulators so that the air is stopped, e.g. p t k, b d g, m n ng)
- fricatives (close approximation of the articulators so that air becomes turbulent, e.g. s sh f)
- approximants (approximation of the articulators but without turbulence, e.g. r j).

Sounds similar in place and manner may be produced with or without voice, e.g. p and b, t and d, k and g. The first of each of these pairs is voiceless and the second is voiced.

Sounds similar in place and manner may also be produced with oral or nasal resonance, e.g. p b and m, t d and n, k g and ng. The first two of each are oral and the third is nasal.

Articulation of vowels

Vowels are specified according to the position of the highest point of the tongue in the vocal tract, and the degree of lip rounding or spreading which gives rise to changes in the resonance of the vocal tract. Notice how the tongue becomes progressively lower and moves further back in the mouth during the following sequence of words: bead, bid, bed, bad, barn, book, boom.

Speech and language therapists are trained to identify all speech sounds and to transcribe them into a symbol using the International Phonetic Alphabet. They may be sound variations used in different languages, sound variations due to different accents within a language, or disordered sounds associated with a speech impairment. This forms the basis of assessment.

Altered anatomy and problems with communication

Normal communication can only be produced if the component parts of the vocal tract mechanism are intact both structurally and in their ability to function in relation to each other. Neurological impairment or altered anatomy of the larynx, pharynx and oral cavity following surgery for head and neck cancer will affect their function and disrupt the normal production of voice and speech.

Impaired voice production is described as dysphonia. Any weakness, slowness or incoordination of speech production is called dysarthria. The effects of treatment for head and neck cancer on voice and speech are described below.

Neurological lesions

In the case of both primary tumours and secondary metastatic tumours within the brain, the normal function of nervous tissue becomes impaired, giving rise to a number of symptoms (Ross Russel & Wiles, 1985).

Lesions along the Xth (vagus) nerve anywhere from brainstem to muscle can cause paresis (weakness) or paralysis (immobility) of the laryngeal muscles and result in dysphonia. The extent of weakness, the position of vocal fold fixation, the unilaterality or bilaterality of weakness, and the degree of voice impairment depend on the location of the lesion along the pathway of the nerve and whether one or both nerves of the pair have been damaged (Aronson, 1990b).

Parotid gland tumours invading the VIIth (facial) nerve, or surgery to resect such a tumour, which necessitates sacrificing the facial nerve, will result in a facial palsy or paralysis, and consequently a dysarthria.

Oral/oropharyngeal lesions

The impact of the treatment of oral lesions on swallowing function is discussed in Chapter 2.3. The potential consequences on speech can be similarly devastating and have serious implications for quality of life.

Oral cancers may present anywhere, but six common sites have been described (Logemann, 1983):

a. anterior or lateral tongue
b. tongue base
c. anterior or lateral floor of mouth
d. hard palate
e. soft palate
f. tonsil.

The location, size, and extent of the tumour will dictate the amount of excision that will be necessary. Tumours of the tongue are most common (Maran et al, 1993), but often adjacent structures are affected and are involved in the resection (Appleton & Machin, 1995b).

Glossectomy refers to a resection of part or all of the tongue. Postoperative speech intelligibility depends on the extent of the lingual excision, the mobility of the residual tongue, the presence or absence of teeth and the type of reconstruction, as well as factors of age, hearing, general health and motivation. Both articulation and vocal resonance can be affected (Casper & Colton, 1993b).

Small tumours require the least extensive surgery and should create the least functional disability. More extensive tumours require increasingly greater resection and will need to be reconstructed with a flap that aims to restore form and function as closely as possible. A reconstructive technique that results in maximum mobility of the residual mass following surgery will be the most beneficial for the purpose of speech (Casper & Colton, 1993b). In fact, the mobility of the residual tongue is more important than enlarging the tongue volume after surgery in terms of retaining speech intelligibility. This is best achieved using a 'radial forearm free flap reconstruction' or a 'split-skin inlay graft' (Imai & Michi, 1992).

Anterior or lateral tongue

The effect of resection of tumours of the anterior or lateral tongue is particularly marked in terms of speech intelligibility. Dental, alveolar and palatal places of articulation may be impossible to achieve, resulting in a severe reduction in speech sounds produced, particularly sounds such as t, d, s, z, n, ch, j and th. It may also be particularly difficult for a client to discriminate between different manners of articulation. Alveolar fricatives may be more easily identified than plosive sounds (Imai & Michi, 1992).

Tongue base

Resections involving the base of tongue, with flap repair, can result in a difficulty elevating the back of the tongue for velar sounds, e.g. k, g and ng.

Anterior or lateral floor of mouth

Tumours confined to the floor of mouth may not affect speech intelligibility if reconstruction does not impair the mobility of the tongue. However, due to the small surface area of the floor of the mouth, they often extend on to the tongue or the mandible, and can still result in speech impairment.

Hard palate

Resections involving the bony structure of the hard palate are less common and may be performed as part of a resection for a nasal carcinoma. Depending on the size of surgical resection, speech may be affected due to impaired tongue-to-palate contact for the palatal sounds ch and j. Resonance will become 'hypernasal' and many sounds will lose their clarity due to 'nasal emission of air'. An obturator is indicated in such cases, because exercises provided by the speech and language therapist will not accomplish improved articulation or resonance.

Soft palate

Similarly, resections for soft palate tumours resulting in palatal insufficiency have such a severe effect on vocal resonance and on the ability to produce many speech sounds that speech may become unintelligible. Sounds requiring a build-up of oral plosion (e.g. p b, t d, k g), will be particularly affected and may be difficult to discriminate from their nasal counterparts (m n ng).

Tonsils

Tumours localized to the tonsil are rare as the disease has usually spread to adjacent structures at the time of presentation (Stafford et al, 1989). They often present with tumours of the soft palate, tongue base or pharyngeal wall with associated speech problems.

Partial laryngectomy

'Conservation surgery' is performed in appropriate candidates to remove the entire cancer while preserving the functions of respiration, swallowing and speech. (The effects of partial laryngectomy on the swallowing function are described in Chapter 2.3.) It usually eliminates the need to perform a permanent tracheostomy, thus allowing speech production to continue in the normal fashion, through exhaled air (Hamaker & Hamaker, 1995).

Voice quality is impaired when the normal structure and function of the vocal folds is altered in any way. Therefore, normal voice quality is compromised after 'vertical hemilaryngectomy', when one vocal cord may be removed completely, and after a 'frontolateral hemilaryngectomy' or 'three-quarter laryngectomy when the anterior portion of the larynx is removed.

Currently there is no generally accepted, standardized approach for the reliable evaluation of voice quality after partial laryngectomy (Giovanni et al, 1996). One study concluded that there is often a significant correlation between measures of physical and acoustic parameters of the voice, and subjective accounts of the voice quality (Ptok & Maddalena, 1990).

A 'near-total laryngectomy' is an effective approach to cancer therapy with cure rates comparable to total laryngectomy. The main limitation of this technique is that voice recovery is unpredictable. Voice quality is difficult to measure, but one study found that of 57 patients, five had 'whispery voices', 25 were difficult to understand in a noisy environment and 27 were easily understood (Zanaret et al, 1993).

Total laryngectomy/pharyngolaryngectomy

Following a laryngectomy, the important functions of the larynx are lost:

1. The respiratory function, resulting in diminished oxygen levels in the blood.
2. The airway protective function during swallowing, such that the open end of the trachea is sewn to the skin at the front of the neck forming a permanent tracheostoma. Aspiration of secretions, food and fluid is thus prevented.
3. The effort closure function, such that the patient may experience a loss of physical stamina, particularly when lifting or pushing. Glottic closure during coughing is not possible, and the laryngectomee must learn to clear mucus from the lungs by rapid expiration followed by wiping away of the secretions from the stoma with a tissue.
4. The phonatory function, such that voice is lost.

Communication after total laryngectomy

This section describes the options available to the patient for alaryngeal communication as a consequence of the loss of the phonatory function. At different times the patient may use different methods. The choice depends on the type and extent of surgery, the patients' social and vocational needs, their determination and perhaps the availability of speech therapy support.

There are several options available to the laryngectomee:

i. non-verbal communication/picture charts
ii. electrolarynx
iii. oesophageal speech
iv. surgical voice restoration.

Non-verbal communication

It is important to realize that the loss of the ability to phonate does not result in the loss of the ability to communicate. All aspects of non-verbal communication are retained, for example, personal mannerisms, gestures and facial expression. Many aspects of verbal communication are also retained; the language used including the dialect, the patient's unique pattern of articulation and accent and *all* voiceless consonants. Only the voiced consonants and vowels are lost.

Immediately postoperatively, the best means of communicating is by writing. Commercially available 'Magic Boards' are convenient and tend to be more confidential since anything written can be erased and does not have to be destroyed. However, some patients prefer to use a pen and paper to communicate, and like to keep their communications as 'memoirs' to look back on!

The written word can be a very powerful method of expression. It is not just the words used that convey meaning and emotion, but the style of writing; whether capital letters, size of writing, neatness, or how firmly the pen is used on the paper — all convey meaning to the 'listener'.

An illiterate patient may be provided with a picture chart in the early stages, but the number of messages possible to convey are fairly few, and tend to be limited to practical requests rather than any expression of emotion.

Artificial electrolarynx

There are two types of electrolarynx available, categorized according to the to the anatomical site at which the sound enters the vocal tract.

The *intraoral electrolarynx* consists of a battery-powered unit that, when activated, produces a tone which is transmitted along a plastic tube directly into the mouth. The plastic tube is usually placed into the corner of the mouth, and between the teeth. The sound is then articulated for speech (Evans, 1990). The volume and pitch can be adjusted appropriately for male and female speakers. This type of electrolarynx is particularly useful for patients who have postoperative facial swelling, lymphoedema, or skin reactions following radiotherapy, and are unable to use the neck-type electrolarynx as described below.

A *neck-type electrolarynx* is one where the unit is placed directly on to the skin under the chin or towards either side of the neck. It can also be used reasonably effectively against the cheek. As the button is depressed, sound is transmitted through the tissue into the oral cavity, to be articulated into speech. As with the intraoral device, the volume and pitch can be altered to the liking of each speaker. Most neck-type electrolarynges can be adapted into an intraoral type for early postoperative use by means of a cap which fits over the vibratory head, and a tube leading from this into the oral cavity.

The use of the electrolarynx may be introduced fairly early on while patients are still in hospital. They allow for rapid communication soon after surgery, resulting in less frustration and less likelihood of developing bad communicative habits such as 'stoma blast' and 'forced whisper'. They can be used over the telephone, above background noise, when the wearer is fatigued, and whilst training for oesophageal speech or waiting for secondary surgical voice restoration.

Though some people reject the use of an electrolarynx in the early stages, particularly if given negative feedback from a listener, the benefits listed above make it an extremely effective means of communication, and well worth persevering with.

Some clients, particularly the more 'chatty' and rapid talkers, choose to use the electrolarynx as a long-term method of communication once they are acquainted with its use. The electrolarynx may also be the preferred option following extensive surgery.

The electrolarynx should *never* be offered as a last resort.

Difficulties can be experienced in the correct placement of the electrolarynx in the oral cavity or under the chin for optimum quality of sound, and with the on–off timing of the device to coincide with speech. Speech training will be necessary initially to overcome these difficulties. These devices also necessitate the use of one hand, limiting the patient to only using one hand whilst speaking (which may consequently make speaking difficult whilst driving, eating, etc.). Some clients reject the electrolarynx, describing it as 'robotic', (due to the absence of inflection), or they experience negative feedback from listeners not acquainted with the sound. It is also difficult to engage in discreet conversations since 'whispering' is not possible when using an electrolarynx. Such patients need support and gentle encouragement to use the communication aid.

Oesophageal speech

The term *oesophageal voice* refers to the sound produced by a moving column of air in the oesophagus, which passes through a narrowing called the pharyngo-oesophageal segment. This is opposed to *laryngeal voice*, which is produced by a moving column of air from the lungs passing through the vocal folds within the larynx (Evans, 1990). The pharyngo-oesophageal segment serves as the vibratory site for oesophageal speech. In 90% of cases it is situated somewhere between the levels C4 and C7 and approximately corresponds to the previous level of the larynx (Edels, 1979).

In order for oesophageal speech to occur, air must somehow pass down from the oral and pharyngeal cavities, through the segment, and into the oesophagus. Then the air must be immediately redirected upward from the oesophagus and pass through the segment in order to create sound (Keith & Darley, 1979) (see Figure 2.5.1). It is this ability to voluntarily achieve rapid air intake and expulsion, into and out of the oesophagus, that is basic to oesophageal speech.

There are two primary methods of air intake: air is either 'injected' or 'inhaled' into the pharynx. It is not produced by swallowing air into the stomach, since swallowed air would be lost to voluntary control and would cause flatulence instead.

During the inhalation method, the patient is instructed to keep his/her mouth and nose open whilst quickly inhaling air in through the stoma. In doing this, a negative pressure is instantly formed within the thoracic cavity, causing a negative pressure within the oesophagus. Air is drawn into the oesophagus to equalize the pressure.

Air can alternatively be injected into the oesophagus using a 'tongue-pumping' motion. During this method the lips are sealed and the soft palate is raised such that the nose and mouth are closed.

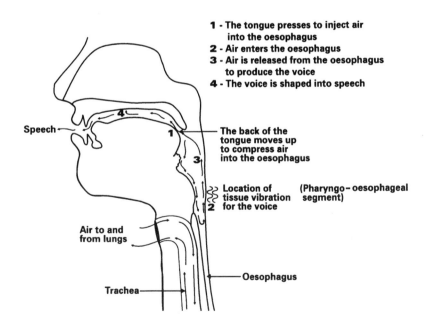

1 - The tongue presses to inject air into the oesophagus
2 - Air enters the oesophagus
3 - Air is released from the oesophagus to produce the voice
4 - The voice is shaped into speech

Speech

The back of the tongue moves up to compress air into the oesophagus

Location of tissue vibration for the voice   (Pharyngo-oesophageal segment)

Air to and from lungs

Oesophagus

Trachea

Figure 2.5.1: Pharyngo-oesophageal segment

A 'pumping' motion of the tongue injects air from the oral cavity into the pharynx and oesophagus.

Whichever method of air intake is used, the trapped air in the oesophagus is released, and during this eructation the patient articulates and produces audible speech.

Oesophageal speech is advantageous in that no hands are required, there is no equipment to maintain and it does not rely on the hospital for the provision of supplies (e.g. replacement batteries, speaking valves, etc.). The sound of oesophageal speech is considered to be more 'natural' compared with that of an electrolarynx, and nearly like that produced by the vocal folds, though of a lower pitch (Casper & Colton, 1993b).

The disadvantages are that it is a technique that must be learned and may take a long time to master. It is estimated that approximately 50% to 70% of laryngectomized individuals are able to learn effective oesophageal speech (Keith et al, 1977), but the remainder cannot due to a number of physical or psychological reasons. The client must be motivated to learn, and must be willing to attend speech and language therapy regularly for up to 6 months. They must have good hearing skills in order to monitor their own speech and they must have clear articulation to aid intelligibility.

Oesophageal speech is also markedly slower than normal laryngeal voice. Even superior laryngeal speakers may only be able to achieve 110 words per minute compared with an average of 165 words per minute for laryngeal speakers. Thus they must not attempt to speak too quickly. They may also have difficulty in speaking against background noise, as oesophageal speech is quieter than normal voice being on average between 40–50 dB, compared with a normal average of between 60–65 dB. These difficulties are due to the limited reservoir of air within the oesophagus (between 40 cc and 80 cc) that the laryngectomee is able to utilize for speech (Edels, 1979).

It is also worth noting that patients who have undergone more extensive surgery may have difficulty in oesophageal voice acquisition. For example, those with lingual or mandibular resections may not articulate clearly enough nor manage the injection method of air intake. Those who have undergone additional pharyngeal or oesophageal resections, repaired with a jejunal graft, may not have the vibratory pharyngo-oesophageal segment, and will have difficulty in producing voice. In this case, it may help to place digital pressure on to the neck over the jejunal graft to create an artificial narrowing, thus aiding voice production. This technique may be introduced to the patient by the speech and language therapist (Casper & Colton, 1993b).

Surgical voice restoration

Tracheoesophageal puncture

This technique has evolved worldwide as an established option for post-laryngectomy voice restoration since its introduction by Singer and Blom in 1980 (Blom, 1995). However, not all departments carry out surgical voice restoration and not all people undergoing laryngectomy are suitable candidates for a tracheoesophageal speaking valve.

The technique involves surgically creating a small fistula through the tracheal wall into the oesophagus. A voice prosthesis in the form of a small one-way valve is inserted into the fistula. This allows air to be shunted from the trachea into the oesophagus and up through the pharyngo-oesophageal segment, thus creating an acoustic wave form and voice (see Figure 2.5.2). It should not allow aspiration of food and fluid from the oesophagus into the trachea.

Since pulmonary air is used as the initiator for voice, it is possible for the speaker to maintain a longer flow of voice and obtain greater volume than that achieved using oesophageal voice. The prosthesis re-routes the air into the oesophagus for voice to be created here. It does not itself create voice (NALC, 1991).

Surgical voice restoration may be done as a primary procedure (at the time of the laryngectomy), or as a secondary procedure (at a later date).

Primary voice restoration may be considered in patients who undergo a total laryngectomy. It is contraindicated if the surgery is extensive, involving separation of the tracheoesophageal wall at the level of the puncture site. An example is total hypopharyngectomy and cervical oesophagectomy, repaired with a gastric pull-up and pharyngo-gastric anastomosis. It must also be discussed with the patient pre-operatively to determine if surgical voice restoration is their preferred option for alaryngeal voice (Blom & Hamaker, 1996).

A 14 French Gauge (FG) catheter is placed within the fistula whilst healing takes place and swelling reduces. The patient is fed via this catheter instead of nasogastric feeding.

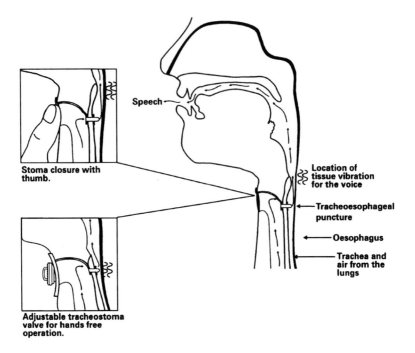

Speech

Stoma closure with thumb.

Location of tissue vibration for the voice

Tracheoesophageal puncture

Oesophagus

Trachea and air from the lungs

Adjustable tracheostoma valve for hands free operation.

Figure 2.5.2: Tracheoesophageal valve.

Placement of the voice prosthesis following primary puncture usually occurs at 8 to 10 days when the suture line competence has been confirmed by a Gastrografin swallow and when nutrition orally eliminates the need for the tracheoesophageal feeding catheter (Blom & Hamaker, 1996). However, voicing should be deferred until 12 to 14 days postoperatively to avoid the potential for fistula formation due to speech airflow and pressure in the reconstructed pharynx, particularly in irradiated patients.

Secondary voice restoration may be considered at any time after laryngectomy as long as the effects from radiation therapy are settled. A technique called 'air insufflation' can be used first to determine the pharyngo-oesophageal segment function, thus reliably predicting voice quality preoperatively. (This is a procedure, conducted under videofluoroscopy, whereby air is blown into the oesophagus to assess for hypertonicity or hypotonicity of the pharyngeal constrictor muscles.) It is not necessary to discuss the surgical technique used for fistula formation in detail here, but it is often a quick procedure, taking about 15 to 20 minutes. It may take a little longer in those patients who have an oesophageal stricture that necessitates dilatation, or patients who have not already undergone a cricopharyngeal myotomy.

A 14 FG catheter is placed into the fistula to allow for healing and swelling to reduce. The voice prosthesis may be inserted from the third day following secondary tracheoesophageal puncture (Blom & Hamaker, 1996).

Voice prosthesis fitting

This is essentially the same following primary and secondary tracheoesophageal puncture.

The first step is to remove the 14 FG catheter placed at surgery and immediately insert a silicone tracheoesophageal dilator into the fistula. This serves to stretch the fistula sufficiently to allow for easy insertion of the voice prosthesis.

Once the fistula is sufficiently dilated a measuring device is inserted into the puncture until it contacts the posterior oesophageal wall. It is tilted down and then withdrawn up and out of the puncture until the retention collar rests against the anterior wall of the oesophagus. The appropriate size can be read from the measuring device. If in doubt, a prosthesis that is one size longer than that indicated may be used to prevent under-fitting of the puncture, which can result in closure of the tract (Blom and Hamaker, 1996).

It is recommended that you refer to the manufacturer's instructions provided with the prosthesis for more detail relating to insertion of the particular valve. Generally it is the responsibility of the medical practitioner, trained ENT nurse or speech and language therapist to fit or change a voice prosthesis. Courses are available aimed at training the professional in valve fitting, care and use. Supervision may also be given from a trained professional within the ENT department for those wishing to enhance their skills in this technique.

Voice prosthesis design

Design of a voice prosthesis falls basically into two categories: the indwelling kind, and the kind that patients can change for themselves.

Indwelling voice prostheses are inserted only by the physician, trained ENT nurse or speech and language therapist. Generally they are 20 FG or 22 FG in diameter, and are consequently 'low pressure' valves since they offer little resistance to airflow through them. They also come in a variety of lengths depending on the thickness of the tracheoesophageal wall.

This type of voice prosthesis is intended for long-term placement in those patients who are unwilling or unable to change their valve themselves. For example, in the elderly, those with poor hand–eye coordination, or those with poor learning skills. Designs vary, but often the ease of insertion of the valve is a significant factor to consider when selecting a valve made by a particular manufacturer.

The valve is cleaned in situ with a purpose-made brush, and is changed perhaps every 6 months by a trained professional, when the one-way valve mechanism fails and fluid begins to be aspirated through the valve (see *Troubleshooting*, below).

The alternative is to provide patients with a voice prosthesis that they are able to change for themselves. These may be 16 FG (duckbill) or a low-pressure 20 FG, and again come in a variety of lengths depending on the thickness of the tracheoesophageal wall.

This type of voice prosthesis is intended to be removed, cleaned and then reinserted by the patient every 2 to 3 days, according to the manufacturer's instructions.

Voicing

Voicing is produced when the patient occludes the stoma with a finger or a thumb in order to speak. This can often be difficult for a patient to master initially since they may not fully occlude the stoma, allowing air to leak whilst speaking. Sometimes they press too hard and occlude both stoma and valve, and many patients feel awkward, positioning their hand inappropriately in front of their face while attempting to speak. Considerable practice is often necessary, with guidance from the speech and language therapist.

Tracheostoma (hands-free) valves

The adjustable tracheostoma valve can be used with a low-resistance voice prosthesis when the patient finds it unacceptable to occlude the valve with a finger, or requires hands-free speech for either social or professional reasons. As they do not use a finger or a thumb to occlude their stoma whilst speaking, less attention is drawn from the listeners to the tracheostoma during speech. This is considered by patients to be an important advance in the successful process of voice rehabilitation (Grolman et al, 1995).

The tracheostoma valve is fixed over the stoma by securing it into an outer tracheostoma valve housing that attaches to the skin using adhesives, or into a modified stoma button placed tightly into the stoma so that air cannot leak around it. With forced expiration the valve closes, causing occlusion of the tracheostoma.

The use of the tracheostoma valve is a valuable addition for a considerable number of patients who have undergone surgical voice restoration. They are often best used in conjunction with a low-pressure voice prosthesis which reduces the 'back-pressure', and is more likely to maintain the airtight seal. However, not all patients persevere with the tracheostoma valve due to discomfort when wearing it. It may also be difficult to create an airtight seal over an irregularly shaped stoma, especially if it is deeply recessed between the sterno-cleidomastoid muscles. Some patients cannot tolerate the extraneous noises whilst speaking. Severe mucus production is also a major contraindication of tracheostoma valve use (Grolman et al, 1995).

In centres where surgical voice restoration is performed, an open-access support service must also be available to the patients at all times. This may be offered by the ENT nurse, specialist nurse in head and neck oncology, or by a dedicated speech and language therapist. Such a service is necessary to educate patients intending to change their own valves, to provide a 'drop-in' advice and support service, to provide supplies of equipment, and to change the indwelling valves for patients who are unable to change their own. Although it is difficult to document statistically, the participation of a well trained 'tracheoesophageal puncture team' seems to be an important factor in achieving a high success rate with this procedure (Wetmore et al, 1985).

Troubleshooting

Members of this team must also be experienced in troubleshooting since tracheoesophageal puncture might appear to be a simple, straightforward method of post-laryngectomy voice restoration, but in practice it requires more than just surgery and insertion of a voice prosthesis. Introduction of the indwelling voice prosthesis has considerably minimized patient instruction in device removal for maintenance. However, users must still be instructed in methods of in-situ cleaning, finger occlusion of the tracheostoma for speech, and the optional use of a tracheostoma valve. Speech and language therapy is also necessary to facilitate intelligible speech of the maximum quality for both face-to-face contacts and for use over the telephone (Blom & Hamaker, 1996).

Tracheoesophageal voice restoration is not always problem-free, and an experienced clinician will be able to diagnose and solve problems that may occur. Some of the more common problems are presented below.

Leakage through a voice prosthesis
Blom & Hamaker, 1996

There are several reasons for fluids to start leaking through a prosthesis. The most common is damage caused by *Candida*, which tends to colonize the porous silicone surface of the valve mechanism and prevents competent closure against liquids. Yeast from the mouth is continuously carried to the voice prosthesis via saliva. This can be avoided by alternating between two 16 FG valves, soaking the most recently used one in a solution of 3% hydrogen peroxide. Colonization of *Candida* may be prevented around an indwelling valve by giving the patient 1 ml of nystatin oral suspension two times per day. It has also been found to be effective to dip the cleaning brush into nystatin suspension or a weak iodine solution, before using it for cleaning the valve in situ.

Another cause of leakage is if the valve abuts the posterior pharyngeal wall, in a patient whose luminal dimension is narrow. This can cause the valve mechanism of some designs of voice prosthesis to fail.

Finally, the voice prosthesis will begin to leak after prolonged use even in the absence of *Candida* colonization. Most prostheses can be expected to last up to 6 months before the silicone becomes more flaccid and the one-way valve starts to allow liquids to seep from oesophagus to trachea. This indicates that a new prosthesis must be fitted.

Some manufacturers of indwelling valves have introduced the 'valved insert'. This is a device attached to a safety neck strap and which inserts into the open end of the voice prosthesis. It can be used to control sudden and unexpected leaks through the prosthesis, whilst still allowing a temporary means of voicing. The 'plug-insert' is a non-valved version used for shorter prostheses (Blom, 1996).

Leakage around the voice prosthesis
Blom & Hamaker, 1996
This indicates that the tracheoesophageal fistula has dilated, allowing fluid to seep around the voice prosthesis as the patient swallows. This usually occurs when the voice prosthesis is too long, causing a piston-like motion during each swallow. This will stop after 24 hours if the patient is resized and a shorter prosthesis fitted. If leakage still does not stop, it can be a warning that the patient has recurrent disease which must be eliminated by the medical team.

Occasionally leakage of fluids around the prosthesis occurs in those patients with a very thin tracheoesophageal wall, or due to radiation necrosis at this site. In such circumstances it may be necessary to remove the prosthesis and allow the fistula to close. This would normally be expected to take approximately 2 weeks, during which time the patient may need nasogastric feeding or thickened liquids to prevent aspiration through the fistula. However, some patients may need surgery using a flap of muscle to repair the puncture site.

Microstoma
Blom & Hamaker, 1996
Very narrow tracheostomas can make insertion and management of the voice prosthesis very difficult. It may be advisable for the patient to wear a stoma button or soft silicone laryngectomy tube to prevent stenosis of the trachea. The stoma button may need to be modified by cutting a wedge out of the outer rim which when worn will still allow air to be shunted through the voice prosthesis for voice production, or a fenestrated laryngectomy tube may be necessary if it impinges on the voice prosthesis.

Tracheoesophageal-related flatulence
Blom & Hamaker, 1996
This is a problem commonly associated with low-pressure valves. It can be reduced by fitting an alternative type of valve requiring increased effort to produce voice.

Flatulence may also be a problem if there is an oesophageal stricture or hypertonicity of the pharyngeal constrictor muscle above the level of the voice prosthesis. This may not easily allow the air to pass through, causing it to be redirected to the stomach instead.

Oesophageal dilatation and pharyngeal constrictor muscle myotomy should be considered, respectively.

Granuloma
Blom & Hamaker, 1996

In a small number of patients a granuloma may form around the fistula. This appears as a ring of thickened tissue, and necessitates voice prostheses of increasing lengths to be fitted as the granuloma increases in size. Eventually it may become so large as to affect ease of breathing, and in such cases it must be surgically removed.

Immediate absence of voice or poor voice
Blom & Hamaker, 1996

It is obviously disappointing to both patient and clinician if voicing fails upon inserting a voice prosthesis for the first time. There are several reasons why this may happen. Firstly, the new valve may be stuck in the closed position. It should be removed, checked and released if this is found to be the case. A faulty voice prosthesis can also be identified if the patient is able to phonate easily through the tracheoesophageal fistula with the voice prosthesis removed. If voicing still fails, ensure that the patient is not applying excess digital pressure against the tracheostoma, since this can often result in effortful voicing. Alternatively, the patient may be inadvertently occluding the valve, thus preventing air from being shunted through it. Finally, poor voice may be caused by pharyngeal constrictor spasm, or hypertonicity above the level of the valve. This can be assessed radiographically.

Delayed deterioration in voice
Blom & Hamaker, 1996

This may be caused by a voice prosthesis in which the valve mechanism is fixed in the closed position, in which case it is necessary to remove the prosthesis, check it and replace it. However, it is occasionally due to stenosis of the oesophageal end of the tracheoesophageal fistula. This can happen if the valve has not been inserted fully, or if granuloma anteriorly has rendered the voice prosthesis too short.

It may be necessary to completely re-puncture the tract surgically. However, if the fistula has not completely closed (which is determined if the patient can still produce some voice with the prosthesis removed), it may be possible for the surgeon to dilate it using a series of soft catheters from 8 FG through to 18 FG. Once dilated the fistula should be stented for 24 hours before fitting the appropriate size of voice prosthesis.

Dislodging of the voice prosthesis

This can occur when the puncture enlarges. For example, a man who had the tracheoesophageal puncture through a pectoralis major flap reconstruction found that the fistula became progressively larger, and it would not shrink sufficiently to prevent the prosthesis from falling out. Initially the patient avoided aspirating or losing his prosthesis by threading suture through the strap of his prosthesis and securing the other end of the suture to his neck, underneath his collar, with tape. Eventually the problem was overcome by having a voice prosthesis made with an enlarged retention collar to fit behind the tracheoesophageal wall.

Occasionally the voice prosthesis is dislodged. An example is that of a patient who dislodged his voice prosthesis when fitting the cuffed tracheostomy tube of a 'swimming snorkel'.

Valves may also be dislodged when swallowing. They will pass harmlessly through the gastrointestinal tract.

If the voice prosthesis is aspirated, encourage the patient to bend forwards and cough the valve out. If this is unsuccessful, refer immediately to the medical team. The valve will be located by chest X-ray and a bronchoscopy will be arranged for removal of the prosthesis from the lungs. If a valve has been dislodged and cannot be found, a chest X-ray should always be performed to exclude aspiration.

Fainting when the valve is fitted

This can be indicative of a vasovagal attack. Refer to the medical team.

Vomiting or excessive coughing on fitting the valve

It is useful to spray the fistula with local anaesthetic prior to changing the valve. The use of anaesthetic should be authorized by the medical practitioner first.

Total laryngectomy has a profound impact on the life of a patient; in particular, the loss of the ability to communicate easily results in disruption of the patient's normal pattern of social interaction. It is a joint decision between the medical practitioner, speech and language therapist, and the informed patient as to which means of communication is best. The use of an electrolarynx, oesophageal speech or surgical voice restoration all have their pros and cons. It is often possible for the client to be able to use two or even all three of these methods. For example, the patient may use tracheoesophageal voice for longer conversational speech, oesophageal voice for shorter responses, and an electrolarynx to speak during mealtimes when it is not possible to swallow food and eruct air at the same time. Whichever method is preferred, it is the responsibility of all staff involved with this client group to provide the patient with unbiased information, encouragement and support at all times.

Psychosocial aspects of communication impairment

Improved medical and surgical techniques have resulted in increased cure rates for cancer. Therefore, greater emphasis is now placed on the rehabilitation of cancer patients — in particular their quality of life.

Survivors of head and neck cancer should have an excellent post-operative physical recovery. However, coping emotionally with this type of cancer can be extremely difficult. Not only do patients have to come to terms with the fear of having a potentially life-threatening diagnosis but, as a result of the disease and its treatment, they might also endure physical alterations to the face and neck appearance, as well as any number of possible alterations to functions such as eating and swallowing, taste, smell, vision, hearing and communication.

The loss of the ability to communicate readily can be devastating to head and neck cancer patients. They can experience intense feelings associated with grief, and frequently feel frustration and isolation. It is not unusual for them to become depressed at some stage, perhaps before their surgery, during their hospitalization, or after returning home when the realization of their surgery occurs.

Their emotional response may be dependent on more than one factor.

Personality factors

The extrovert is said to be more motivated towards speech rehabilitation, demonstrating force, determination, perfectionism and good humour in their initial attempts to communicate. They may learn sooner and better, and take immense pride in their new skills, and may serve as an inspiration for beginners, for example as a laryngectomee visitor.

The introvert may have fears of failure, and will need more encouragement and reassurance. Introverts may resent their situation and oppose speech training (Lauder, 1997).

Gender of patient

Though there are an increasing number of females, the laryngectomy population is predominantly male. However, it has been found that the gender of the laryngectomee is perhaps less significant than such characteristics as personal pride, inability to accept defeat, and the need to return to work when adjusting emotionally.

Some female laryngectomees have an initial intolerance of the sound of their pseudo-voice. They often reject the electrolarynx in the early stages and find the lower pitch of oesophageal and tracheoesophageal voice too masculine. The speech and language therapist can help in facilitating a more feminine-sounding voice.

Family attitude

Clinical observations support the theory that the families that are helpful, understanding and patient tend to help the patient attain success (Lauder, 1997).

Vocational and social activities

Many patients with a communication difficulty have initial concerns over returning to work, particularly if they have a vocally demanding job. However, with the cooperation of an understanding employer, and a few modifications to the work environment, it may be possible for them to return to work. For example, the use of a fax machine or e-mail can replace the use of the telephone.

Some social activities may also be difficult, though again with a little imagination the resourceful patient can often find ways of overcoming such difficulties. An example is using a bell to 'call out' at bingo.

No matter how the individual client reacts to his or her communication difficulty, it is crucial that head and neck cancer patients and their families seek a programme of support from the preoperative stage onwards. This support may be provided by the members of the multidisciplinary team, in particular the speech and language therapist who has experience of working with this client group. Self-help groups may also provide welcome support.

A referral to a psychiatrist, psychologist or other skilled counsellor may be necessary if the patient is unable to deal with their feelings of depression, since this itself may interfere with successful speech rehabilitation, and consequently their psychosocial adjustment.

More information on psychosocial problems and their management is given in Section Three.

The role of the speech and language therapist

Preoperative role

It is very important for the patient to be seen by the speech and language therapist prior to their surgery for a number of reasons:

1. To review what the patient knows, and to correct any misunderstandings.
2. To provide information about what to expect in the postoperative period and to discuss any difficulties anticipated with communication. Prior to laryngectomy, the speech and language therapist plays a role in helping the patient make an informed choice about which method of alaryngeal communication they wish to use.
3. To discuss postoperative therapy, and to emphasize the patients' own responsibility towards their rehabilitation. Speech and language therapy is a joint effort between patient and therapist. The therapist can instruct patients on various ways in which they can improve their communication, but it is up to the individual patient to work at it with determination and commitment.
4. To assess the patient's preoperative communication. For example: to check for any existing disorders of articulation that may not be alleviated postoperatively, to check their hearing, and their dentition (and whether they will undergo a dental clearance during their surgery).
5. Preoperative counselling should also be directed towards the carer and family of the patient. It has been found that the most immediate concerns of the carer are: whether patient will survive the surgery, whether they will be cured of cancer, whether they will be able to communicate, how they will react to the effects of surgery and the effect on their general morale (Salmon, 1979a).

6. Both the patient and the carer should be given an opportunity to meet a laryngectomee and his or her carer, and they should be provided with information regarding local support groups and laryngectomee clubs.

Postoperative role

All patients have the right to return to some form of communication in the shortest time possible, as long as it does not interfere with their medical condition or jeopardize their recovery from surgery. It is important to begin rehabilitation promptly, because the longer the time between surgery and the beginning of therapy, the poorer are the prospects for a good result. It is particularly important for patients to have some effective means of communicating, other than writing, prior to radiotherapy if at all possible because a lack of such a means of communication may interrupt or retard their progress, leading to feelings of isolation, depression and frustration (Casper & Colton, 1993b).

The nature of the initial postoperative contact depends on several factors: whether this is the first contact, whether the patient is in hospital, at home, or at their first appointment at the head and neck combined clinic. It also depends on whether other family members are present, and of course whether the patient has undergone primary surgical voice restoration (Casper & Colton, 1993b).

If the patient was seen preoperatively, then the speech and language therapist would normally wait until at least the fifth post-operative day, since the patient's nursing needs are a priority up until then. After consulting the operation notes for the details of the surgery performed, and checking with the medical team that there are no medical complications that would contraindicate a visit, the speech and language therapist will make contact with the patient with the following aims:

1. To review what the patient knows, and to correct any misunderstandings. Even if this was done during the preoperative visit, it may be useful to clarify the facts once again for the patient.
2. To assess the extent of the communication impairment.
3. To provide information about the nature of the client's difficulty and introduce some very early non-invasive therapeutic procedures. For example, suggesting some very gentle articulation exercises, encouraging the laryngectomee to gently mouth words

but not to develop forced whisper. It would also be appropriate to demonstrate the use of an electrolarynx at this stage.

4. A visit by a previously laryngectomized individual can be arranged if the patient agrees.

5. The spouse and family's concerns should be addressed. Concerns may relate to physiological issues such as stoma care, coughing and suctioning, or mouth-to-stoma resuscitation. They may relate to psychosocial issues, for example returning to work, financial concerns, marital and sexual issues, or how to deal with depression, etc. It is also very important to advise on how to make communication easier between spouses. When spouses were asked to indicate some of the things they thought should be mentioned prior to discharge from hospital, numerous items were suggested:

- try to remain cheerful and do not panic
- be patient and understanding
- resist the urge to 'baby' or pity the patient
- provide lots of love and encouragement
- pay close attention when the patient attempts to communicate, and encourage their speech rehabilitation
- continue a normal life as far as possible, i.e. maintain social contacts
- keep the patient busy
- expect frustration and depression
- look forward to better days ahead.

It is of course essential to provide the carer with information relating to voice and speech rehabilitation, since it is often of primary concern (Salmon, 1979b).

Assessment of communication problems

The assessment of the patient who has undergone surgery for an oral cancer will be different from that of the laryngectomee. Following a resection for oral cancer, the client will experience problems with articulation. The aims of assessment with such patients are as follows:

1. To complete a phonological assessment of sounds that the patient is able to produce, and those that are difficult.

2. To assess lip closure, the range and speed of tongue movement, and soft palate function.
3. To establish compensatory sounds that approximate the target sound, and substitutions to replace those that the patient cannot attempt.
4. Many patients undergo a dental clearance, reducing their repertoire of sounds further. A referral to the dental prosthetics team should be considered.

The speech and language therapist may decide to complete a formal phonological assessment of the patient's sound system, including the use of a tape recorder to record sounds for phonological transcription and detailed analysis (using the International Phonetic Alphabet described in the section on the anatomy of voice and speech, at the beginning of this chapter).

Periodic assessment of the laryngectomee is essential throughout therapy. With regard to the patient using an electrolarynx, it is necessary to ensure that they are using the most appropriate aid. For example, a patient who may only have been able to use an intraoral device due to swelling around the neck and chin, might be able to use a neck-type aid as the swelling reduces. Electrolarynges produced by different manufacturers can also have slightly different tones. It is often worth experimenting to ensure that the sound produced is the most pleasing to both speaker and listener. (Some departments may not be able to keep a selection of aids available for trial due to restrictions on their budget.)

Assessment of the use of the electrolarynx should also include whether the patient places it correctly under the chin or against the cheek. Other important considerations are whether they use efficient on–off timing using their finger or thumb, whether they phrase appropriately, and whether they have the aid preset at the best pitch and loudness levels according to their environment. It is also necessary to check that the patient has the confidence to use the electrolarynx while talking on the telephone, and that they hold the mouthpiece of the telephone directly in front of their mouth and not lower in front of the electrolarynx, thus maximizing speech intelligibility over the phone.

Periodic assessment of oesophageal speakers is also necessary to ensure that they are developing their skills and have not plateaued at an unacceptable level. Several objective assessments are available for the clinician to use, but guidelines have also been provided for the speech and language therapist who does not have access to formal assessment techniques. These use measures of voice quality, fluency, and clarity to improve their clients' performance in oesophageal speech (Keith & Darley, 1986).

Tracheoesophageal speakers should be similarly monitored in terms of voice production. However, it is also important to check their ability to finger occlude effectively, or their proper use of the tracheostoma valve for hands-free speech. It is also necessary to ensure that they are able to clean or change their tracheoesophageal speaking valves safely and effectively.

Management decisions

Management of the patient with head and neck cancer by the speech and language therapist begins upon referral of the patient to the service. It encompasses the overall care of the patient and their spouse, both pre- and postoperatively. It includes the provision of specific rehabilitation of the voice or speech disorder, and tackling the wider psychosocial issues resulting from the communication impairment.

Therapy for such patients may be categorized as direct or indirect. The former refers to specific techniques that can be used to treat particular communication impairment. For example, giving exercises to maximize the patient's residual function, working on appropriate compensatory techniques, suggesting substitutes for sounds impossible to achieve, or providing appropriate communication aids (Appleton & Machin, 1995b).

Indirect therapy refers to counselling the patient and carer about all aspects of communication, and adapting to any communication difficulty that they may have incurred. The speech and language therapist must also decide whether referral to other professionals and support groups is indicated.

How to help the patient with a communication problem

Ideally, a means of communication should be worked out in advance of surgery to prevent unnecessary frustration. Pen and paper can be provided, or some sort of sign language might be agreed upon.

A small number of laryngectomees never acquire a voice and are unable to use an electrolarynx, perhaps because of lymphoedema creating swelling around the chin and cheeks, trismus affecting the use of an intraoral electrolarynx, or glossectomy. They may need to communicate by attempting to silently articulate words or use some means of non-verbal communication. The following hints and tips may be considered when communicating with such patients, to reduce their frustration and your embarrassment should you fail to comprehend them.

1. Do not assume that alaryngeal patients cannot hear. They may not be able to communicate readily with you, but they are not necessarily deaf.
2. Do use a normal tone of voice when communicating to a laryngectomee. Avoid raising your voice when speaking to a laryngectomee, or writing to communicate back to them.
3. Do not assume that the laryngectomee cannot communicate with you. Direct your speech towards the person, maintain eye contact whilst you are talking, and avoid questioning the patient's relatives instead of the patient. Include the laryngectomee in your conversations.
4. Do give the laryngectomee or speech-impaired patient plenty of time to speak. Try not to hurry such patients, as pressure will considerably affect their ability to communicate.
5. Do not anticipate what the speech-impaired patient or laryngectomee is going to say, and resist finishing off their sentences for them. This reinforces their difficulty and takes away any satisfaction they would achieve after successfully communicating their message.
6. Do listen and observe the patient during his or her attempts at communicating. Extra visual cues can be obtained from lip reading and watching facial expressions.
7. Do not pretend you have understood the patient if you have not. Admit that you are having difficulty understanding and ask the patient either to rephrase their statement, to use a key word to give you the context, or to write their message down.
8. Do take an interest in speaking to the communication-impaired patient.
9. Do not make fun of the speech-impaired.
10. Do listen to someone with communication impairment over the telephone. Be patient if they are struggling. It is possible to communicate successfully with someone who has very limited

communication or even no voice at all, by asking closed questions. The patient can tap once or twice on the telephone to signify 'yes' or 'no', respectively. It is also useful to provide such patients with a telephone aid, the Claudius 2. These can be preset with up to 48 messages for the laryngectomee to use when answering the telephone. The Claudius 2 is available from British Telecom. A recent innovation, also from British Telecom, is the TalkType System.

Ward personnel working with this client group should be prepared for the patients' frustrations and fears about their lack of communication. Regardless of which early communication methods will be chosen, the patient will need a means of communicating in the very early postoperative days (prior to their attempts at verbal communication), and should be armed with a means of calling for assistance should they be in distress. Patients often report that one of their overwhelming fears after head and neck surgery is of choking and being unable to call for help (Rigrodsky et al, 1971). Personal attack alarms can be carried by the laryngectomee for this purpose.

Summary

As with the dysphagic patient, rehabilitation of the head and neck cancer patient who experiences a difficulty in communicating, starts in the preoperative stage and continues for many months postoperatively. Though the process is guided by the speech and language therapist to optimize the patient's communicative function, it is the responsibility of everyone, whether within the patient's professional-medical or within their domestic, social or working environments, to encourage and facilitate communication.

'How a person speaks — voice quality, pitch, loudness, stress patterns, rate, pause, articulation, vocabulary, syntax, and ideational content — qualifies as a trait of personality' (Aronson, 1990c). It is essential that we look beyond the impairment to these features, to see the person beneath.

Chapter 2.6
Skin care for patients undergoing radiotherapy

JACQUI CAMPBELL

Introduction

Patients undergoing radiotherapy require a comprehensive skin care regime. Any degree of radiotherapy skin reaction can be a source of discomfort, pain, embarrassment and distress to the individual. A research-based skin care protocol is an important part of the patient's care when undergoing radiotherapy.

The effects of radiotherapy on the skin can be highly unpleasant; inhibiting the production of keratinized epithelium by damaging the dividing cells in the basal layer of the skin, at times causing a painful reaction with symptoms that resemble those of moderate to severe sunburn that may take several weeks to resolve (Thomas, 1992). In the early years of radiotherapy the effect of radiation on the skin was often the only available guide to the patient's ability to tolerate the treatment (Bernstein et al, 1993). The development of modern mega-voltage radiotherapy machines (linear accelerators) has now reduced the frequency and severity of skin reactions. These machines deliver their maximum dosage below the surface of the skin.

Causes of skin reactions

The skin is a radiosensitive tissue that undergoes rapid mitosis. Ionizing radiation causes biochemical changes within the cells as DNA molecules are susceptible to radiation damage during mitosis. The surface layer of the skin, the epidermis, consists of stratified squamous cells which are renewed by constantly dividing basal cells that lie adjacent to the dermis. Following radiotherapy, the basal cells are damaged and mitosis is suppressed. Cell renewal time of the epidermis is 2–3 weeks, therefore skin reactions take this amount of time to become apparent, and continue for a similar period once treatment is completed.

Radiotherapy damage to the skin leads to loss of moisture in the surface corneocytes and intracellular lipids, which leads to reduced pliability, dryness, cracking and scaling. The dry scales activate nerve fibres causing itching and the cracking may lead to pain and infection (Spencer, 1988). It is the skin directly in the treatment beam that is affected, but in addition it is important to remember that there will be both an entry and exit site of this beam.

Radiosensitivity of the skin's tissues varies between individuals and between the various skin structures, and a number of factors can affect the potential for skin reactions (Hilderley, 1983). These include:

- the total dose of radiation administered
- the fractionation schedule
- the volume of tissue irradiated
- the energy or type of radiation given
- the use of radio-sensitizing drugs e.g. 5-fluorouracil, adriamycin, methotrexate
- the area treated — areas where friction occurs e.g. axilla, groin, breast — are more likely to be affected
- treatment techniques, such as bolus materials which increase the dose to the skin.

Levels of acute skin reactions

The acute damage to the skin during radiotherapy is usually temporary and reversible (Stucchi et al, 1987). There are varying degrees of acute skin reactions, which are categorized as follows (Strohl, 1988; Thomas, 1990):

- Erythema. The area becomes pink or reddened and may tingle and feel warm; there may be slight inflammation.
- Dry desquamation. The area remains slightly inflamed and becomes dry and scaly. Superficial flaking of the epidermis occurs and the area may itch and burn.
- Moist desquamation. The inflamed epidermis blisters and sloughs, leaving a denuded, painful area of dermis that may exude serum.

Chronic (late) reactions, such as skin necrosis, are now rare occurrences in UK radiotherapy centres due to the use of modern megavoltage therapy machines. However, with high doses of radiation where treatment is given by superficial beams (such as electrons), permanent effects may occur such as hyperpigmentation, telangiectasis of subcutaneous blood vessels and fibrosis of the subcutaneous tissues.

Ritualistic skin care practice

Over the years various skin care practices have developed in conjunction with the use of radiotherapy, but many of these are of limited value as there is little evidence to support their use. In addition, there are considerable differences in skin care practice between radiotherapy centres and even variations within the centres themselves (Thomas, 1992; Lavery, 1995). Custom and practice or personal preference are not sufficient reasons for using particular products or giving particular advice (Ford & Walsh, 1989). The effectiveness of many radiotherapy skin care practices are of concern, and the use of the following agents or practice needs to be questioned:

1. Talcum powder or corn starch. This may dry the skin further. Powders can block hair follicles and sweat pores, increasing irritation and the risk of bacterial or fungal growth (McGowan, 1983).
2. Gentian Violet. This is no longer recommended for application to mucous membranes or open wounds (DHSS, 1987; BMA, 1994) as it may be carcinogenic and systemic absorption can occur through broken skin or mucous membranes (Littlefield et al, 1985).
3. Hydrocortisone cream. This may result in thinning of the skin and increased susceptibility to injury (Hilderley, 1983). Therefore it should not be used routinely or applied to moist desquamation as this may delay healing time.
4. Flamazine. This has often been used following completion of treatment. However, its use is only indicated for full-thickness wounds, which rarely includes radiotherapy skin reactions. In addition, it should only be used with an occlusive dressing otherwise it will oxidize (Fowler, 1994).
5. Antibiotics. Asymptomatic wound infections which culture *Staphylococcus aureus* should not be treated routinely with

antibiotics as this is a normal occurrence [unless culture and sensitivity shows the presence of pathogenic bacteria (Bernstein et al, 1993)].

Evidence-based skin care

The shortcomings in the care of radiotherapy skin reactions appear to stem from limited utilization of the evidence regarding wound healing and care of damaged skin. Much enlightening research has been carried out regarding wound healing and the appropriate use of dressings (Thomas, 1990; Morgan, 1994).

Wound healing occurs best in a warm moist environment, and 37°C is most suitable for mitotic activity to take place (Thomas, 1990). Wounds heal more rapidly when kept moist than when exposed to air or covered with traditional dressings. This is because the epithelial cells can move across a moist surface more easily (Thomas, 1990). The wound exudate contains nutrients, oxygen and white blood cells, which are important for healing (Quick, 1994).

Table 2.6.1: Characteristics of ideal dressings (Morgan, 1994)

1. Provide the optimum environment for wound healing — a moist environment at the wound interface
2. Allow gaseous exchange of oxygen, carbon dioxide and water vapour
3. Provide thermal insulation — wound healing is temperature-dependent (37°C)
4. Impermeable to micro-organisms (in both directions)
5. Free from particulate contaminants
6. Non-adherent
7. Safe to use
8. Acceptable to the patient
9. High absorption characteristics (for exuding wounds)
10. Cost effective
11. Carrier for medications
12. Capable of standardization and evaluation
13. Allow monitoring of the wound
14. Provide mechanical protection
15. Non-inflammable
16. Sterilizable
17. Conformable and mouldable
18. Available (hospital and community in a range of sizes)
19. Require infrequent changing

Due to the drying effect on the skin following radiotherapy, the use of a simple moisturizing cream such as E45 or aqueous cream in the treated area would appear to be the most appropriate care. The benefits of such creams are as follows:

1. They provide a large dose of water that hydrates the skin during application.
2. They form a barrier over the skin's surface that reduces transepidermal water loss.
3. They provide the stratum corneum with humectants that have the capacity to retain water, thus promoting pliability and flexibility.
4. They contain a lubricant to reduce friction damage to the skin.
5. They assist in retaining the skin's normal pH, thereby providing an environment in which the lipid bilayer in the skin can more readily normalize and re-establish its capacity to bind corneocytes together and to maintain moisture in the intercellular spaces (Quick, 1994).

Patient hygiene has been an issue in radiotherapy centres for many years. Many centres have prevented patients from washing the treated area, although there is no evidence to say that washing is detrimental to radiotherapy skin reactions. The effect of not washing may in fact cause such problems as skin infections, as well as being socially unacceptable and distressing for the patient (Webb, 1979). On the contrary, there is evidence to suggest that washing may in fact reduce the skin reaction, and that there is little difference between washing with soap and water or water alone (Campbell & Illingworth, 1992).

Skin care practice guidelines

Nursing care should be directed towards maintaining the skin's natural integrity, preventing augmentation of radiation-induced effects, and reducing irritation (Thomas, 1992). Therefore, it is appropriate that a skin care regime allows for optimum healing, pain reduction, maintenance of daily activities and reducing risk of infection (Quick, 1994).

Assessment

The patient's skin needs to be assessed daily; this is usually done by the radiographers. In addition, patients will require regular nursing assessments once or twice per week. At these times, reinforcement of their skin care is vital in supporting them through their treatment.

An initial assessment at the start of radiotherapy will include assessment of the patient and carer's knowledge of the expected skin reaction and the rationale of care, the patient's willingness to participate in his/her care; the integrity and susceptibility of the patient's skin.

Rationale

- Patient and/or family may have fear of 'radiation burns'.
- Often patients or their carers may not wish for, or be capable of, involvement in their own care.
- Certain predisposing skin conditions and types, or other medical conditions, may exacerbate skin reactions.

General advice

Preparation of the patient for the onset and likely duration of anticipated skin reaction is vital. Patients having a radical treatment to their head and neck should be advised to use moisturizing cream or aqueous cream. This to be applied at least twice daily to the treated area from the commencement of treatment. The frequency may be increased as the skin becomes drier. Patients should be advised to treat the area carefully and gently. Provide the patient with both verbal and written information and advice.

Rationale

- Information regarding their care will give patients a degree of control.
- Moisturizing the skin will ensure that it is in optimum condition during radiotherapy and help prevent dry desquamation occurring.
- Further trauma to the irradiated area must be avoided to prevent exacerbation of the reaction as the epidermal cells are further eroded by friction.

Hygiene advice

All patients should be advised to keep the area as clean as possible. The treated area may be washed carefully. It should be patted and not rubbed dry. If patients find that the soap irritates their skin, they should be advised to change to a mild brand or wash with water alone. The water used for washing the treated area should not be extremely hot or cold. An electric razor should be suggested if patients wish to continue shaving. They should be advised not to use aftershave lotions that contain alcohol.

Rationale

- To enhance patients' feelings of wellbeing and overall quality of life.
- To prevent increased aggravation of the epithelium and build-up of bacteria.
- To prevent increased irritation and physical trauma to the skin causing exaggerated skin reactions.

Clothing

Clothing covering the treatment area should not cause a shearing force, such as tight-fitting shirt collars and ties.

Rationale

- To prevent increased friction and trauma to the treated skin.

Erythema management

When skin reactions become apparent and increase in severity, assessment of the skin needs to become more frequent. The patient may become anxious or distressed by the appearance and discomfort of their skin reaction. Greater nursing support is required at this stage to ensure the patient will comply with the advice and care provided. Reassurance is required that the reaction will heal within 2 to 3 weeks of completion of treatment. The patient should continue to apply moisturizing cream. Increase the frequency of use if the reaction becomes more marked.

Rationale

- To help retain the skin's integrity and prevent water loss from the skin which leads to dryness, itching and scaling.

Dry desquamation management

Dry desquamation should not occur if the patient is applying sufficient moisturizing/aqueous cream.

Pruritis management

Discourage patients from scratching or rubbing their skin. For patients with intractable pruritis 1% hydrocortisone cream may be used sparingly after the moisturizing cream. The use of antihistamine medications may be more effective in severe cases where the patient is scratching the skin.

Rationale

- To prevent further trauma to the skin which may increase the risk of infection.

Moist desquamation management

The patient may experience lightly exuding moist desquamation or heavily exuding moist desquamation.

All patients should have their reaction assessed in terms of severity and pain to decide on the most appropriate dressing in terms of ease of application, patient comfort and healing properties. If the area requires cleansing then normal saline solution should be used; cleansing should, however, be kept to a minimum as it lowers the wound temperature and causes mechanical damage to the delicate new epithelial cells. The greenish exudate produced by the damaged skin is serum containing white cells and enzymes which promote healing. Antibiotic treatment is not indicated unless there is microbiological evidence of pathogenic organisms. The area should not be cleaned with antiseptic agents, which may cause further irritation and trauma. No tape, or adhesive dressings such as Opsite and Tegaderm should be applied directly in the treated area.

In the case of lightly exuding moist desquamation, continue to apply moisturizing cream, and cover with a non-adherent dressing. Consider non-adherent dressings such as Jelonet or Mepitel with a non-adherent secondary dressing.

In the case of heavily exuding moist desquamation, reactions should be covered with dressings that are non-adherent, highly absorbent, and provide the optimum healing environment. Dressings such as Allevyn are useful as they have a high absorbency, are non-adherent and are rigid enough to stay in place around the neck when secured by light bandaging. Dressings should be left in place for as long as possible. After 10 to 12 days from treatment completion, islands of epithelial cells will become apparent on the damaged area (whitish patches). These quickly grow to re-epithelialize the entire area by around day 14 if they are kept moist and undisturbed.

Rationale

- To minimize pain and risk of infection.
- To prevent further skin trauma and to promote healing.

Sun protection

The skin in the area will be very susceptible to sun damage after radiotherapy treatment and the patient should be instructed to apply total sunblock to the area before going out into the sun and preferably also to keep the area shaded from the sun by a hat/clothing. There is no information in the literature as to how many years this should continue. Even after many years, the skin in the treatment area will tend to tan a darker colour than the rest of the skin.

Summary

In the past 'personal preferences' and 'good judgement' have given direction to skin care in radiotherapy as practice has relied upon unproved rituals and traditions. Despite the wealth of evidence regarding healing and wound care, as demonstrated in this chapter, there remain variations in practice amongst radiotherapy centres. An evidence-based skin care protocol is an important tool for audit, evaluation, teaching and future research as it provides a baseline from which to work. A clear protocol helps healthcare professionals select the appropriate treatment for their patients and it ensures consistency of care.

Strategy for practice

- Ensure your unit has an evidence-based radiotherapy skin care protocol.
- Prevent dry desquamation by asking the patient to apply a moisturizer from day 1.
- Manage moist desquamation according to proven wound care research: provide a non-adherent dressing that maintains a warm, moist environment at the wound interface.

Chapter 2.7
Wound care after head and neck surgery

CLAIRE JONES AND DEBBIE ROBINSON

Introduction

Following surgery to the head and neck, restoration of form and function have always been of prime importance. Prior to the development of sophisticated reconstructive methods, patients undergoing surgical obliteration of their cancers were left with marked deformities. This in turn led to additional aesthetic, functional and emotional difficulties associated with communication and eating. Also previously irradiated skin often led to decreased vascularization and inadequate tissue healing.

There are many flaps available to reconstruct the defects left after excision of malignant disease in the head and neck region. Historically the forehead and deltopectoral flaps were widely used, but the 1970s saw the advent of the myocutaneous flaps, particularly the pectoralis major, latissimus dorsi, trapezius and sternomastoid flaps. The pectoralis major flap remains the prominent flap used in many head and neck centres. The 1980s saw great advances in microvascular surgery and with this development the use of free microvascular transfer of tissue became popularized, resulting in free flaps. This technique is used to reconstruct defects that cannot be repaired by traditional methods using local adjacent tissue. This modality of treatment has greatly enhanced the field of reconstructive surgery following the ablation of head and neck cancer.

An overview of flaps and grafts

A surgical skin flap is the transfer of tissue from one area of the body to another, often retaining an attachment and direct blood supply from the donating tissues (Coull, 1992). Janecka (1988) suggests that 'microvascular tissue transfer is the most dramatic and extremely versatile technique of reconstructive surgery'. The technique involves transfer of the flap and in addition arterial input and venous outflow which are anastomosed to suitable vessels in the recipient site. The principle of microvascular anastomosis is to re-establish flow from the recipient to the donor vessels and thus ensure the survival of the newly transplanted tissue in its new site.

It is important to differentiate between the muscle/free flaps and skin grafts used in reconstructive surgery of the head and neck. Although many patients have both, grafts and flaps are used in different ways (Rodzwic & Donnard, 1986). There are two different types of skin grafts: full thickness and split thickness. In full-thickness grafting, the entire epidermis and the full thickness of the dermis are removed and grafted. In split-thickness grafting the epidermis and a variable quantity of the dermis is taken. Split-skin grafts are described as thin, intermediate or thick depending on the amount of dermis included (McGregor, 1991). The thickness of the graft taken depends on the type of defect to be covered. The donor site for the removal of a split-skin graft is usually the thigh, arm or lower buttock. The healing of this site occurs spontaneously by secondary intention and usually takes about 10 days. (Care and management of these sites will be covered later in this chapter.) Full-thickness skin grafts are usually harvested from the post auricular, abdominal or supra-clavicular region with primary closure at the site usually by sub-cuticular suturing.

Management of flaps and grafts in the initial postoperative period

After many hours of surgery it can be all too easy to undo the many hours of hard work performed by the surgical team. Careful transfer of the patient from the operating table to the recovery area or the high-dependency setting is mandatory. Maximum effort is made throughout the anaesthetic to create optimum conditions for surgery: the patient is kept warm, haemodilated, paralysed, well oxygenated and pain free. This effort must continue postoperatively in order to give the flap the maximum chance of survival.

Temperature maintenance

Initially, when the surgeon has finished operating and the team have moved away from the operating table, the priority is to maintain the patient's body temperature. A slight drop in patient temperature results in vasoconstriction; if the vessels constrict then there will be a reduced blood flow to the flap and this may result in flap failure. A decrease in core temperature also causes the release of serotonin. This hormone stimulates platelet aggregation and thrombus formation at the anastomosis site (Dinman & Giovannone, 1994; Truelson & Pearce, 1997). The use of overwarming blankets and warmed intravenous solutions helps to eliminate this problem. The environmental temperature is regulated by the patient's core body temperature, being increased or decreased accordingly.

Transfer from the recovery room to the high-dependency setting

In addition to keeping the patient warm, the transfer of the patient from the theatre must be carried out with utmost care to prevent any adverse effects on the flap. The transfer of equipment with the patient (intravenous infusions, pumps, ventilation equipment, etc.) must be organized so that when transfer takes place the equipment in use will not pose any significant problems. To assimilate an effective transfer any non-essential equipment is removed and as much of the equipment as possible is attached to a single dripstand. (Remember that a member of the team will have to transfer the dripstand, so ensure that it does not become too 'top heavy' as it will contravene health and safety regulations.) It is also important to ensure that the catheter bag, intravenous fluid bags and drains are lifted clear during the transfer to prevent tension being exerted on any of the lines.

Prior to the transfer the anaesthetist may give a bolus of drugs to prepare the patient for a smooth and uneventful move. A combination of any of the following may be given: Propofol (induction agent), a muscle relaxant and an opiate for pain relief. This practice prevents arousal and movement of the patient. Movement may result in flap failure, especially if it results in coughing or jerking as this may result in kinking of the anastomosis and provoke a rise in blood pressure, creating a surge of blood to the flap. The anaesthetist may also apply suction to the tracheostomy (if there is one in situ) prior to the transfer.

When actually transferring the patient from the operating table to the bed, there is a requirement for all the team to participate. The surgeon will check the flap for colour, tension and temperature; this will provide an accurate measure for comparison when the transfer is complete. In some centres a Polaroid photograph is taken of the flap to document how it looked immediately after surgery (Dinman & Giovannone, 1994); this provides a useful comparison for the nurse in the recovery/high-dependency setting. One person is responsible for the monitors and the transfer is achieved using a transfer device. Throughout, the anaesthetist maintains the patient's head in a neutral position.

Once the patient has been transferred to the bed or trolley, the flap is checked again before moving on to recovery or a high-dependency setting; the rationale for this is that it is far easier to correct any problems whilst still in the theatre suite, with the surgical team and the anaesthetist on hand. When the destination has been reached, a hand over to the nurse who will be caring for the patient is conducted, and the flap is observed to ensure that it remains viable and has not been traumatized in the transfer.

Pain control

Good pain control is essential. Surgery causes severe nociceptive pain (see Chapter 2.11) and the pain response may have a negative impact on flap survival; peripheral blood vessels constrict, blood coagulation increases, and adrenal corticosteroids are secreted (Dinman & Giovannone, 1994). Intravenous opiates are the analgesics of choice to manage this level of nociceptive pain. Muscle relaxants may also be used.

Management of the flap from surgery to discharge

Flap monitoring

The initial postoperative period is paramount for flap viability. The flap is monitored closely every half hour for up to 36 hours as arterial occlusion may still be detected at this late stage (Coull, 1992). Flap observations should be recorded as graphically and precisely as possible. Figure 2.7.1 shows an example of a flap observation chart. Ideally, the same nurse should perform the observations for an entire shift and hand over to the next shift at the patient's bedside so that continuity can be maintained and subjectivity kept to a minimum

(Coull, 1992). It is important also to remember that lighting can alter the appearance of a flap, so time of day must be considered when conducting flap observations, that is, whether it is being assessed in natural or artificial light. Intraoral flaps should be observed using good torchlight. Secretions may be removed first, with careful use of suction.

Name:

Flap type: please circle Intraoral/external/fasciocutaneous/ composite/myocutaneous		Donor site: please circle Right radial forearm/ left radial forearm latissimus dorsi/ pec major
Date		
Time		
Colour	1	
White	2	
	3	
	4	
Pink	5	
	6	
	7	
Purple	8	
	9	
Black	10	
Capillary refill	No blanch	
	> 3 sec	
	3 sec	
	< 3 sec	
	No refill	
Texture	Spongy	
	Soft	
	Firm	
	Hard	
Temperature	Cold	
	Cool	
	Warm	
	Hot	
Comments		

Figure 2.7.1: Flap observation chart

Accurate monitoring of general and local responses is essential to ensure that the general wellbeing of the patient is not compromised and that perfusion of the flap is sustained. The clinical signs used in assessment of flap viability are:

1. colour
2. capillary refill (blanching)
3. tissue turgor
4. temperature.

A healthy flap should be:

- colour — pink
- capillary refill — 1–3 seconds
- tissue turgor — soft to the touch
- temperature — warm.

If the venous supply to a flap is occluded the flap will be:

- colour — blue/purple
- capillary refill (blanching) — < 1 second
- tissue turgor — distended
- temperature — warm or cool.

If the arterial supply is occluded the flap will be:

- colour — pale or mottled
- capillary refill — > 3 seconds
- tissue turgor — shrivelled/dehydrated
- temperature — cool.

Swelling

All free flaps swell in response to ischaemia during their transfer. However, flaps that suddenly become grossly swollen, particularly with a blue or mottled appearance may have suffered a thrombosis of their venous drainage. The flap will fail to blanch and cooling will occur.

General postoperative flap care

1. Maintain adequate blood pressure — if the patient is hypertensive there will be an increased risk of bleeding and formation of a haematoma. If the patient becomes hypotensive then this will lead to inadequate perfusion of the flap.
2. Oxygen saturation — a reduced oxygen saturation leads to poor oxygenation of the tissues and poor perfusion of the flap. Therefore half-hourly pulse oxymetry readings are advised and oxygen should be administered as prescribed.
3. Haemoglobin — a low haemoglobin reduces the amount of oxygen carried in the blood, therefore poor oxygenation will delay wound healing.
4. Temperature — it is vital that the patient and the flap are kept warm. Hypothermia causes vasoconstriction, which can lead to poor perfusion and flap necrosis. If the patient develops a pyrexia this may indicate signs of infection, which will delay the healing process and may cause flap necrosis. In this case the prescribed prophylactic antibiotics should be administered.
5. Haematoma formation — early detection of haematoma formation can prevent flap necrosis. It is of paramount importance that all drains remain suctioned and are removed when drainage becomes minimal.
6. Dressings — if at all possible, all flaps and associated suture lines should be left exposed for close, regular observation. Suture lines should be cleaned with an aseptic technique if contaminated by secretions or crusting. Antibacterial ointments such as chloramphenicol are applied to all suture lines and exposed flaps as prescribed; this intervention is credited with prevention of infection, promotion of wound healing and assistance with suture removal in the literature (Reese, 1990; Truelson & Pearce, 1997).
7. Nutrition/fluid balance — the patient will often be fed via a nasogastric tube in the initial postoperative period. A high protein intake must be maintained. A lowered level of plasma proteins will reduce osmotic pressure, which can lead to a build-up of fluid in the tissues and prevent flap adherence leading to flap necrosis. Fluids containing caffeine, e.g. tea and coffee, must also be avoided as they act as vasoconstrictors. An accurate fluid

balance must be maintained as dehydration can cause reduced flap perfusion which can lead to necrosis.

8. Smoking and nicotine patches — nicotine is a vasoconstrictor which will decrease capillary blood flow, distal perfusion and flap survival. The patient should ideally have stopped smoking at least 1 week before surgery, and nicotine patches should be removed 24 hours prior to surgery (see Chapter 1.3).

Factors causing flap necrosis

1. Tension and kinking — affects the circulation of the flap by stretching the smaller blood vessels. This is often a result of poor design, such as failure to allow for shrinkage. Positioning the patient's head with pillows prevents the flap being kinked or stretched. The head should also be elevated 30 to 45 degrees to allow gravity to reduce oedema formation (Reese, 1990).

2. Haematoma — this is when blood collects underneath the flap causing pressure which compromises blood supply, which in turn can lead to infection.

3. Pressure — external pressure from dressings, tracheostomy tapes or oxygen masks may occlude the blood supply. The flange of the tracheostomy tube may be sutured in place to avoid the use of ties (Reese, 1990).

4. Venous congestion — leeches can be applied to relieve venous congestion (Adams & Lassan, 1995). One of the main complications of leech therapy is infection, and prophylactic antibiotic cover is given. Adams and Lassan (1995) give a comprehensive overview of the use of leeches for those who would like more information.

It must be stressed that a flap can deteriorate very quickly, so if there is any doubt regarding the viability of a flap the surgeon must be called immediately.

Intraoral flaps

Intraoral wounds present a particular risk of infection and scrupulous oral hygiene should be performed. An evidence-based oral care protocol should be used. See Chapter 2.2 for detailed information on oral assessment, protocols, rinses and tools.

The patient is fed via a nasogastric or gastrostomy tube until the wounds heal, over 5 to 7 days, in order to reduce disruption of the wound and risk of contamination by food. Some centres restrict the patient's diet to avoid the oral intake of milk or milk products in order to minimize bacterial colonization of oral wounds.

Suture removal

The timetable for suture or clip removal varies depending on the site of the incision, type of wound and general condition and age of the patient. The surgeon is usually responsible for this decision. Absorbable sutures are usually used for intraoral wounds. Failure to remove sutures at the appropriate time can contribute to scar formation (Smith & Aston, 1991). Removal is via an aseptic technique. It is very important to ensure that a good light is available. A magnifying glass may be useful. Cleansing of the suture with saline ensures a clear view and facilitates easy removal. Fine iris forceps and sharp scissors are the most useful tools (Edwards, 1998). When removing single suture loops, disruption of the wound edges is avoided by gently pulling the suture towards the incision to reduce tension on it. When removing a continuous intradermal suture, only one end should be cut, then the other end of the suture is firmly pulled whilst a finger is placed on the incision line to prevent pressure on the incision (Reese, 1990).

Management of the donor sites

Radial forearm free flap donor sites

The radial forearm free flap is a popular and versatile method of reconstruction following major ablative surgery in the head and neck and has become the flap of choice for microvascular reconstruction of oral and oropharyngeal defects. It is based on the radial artery and vein and is considered a fasciocutaneous flap. The possible incorporation of a portion of the radius with this flap increases its versatility primarily for the reconstruction of segmental mandibular defects (Janecka, 1988).

Following the harvest of the free flap, the distal defect is grafted using a full-thickness skin graft raised earlier from the proximal forearm (see Figure 2.7.2). The wound is dressed in theatre using an

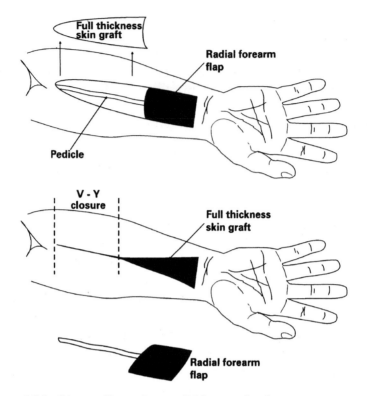

Figure 2.7.2: Diagram illustrating a radial forearm free flap.
Reproduced with kind permission of Chambers et al (1997).

appropriate dressing (see below). The wrist is then hyperextended in
a plaster of Paris backslab to maintain immobilization and thus
prevent the graft shearing from the newly forming vessels (Netscher
& Clamon, 1994). As oedema can destroy neovascularization, a
Bradford sling is used to elevate the arm during the first 48 hours of
the postoperative recovery (Netscher & Clamon, 1994). Circulatory
observations are carried out on a half-hourly basis to ensure good
perfusion of the hand (Chambers et al, 1997). The dressings remain
in place for 10 days; at this stage they are removed with great care to
expose the skin graft for examination. If satisfactory healing has
taken place, the sutures will be removed and chloramphenicol cream
applied to the healing margins of the graft. A suitable dressing is then
applied and the patient advised to use the affected limb gently, but to
avoid strenuous activity.

In some cases the graft may fail and the patient may be left with
an extensive area of exposed tendon. Despite this, a deficit in hand

function does not usually occur. The exposed area is treated with the most suitable dressing (see Table 2.6.1); a hydrocolloid dressing is commonly used. With patience, the exposed tendon will be found to granulate slowly and heal spontaneously (McGregor, 1991).

Split-skin graft donor sites

Care of the donor site is one of the less satisfactory aspects of skin grafting (McGregor, 1991). The removal of skin for grafts leaves a clean, superficial wound at the donor site which should, in theory, heal by secondary intention if left undisturbed for 10 to 14 days. In reality, the donor site can present difficulties for both nurses and patients which can result in delayed healing and uncomfortable, prolonged treatment time.

The skin contains more sensory nerves than any other organ of the body. When a thin layer of skin is excised nerve endings are left exposed, resulting in acute nociceptive pain which the patient will often describe as more painful than any other aspect of their head and neck surgery. This factor must be taken into account when re-dressing a donor site and appropriate, prescribed analgesia must be administered (see Chapter 2.11) approximately 30 minutes prior to the dressing change.

The donor site is dressed in theatre with a non-adherent dressing and multiple layers of crepe bandage. Left undisturbed in warm and moist conditions, this type of shallow wound, although fragile, should heal in about 10 to 14 days depending on the site and depth of tissue loss and the condition of the patient (Wilkinson, 1997).

Dressings

The main problem associated with the care of a split-skin graft donor site is the adherence of the dressing to the raw wound bed. Custom and practice seems to dictate wound care in many centres, with the most widely used dressing being paraffin gauze (Wilkinson, 1997). However this product has a tendency to dry out, causing tissue damage on removal even after soaking. On occasions granulation tissue may begin to grow up through the spaces in the dressing causing significant trauma and bleeding on removal. Paraffin gauze can also slip, causing slippage of the graft, and exposing nerve endings (Edwards, 1998). Table 2.6.1 gives the characteristics of an ideal dressing. Paraffin gauze can be seen to fail to meet these characteristics, because if allowed to dry out it adheres to the wound and sheds fibres, causing particulate contamination. It does not protect the wound from bacteria. Other disadvantages include the bulkiness of the dressing and the fact that the patient cannot bathe with it in situ. It cannot, therefore, be recommended as the dressing of choice.

Recently a new non-adherent silicone dressing, Mepitel (Molnlycke) has been introduced (Williams 1995). It is made of medical-grade silicone gel bound to soft, pliable polymide net. The open structure allows exudate to pass directly through to secondary absorbent dressing. This also allows topical medication to be applied without disturbing the wound. It prevents the problem of donor slippage as it adheres to adjacent healthy skin. It can be left in place for several days, during which time secondary dressings can be replaced without the risk of damaged new epithelial tissue. It does not shed fibres. A number of authors support the use of Mepitel as superior to paraffin gauze as a skin graft dressing (Vloemans & Bankras, 1991; Vloemans & Kreis, 1994; Platt et al, 1996).

Other dressings recommended in the literature for donors sites include:

Polyurethane film (e.g. Opsite, Tegaderm) is recommended by some authors (Reese, 1990; Brotherston & Lawrence, 1993) as it is bacteria-proof and reduces pain. However, it is difficult to use and exudate can collect underneath, causing leakage and appearing unsightly to the patient (Edwards, 1998).

Hydrocolloids promote healing well, leaving donor sites soft, pink and supple (Doherty et al, 1986; Reese, 1990). They are simple to change and cause minimal disruption to new epithelium. They promote comfort, prevent bacterial contamination and increase healing rates (Edwards, 1998). As they are waterproof, the patient is able to bathe freely.

Many other innovative, but anecdotal, alternatives are described within the literature to minimize the pain of dressing removal, including using a solution of 15% beeswax and 87% liquid paraffin applied directly to the donor site (Robinson et al, 1983). Dattatreya et al (1991) describe the use of boiled potato peel to dress full thickness skin loss sites. This works on the principle that potato skin prevents water loss and thus aids the newly formed epithelium in its migration across the wound. It is also thought to act as a bacterial barrier as it contains small amounts of steroidal glyco-alkaloids (Wilkinson, 1997).

Aftercare

The patient should be reviewed on a regular basis until satisfactory wound healing has taken place. While complete wound healing may not occur for up to 1 year, the scar tissue will gradually become paler and may disappear after 6 months if managed correctly (Wilkinson, 1997). A common problem is raised, red scar tissue due to the whorl-like pattern of collagen which is laid down. This can be greatly reduced by daily massage using moisturizing cream and firm, small circular motions (Edwards, 1998).

Grafted skin does not produce oil or sweat as sebaceous glands are sacrificed when the graft is harvested. Patients often complain many months after skin grafting of a red/itchy donor site. Regular moisturizing with an aqueous-based cream will help keep the affected area moist and supple and reduce the incidence of hyper-trophic scarring (Reese, 1990; McGregor, 1991). The area should be protected from the sun, using total sun block, for the first 12 months (Young & Fowler, 1998).

Unfortunately, mismanagement of these types of wounds is not uncommon and this can often lead to prolonged healing times and deeper scarring. Optimal, evidence-based wound care is essential, and can be achieved through nurse-led wound management clinics and good liaison with the community nursing team.

Maxillectomy wounds

Post-maxillectomy, the surgical site is reconstructed using a skin graft. The purpose of the graft is to provide a base for a prosthesis (the obturator) which is resistant to abrasion. It also decreases contraction of facial tissues during healing. Packing is usually placed in the surgical site to hold the skin graft in place during the initial healing period. The obturator, made prior to surgery, is placed over the packing to restore the contour of the oral cavity. The obturator and packing are removed on days 5 to 7. An 'interim' obturator is inserted to correct the defect, and over a period of months this is adapted by the prosthetics team, as the defect changes shape during healing. Once the surgical site has stabilized, a permanent prosthesis is made (Martin et al, 1994).

Good oral hygiene is essential during the postoperative period (see Chapter 2.2). After the initial packing has been removed, the patient must be taught how to remove and clean the obturator, as well as how to clean the maxillectomy cavity. The cavity can be cleaned by irrigation with saline, and gentle mechanical cleansing using pink foam sticks. The obturator should be cleaned thoroughly with soap, and rinsed with water each time oral cavity hygiene is performed (Martin et al, 1994).

The maxillectomy patient is at high risk of trismus. Trismus in these patients is devastating, as it makes prosthetic rehabilitation difficult, if not impossible. It should be prevented at all costs. Preventative exercises should start immediately after surgery. See Chapter 2.2 for more information.

Osteoradionecrosis

Necrosis of the mandible can occur after radiotherapy. This presents as an ulcerated, painful area. Early stages may respond to conservative treatment with antibiotics and hyperbaric oxygen (McKenzie et al, 1993; Neovius et al, 1997). Hyperbaric oxygen treatment consists of a course of 'dives', with 100% oxygen being inhaled by the patient at an increased atmospheric pressure (2.0 to 3.0 bar). This raises oxygen levels in hypoxic tissue, stimulates angiogenesis and fibroplasia, and has antibacterial effects on anaerobes. Smoking cessation can also enhance resolution of necrosis.

Advanced osteoradionecrosis requires resection of the necrotic bone and reconstruction with a free flap (Maksud, 1992).

Problem wounds and fistulae

There are multiple predisposing factors leading to healing problems in the head and neck cancer patient. These factors include prior radiotherapy, chemotherapy, tumour size, compromised nutrition, poor physical condition, and preoperative use of nicotine (Harris & Komray, 1993; Soylu et al, 1998). Radical neck dissection, which compromises lymphatic drainage, may contribute to poor healing and infection. The resulting wounds present a challenge for the nurse; a good knowledge of wound care products and creative dressing techniques are required. See Chapter 2.12, Figures 2.12.1 to 2.12.5 for an overview of wound care products.

Hotter & Warfield (1997) describe the packing of a deep, complex tracheostomy wound with Mesalt ribbon. Purulent secretions and odour reduced after 2 days, and the wound had granulated after 11 days. Harris and Komray (1993) describe the management of pharyngocutaneous fistulae using Mesalt to pack the wound, with a suction catheter attached to continuous low suction (60 mmHg) fixed into place in the pharyngo-fistula junction with semi-permeable film membrane holding it in place on the neck. As the wound exudate reduced, the Mesalt was replaced by a hydrogel.

More traditional methods of managing fistulae include:

- containing the leakage using a high absorbency dressing
- containing the leakage using a wound drainage or ostomy bag
- protecting the surrounding skin from excoriation by using a skin barrier (e.g. Clinishield, Cavilon).

Until the fistula heals, leakage is minimized by avoiding oral intake completely, providing nutrition via a nasogastric or gastrostomy feed.

Wound breakdown and pharyngocutaneous fistula predisposes the patient to the risk of carotid haemorrhage. See Chapter 2.8 for management of carotid haemorrhage.

Summary

Wound management is a never-ending challenge which tests the aptitude and skills of nurses across all specialities. However, caring for wounds specific to the head and neck provides nurses with an even greater challenge. Observational skills are paramount; recognition of subtle alterations and early reporting of changes within the assessment guidelines when caring for a flap can prove to be critical if the reconstruction is to be saved. In order to maintain the viability of a flap from the initial postoperative phase through to managing problem wounds, the nurse must have a good knowledge of the necessary nursing interventions and wound care products.

Bale (1997) points to several factors that may cause problems in wound care. Therapeutic traditions, strongly held by practitioners in positions of influence, can make it difficult to use new products. The responsibility for wound care is blurred; many professionals are involved, including theatre staff, medical staff, pharmacy staff, ward staff, supplies departments and community staff. The economics of wound care are complex. Many modern dressings have a high unit cost but require infrequent changes, thus being more cost-effective and convenient to both patient and nurse. Evidence-based wound management protocols are needed and should be addressed by a working party consisting of all team members. Evaluation of protocols needs to incorporate all the characteristics of ideal dressings.

Strategy for practice

- Ensure that all possible measures are taken to reduce flap morbidity. This includes helping patients to stop smoking prior to surgery.
- Ensure flap observation is continuous and documented.
- Ensure wound care practice is based on up-to-date evidence.
- Develop an evidence-based wound care protocol for your unit.
- As many wounds are intraoral, an evidence-based oral care protocol is essential.

Chapter 2.8
Carotid haemorrhage

Introduction

Carotid artery rupture, or carotid 'blow-out' occurs when the wall of the carotid artery is ruptured, producing major haemorrhage (Casey, 1988). The common carotid artery arises from the aorta on the left, and from the innominate (or brachio-cephalic artery) on the right. They run upwards on either side of the neck and divide at the level of the hyoid bone into the internal and external carotids. It is at this bifurcation that the vessel wall is thinnest, and most vulnerable to rupture. The artery is protected by the adventitia and nourished by the vasovasorum, which provides 80% of nutrition to the arterial wall (Lesage, 1986). When this essential nourishment is interrupted, destruction of the arterial wall occurs over 6 to 10 days. This process begins with the loss of the adventitia through desiccation, irradiation, bacterial invasion, tumour invasion or surgical removal.

More than 10% of deaths from head and neck cancer are caused by haemorrhage, and 20% of recurrent cancers bleed (Shedd et al, 1980). Carotid blow-out is dramatic, and exsanguination can occur within minutes if the vessel is badly damaged. The nurse is usually the first person on the scene when a haemorrhage occurs.

See Figure 2.8.1 for the main arteries of the head and neck.

Causes of haemorrhage

There are several factors predisposing the patient to haemorrhage:

- Surgery. The arteries in the area of surgery are exposed to potential damage or weakness. Excision of the tumour may involve removal of some of the adventitia.

245

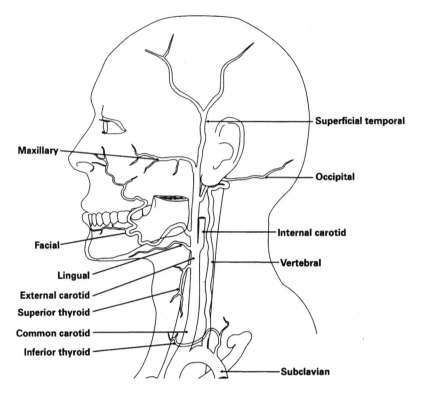

Figure 2.8.1: Main arteries of the head and neck.

- Postoperative healing problems. Wound healing may often be impaired after head and neck cancer surgery due to preoperative radiotherapy, and to the excision of lymphatic chains causing lymphoedema and wound infections. The resulting wound breakdown causes exposure of the carotid artery; flap necrosis allows bacterial invasion and desiccation of the adventitia. Pharyngocutaneous fistula results in the adventitia being bathed in saliva, which is bacteria-laden and destructive to the adventitia (Shumrick, 1973; Swain et al, 1974; Heller, 1979; Lesage, 1986).
- Erosion of the arterial wall by a tracheostomy tube (see Chapter 2.1).
- Radiotherapy. Neck irradiation has been implicated as a major factor in haemorrhage; it has been shown to reduce the blood supply to the adventitia (McCoy & Barsocchini, 1968; Shumrick, 1973; Huvos et al, 1973).
- Tumour invasion of the vessel wall.

Sentinel bleeds often herald a carotid artery rupture, and appropriate treatment should be selected for the individual depending on prognosis.

Postoperative bleeds

For postoperative bleeds, resuscitation will be appropriate for most patients. The aim of management is to maintain the airway, control bleeding, replace fluid loss and return the patient to theatre for ligation of the damaged artery. It is vital that the nurse clarifies the resuscitation status of the patient with the surgeon postoperatively in order to avoid inappropriate resuscitation.

Patients at risk of carotid bleed postoperatively should be identified to the whole team and all staff should be aware of the resuscitation procedure. Lesage (1986) suggests the patient's nursing notes or bedside chart are labelled 'Carotid Alert Precautions'. Emergency equipment should be kept at the bedside (Yuska & Blendowski, 1997) (see Figure 2.8.2). A wide-bore venous access device may be placed in advance to allow rapid infusion of IV fluids. The patient should be grouped and cross-matched and have 2 to 4 units of blood readily available (Lesage, 1986). The activity of high-risk patients should be restricted as heavy physical activity such as lifting, straining to defecate and excessive stair climbing cause a rise in blood pressure, and thus exert pressure on the damaged vessel (Lesage, 1986). Haemorrhage may often be precipitated by increased pressure within the artery, such as that caused by coughing (Johantgen, 1998). Because of the large volume of blood that can be lost, it may be most appropriate to nurse patients at risk in a single room.

All these procedures and their rationale should be carefully explained to the patient; the high-risk patient and significant others should be given a realistic portrayal of the possible event (Johantgen, 1998). Lesage (1986) suggests that the patient should be taught how to apply digital pressure him/herself.

Bleeding may start as a trickle from the wound or airway, and progress to a rapid, pulsating flow. In the presence of active bleeding, direct pressure should be applied to the site immediately, using sterile dressing pads and gloved hands. If the bleed is from the tracheostomy, the airway should be protected using a cuffed tube, which will also exert pressure on the bleeding point. Suction should be used to clear the tracheal or oral airway. Oxygen therapy should

- Box of gloves
- Plastic aprons, goggles/face shields
- Large sterile dressings
- Suction equipment
- Cuffed tracheostomy tubes (if appropriate); same size and one size down, syringes for cuff inflation
- Intravenous cannulae (wide bore)
- Syringes
- Giving sets
- Normal saline for infusion
- Oxygen
- Bath towels
- Drugs for sedation (midazolam 10 mg IM/SC)
- Clinical waste disposal bags

Figure 2.8.2: Emergency equipment for resuscitation.

be provided. Hypovolaemic shock should be treated with volume expanders and/or blood products. The patient should be placed in the Trendelenberg position.

Haemorrhage is an extremely frightening experience for the patient. A staff nurse describes a critical incident with a patient: 'He was so frightened ... He was conscious all the time and he gripped my arm so hard that I had bruises on it for days afterwards'.

Emotional support should be provided, and the nurse should explain all activities in a calm, reassuring manner. The patient can be sedated whilst surgery is organized for ligation of the artery. Midazolam is a useful drug for sedation purposes; it has a rapid onset, short duration of action and produces retrograde amnesia. It can be administered by intramuscular injection to spare patients memories of distressing events (Forbes, 1997).

Once the patient has been haemodynamically stabilized, he or she can be returned to theatre for arterial ligation. Unfortunately, ligation of the carotid has a high complication rate: death in 32% to 77% of cases, and permanent neurological defects in 12% to 50% of cases (Fortunato & Ridge, 1995).

Haemorrhage in terminal care

However well the family are prepared for death in terminal illness, the actual event often appears to them as an emergency. In the emergency event, management includes making the patient comfortable, thinking of the needs of other patients and relatives observing the event, explaining what is happening and is being done and communicating reassurance to the patient and relatives as well as to other observers (Smith, 1994). This is nowhere more relevant than in the management of the head and neck patient who haemorrhages.

Most episodes of haemorrhage in the terminal patient will be preceded by a 'herald' or 'sentinel' event (Forbes, 1997). The goal for management in this situation is to provide an atmosphere that minimizes anxiety and ensures death with dignity. A plan to manage episodes of bleeding should be discussed with the patient, their relatives and staff before the emergency occurs.

The hospital or hospice setting

Equipment should be kept at the bedside in preparation (see Figure 2.8.3). Because of the large volume of blood which can be lost, it may be most appropriate to nurse patients at risk in a single room.

The community setting

Many patients may wish to spend as much time as possible at home. They may not want to stay in the hospital or hospice setting 'waiting to bleed'. It may be very difficult for the nursing and medical team to decide how, or even whether, to inform the patient of the risk of haemorrhage and to discuss a management plan with the family.

- Box of gloves
- Plastic aprons, goggles/face shields
- Large dressing pads
- Bath towels to absorb blood loss; dark-coloured towels disguise the alarming blood loss to some extent
- Cuffed tracheostomy tubes (if appropriate); same size and one size down, syringes for cuff inflation
- Suction equipment
- Drugs for sedation (midazolam 10 mg IM/SC). If bleeding remains uncontrolled, sedation can be continued until the patient's death to avoid distress. This can be administered by repeated injections, or a subcutaneous infusion device (Forbes, 1997). However, exsanguination is often so rapid that there is insufficient time for drugs to act, and the only sensible intervention is to stay with the patient

Figure 2.8.3: Emergency equipment for palliative management.

However, although this may make the patient and family apprehensive, in most cases haemorrhage may already be an unexpressed fear. An empathetic and knowledgeable approach by the nurse can do much to facilitate a calm atmosphere at the time of death (Yuska & Blendowski, 1997). The nurse should discuss a management plan for haemorrhage at home with the patient, family and primary healthcare team. The district nurse plays a key role in this situation and the GP and community palliative care nurse specialist will need to be closely involved. A case conference is the ideal forum for this to happen.

A pack of emergency equipment, old towels and a bowl should be kept near the patient. The local ambulance service should be alerted: they may be willing to provide emergency support without resuscitation.

The following descriptions of actual family experiences of carotid haemorrhage at home demonstrate the difference that preparation can make.

Case examples

Case one: Gerry

Gerry was a 59-year-old man living with his elderly, but very fit, mother Joan. He had a recurrent fungating lesion in his right neck, invading his carotid artery. Gerry was admitted to hospital after a bleed from his lesion which had stopped spontaneously. He wanted to go home.

Gerry was told: 'The cancer has damaged the artery in your neck and there is a good chance that it will bleed again. Because it is a major artery, there will be a lot of blood loss that may well lead to your death. We need to talk about how you feel about being at home in this situation, and also how your mother feels about it'. The nurse discussed the situation with Gerry and Joan. Gerry was very concerned about causing 'a mess' in the house. Joan was adamant that she would much prefer Gerry to be at home, and the options for managing a haemorrhage at home were discussed. Joan decided she would be able to handle the situation if she had the equipment nearby and the backup of the district nurses and GP.

Gerry was discharged home after the district nurses had been contacted and the management of the situation discussed. The district nurses were able to provide a high level of support, visiting every day to check on the wound. Joan had their 24-hour emergency phone number by the phone. She decided that if the haemorrhage did happen, she would not call an ambulance, as she did not want Gerry to die in an ambulance or a strange place. A stock of large dressing pads, gloves, and a vial of midazolam and injection equipment were provided and were kept with several bath towels and a blanket in a box near to Gerry in the house. Gerry and Joan hoped that the wound would not bleed, but felt well prepared if it did.

A few weeks later, Joan phoned to say that Gerry had haemorrhaged the previous day and died.

'I was in the kitchen and I heard him banging his stick on the floor, like he does when he wants me. I went into the sitting room and there was blood spurting out of his neck on to the wall and the chair. I grabbed the towels and held them over his neck like we said. I could see he was going quickly so I put my arms round him and I said 'It's all right love, I'm here, I'm with you'. And a few minutes later he had gone. I covered him with the blanket and rang the nurse and she came with the doctor. The worst thing was the blood everywhere. The carpet and wallpaper are ruined. I'm so glad he was at home and I could hold him, it made it all worth it ... I don't think he suffered, it was so quick. The nurses and my GP were brilliant, they phoned the funeral director and they helped me clean up. I just couldn't have managed without them. The district nurses still call in to have a cuppa with me'.

Case two: Ted

Ted was 65 when his cancer of the larynx recurred. He had extensive disease, invading his carotid artery. He and his wife June were very anxious. The team caring for them did not want to make them more anxious by telling them he might bleed to death; they felt this would ruin the rest of their days together.

June describes Ted's haemorrhage and death:

'On Saturday morning, he was in the bathroom for ages. I went to find him, and he was there with all these tissues covered in blood. He said, it's OK, it's stopped now. I took him down to the GP because I was very worried about it. I wanted to take him back to the hospital, but he refused to go. The GP said it would probably be OK, but we should contact the hospital if it happened again.

We got home from the GP at 11 am. At lunchtime he went in the kitchen to make a drink. I remember going in the kitchen and seeing him stood over the sink. There was blood everywhere; the window, the tops, the floor. There was blood everywhere. His legs gave way and he fell to the floor. I have never seen such a look of fear on his face before. I just panicked. I'd never seen anything like it before. I grabbed a tea towel — it's all there was; it was no use. I ran to the phone and called an ambulance. I couldn't even find a blanket to cover him up. There was nothing to soak up all this blood. I felt so useless.'

Ted died the next day, having been resuscitated by the paramedics, taken to the local casualty at a hospital where he was not known, and then transferred to an intensive care unit in the next town due to unavailability of intensive care beds in his home town. June was not with him. If Ted, June and their GP had been prepared for this event, they could have taken Ted to the head and neck unit where he was well known when the herald bleed occurred, and Ted could have been managed palliatively there. Alternatively, they may have decided to stay at home, as Gerry did. The inappropriate resuscitation attempts would have been avoided. More importantly, June would have had the practical knowledge of what to do, and the equipment at hand to deal with it. She would also have had the support of the district nursing team.

It should be noted that if an ambulance is called to a patient who is haemorrhaging, the paramedics are legally bound to resuscitate the patient unless they have medical instructions otherwise. The same applies to the receiving team in the casualty department. It is therefore worth considering giving the family a doctor's letter which clearly states that the patient is not for resuscitation.

Summary

Carotid haemorrhage is probably the most dreaded of all events in head and neck cancer. It is traumatic and distressing for all concerned; patient and significant others, as well as nursing and medical staff. The image of the dramatic blood loss remains in everyone's memories forever. There is no literature on the psychological effects of this event on significant others and healthcare professionals. The authors cited seem to support the practice of preparing high-risk patients for the event, but again there is no evidence on the psychological advantages and disadvantages of this strategy. Carotid haemorrhage is therefore an area of head and neck cancer care which nursing research needs to address.

Strategy for practice

- Identify at-risk patients to the whole team, clarifying their resuscitation status.
- Ensure that the whole team is fully conversant with the appropriate management of carotid haemorrhage.
- Ensure a management plan is discussed for at-risk patients in the community; sensitive discussion should take place with the patient and family so that they are prepared for the worst. A case conference may be required.
- More research is required on the management of haemorrhage at home and the advantages and disadvantages of preparing the patient and family.

Chapter 2.9
Lymphoedema

Introduction

Lymphoedema results from insufficient transport of water and protein from the skin, subcutaneous tissue, mucous membrane and oral structures. The abnormal collection of protein-rich fluid in the interstitial spaces results in chronic inflammation and fibrosis of the surrounding tissue (Humble, 1995).

A literature search on CINAHL and MEDLINE revealed no English language literature specifically addressing the problem of lymphoedema in head and neck cancer. Three articles in German were found. However, there are numerous papers describing lymphoedema of the arms after breast cancer treatment. This section will therefore examine the general principles outlined in the literature on the management of lymphoedema and relate this to the management of lymphoedema in the head and neck.

Physiology of the lymphatic system

The lymphatic system is made up of capillaries, vessels and nodes. It is a one-way drainage system that transports lymph from the tissues to the vascular system. The peripheral lymphatic vessels continuously remove water, electrolytes, plasma proteins, cells and debris from the interstitial fluid. They drain into larger vessels which flow into major lymphatic trunks. These vessels drain the material through groups of lymph nodes and finally form two large lymphatic trunks, the thoracic duct and the right lymphatic duct. These drain into the large veins at the base of the neck (Williams, 1997). Lymphatic drainage of the head and neck is shown in Figure 2.9.1.

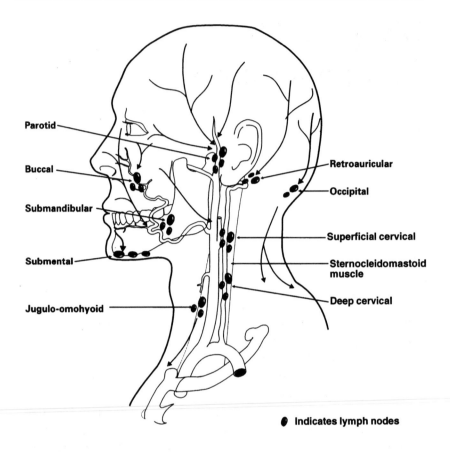

Figure 2.9.1: Lymphatic drainage of the head and neck.

The fluid dynamics within the capillary bed are maintained by the pressure gradients that are created by the capillary plasma hydrostatic and plasma colloid oncotic pressures and the interstitial fluid hydrostatic and colloid oncotic pressures. The pressure gradient supports filtration of serous fluid and proteins from the intravascular circulation to the interstitial space and reabsorption by the lymphatic capillaries, which then drain into larger vessels. The lymph moves through the lymphatics as a result of negative intrathoracic pressure during inspiration, local muscle contractions, the suction effect of high-velocity blood flow of the venous system in which the lymphatics terminate and the rhythmic smooth muscle contractions of the lymphatic vessel walls. It is returned to the intravascular space via the right and left subclavian veins. One-way valves in the lymphatic system prevent backflow of lymph (Humble, 1995).

Pathophysiology of lymphoedema

Insufficiency or blockage of the lymphatic vessels can result in an increase in the hydrostatic pressure within the regional lymph vessel, which leads to a decrease in the vessel wall integrity and in the patency of the one-way valve. This pressure increase results in a backward flow of lymph, causing proteins and fluid to leak out into the interstitial space. Protein accumulation in the tissues results in an increase in the interstitial colloid oncotic pressure, leading to more fluid leakage. Increased levels of fibroblasts and globulins, in conjunction with decreased levels of collagenase and other proteolytic enzymes within the leaked fluid, may lead to deposits of collagen-type substances in the tissues, which produce an inflammatory reaction that results in subcutaneous tissue fibrosis. The accumulated fluid can become a superb medium for bacteria, resulting in an increased risk for cellulitis and lymphangitis. Infections will result in increased blood flow, which causes increased hydrostatic pressure and capillary permeability, both of which will worsen the lymphoedema (Humble, 1995).

Causes of lymphoedema in the head and neck

Patients who have neck dissection to remove the cervical lymphatics, or have radiotherapy to the cervical lymphatics, may develop lymphoedema. Acute lymphoedema occurs after surgery and resolves within 2 weeks to 3 months. It is characterized by pitting oedema without skin changes (Humble, 1995). Chronic lymphoedema is diagnosed if it has been present for at least 3 months. Some skin changes are evident, and less pitting occurs. Lymphoedema can occur at any time after lymph node dissection, typically within days to weeks after surgery.

Radiotherapy damage to the lymphatics is expressed much more slowly as lymphatics have a slow cell turnover; it becomes most apparent around 3 months post-treatment when scarring and fibrosis occurs in the lymphatic vessels. Patients who develop unilateral lymphoedema could potentially respond very well to manual lymphatic drainage aimed to move lymph across to the contralateral side, as there is an extensive collateral system leading to this side (Hollo, 1993). Patients who have bilateral radical neck dissection, or bilateral neck irradiation, will experience severe and distressing lymphoedema of the head and neck which is much more difficult to control.

Late occurrence of lymphoedema is usually a result of an infection, inflammatory process, or recurrence (Brennan & Weitz, 1992).

Impact of head and neck lymphoedema

Lymphoedema of the face can be grossly disfiguring, causing distress, embarrassment, self-consciousness and social avoidance. It also causes severe functional problems:

- impaired speech, eating and swallowing if the intraoral structures and lips are affected
- impaired airway if submental oedema occludes the tracheostomy
- impaired, or even total prevention of, use of electrolarynges
- impaired vision due to oedema of the eyelids, optic disc oedema and raised intraocular pressure (Hollo, 1993)
- unpleasant feelings of tightness, tension and hardness in the skin (Casley-Smith et al, 1993).

Lymphoedema also causes worries about cancer recurrence. A common example of this is the firm, hard submental lymphoedema which occurs up to 3 months after radiotherapy to the larynx. This never fails to alarm patients, who should always be warned that it will occur.

Management of lymphoedema

There are no cures for lymphoedema — simply measures to control it (Gillham, 1994). Conservative management of lymphoedema is a multi-element treatment based on principles of massage, exercise, skin care and use of compression garments (Williams & Venables, 1995). Applying increased pressure on the affected area helps mobilize fluid in the tissues. This helps to correct the disturbed equilibrium between the lymphatic protein load and lymph transport capacity by increasing the latter and thereby facilitating the removal of excess protein from the tissue spaces. Conservative management of lymphoedema is successful in approximately 60–80% of patients with lymphoedema of the upper or lower extremities (Pappas & O'Donnell, 1992).

Manual lymphatic drainage (MLD)

MLD is the cornerstone of lymphoedema management. It consists of butterfly-light massage to the skin surface to promote fluid movement along the skin and subcutaneous lymphatics, bypassing the lymph system obstruction (Williams, 1997). In head and neck lymphoedema, it can also be used on intraoral surfaces. Massage is always performed in a distal to proximal direction so that the distal area is emptied to make room for fluid movement in from the proximal end. Thus massage should start at the axillae, working gradually upwards towards the affected area.

One of the best MLD techniques for the face is stationary circles. This involves placing the pads of the fingers on the skin and gently pushing the skin in the same place in a downward direction towards the neck base. The circle is completed by relaxing the pressure as the fingers move in an upward direction to repeat this gentle pumping movement. This is repeated five times in the same place, before moving approximately 1 cm further up. The pressure is very gentle, allowing the skin to spring back when released. No erythema or pain should occur (Humble, 1995). Gentle effleurage (stroking movements with the hands) may also be used (Gillham, 1994).

Einfeldt et al (1986) demonstrate the use of MLD in the head and neck using a case history with pictorial records and conclude that 'therapeutic drainage of lymphoedema can alleviate facial and cervical edema after surgery or irradiation. It is fully justified even in a malignant tumour with a hopeless prognosis'. They describe twice-daily MLD for 14 days to a patient who has recurrent disease and massive facial lymphoedema after extensive excision of a T4N2 cancer of the epiglottis, followed by radiotherapy and chemotherapy. MLD was performed on the front and back of the head and neck, including the trapezius muscle, down to the axillae. The oral mucosa was also covered, including the hard palate. The whole face was treated, especially the temples. The time taken to perform this procedure is not noted. There was a noticeable improvement after 14 days.

Some authorities have expressed concern that MLD promotes metastatic spread and in order to evaluate this Preisler et al (1998) compared 100 head and neck cancer patients who received MLD to a control group who did not. They found no evidence that MLD increased the rate of recurrences.

Hildmann et al (1987) recommend that MLD for head and neck lymphoedema be started as early as possible in order to control the progression of the condition.

Exercise

Exercises of the affected areas (shoulders, neck, tongue, periorbital muscles) promote muscle contraction, putting pressure against lymph channels, and promoting collateral drainage (Wilson & Bilodeau, 1989). Exercises of the arms, shoulders and neck particularly promote lymph flow; muscular activity has a massaging effect on the large lymphatic vessels and surrounding tissues in the upper chest and neck.

External compression

External compression (> 40 mmHg) is an important part of lymphoedema treatment. Its application limits blood capillary filtration by raising interstitial pressure, opposing tissue pressure and improving striated muscle pump efficiency (Williams, 1997). High-pressure garments such as elastic sleeves or bandaging are used after massage to maintain displaced fluid in arms and legs (Humble, 1995). This intervention is much more difficult in the head and neck; an elastic bandage such as Tubigrip, applied over a thin layer of foam balaclava-style, can be used on the face, but this is very difficult for the patient to tolerate for any length of time. Special facial masks are used in continental Europe but are not available in the UK. It is emphasized that compression cannot 'treat' lymphoedema but is a method used to conserve a state free of oedema achieved by successful therapy (Foldi et al, 1989).

Skin care

Skin problems in lymphoedema include dry skin, fungal infections, hyperkeratosis, acute inflammatory episodes (infective and non-infective) and contact dermatitis (Williams & Venables, 1995). Good skin care is therefore crucial and has two main aims — to keep the epidermis and dermis hydrated and supple, and to prevent infection.

The basic regime should include:

- careful daily cleansing of the area using soap and water
- careful observation of the skin condition, being alert to any changes
- daily application of moisturizing cream
- avoidance of skin damage (e.g. shaving, sunburn, insect bites)
- prompt treatment of any injury with judicious use of antiseptics
- avoidance of tight collars
- use of appropriate dermatological preparations for specific skin problems.

Patients are initially given an intensive phase of treatment by the therapist over a 2- to 4-week period. The second phase of treatment aims to maintain the improvements in skin condition and oedema reduction. These techniques are taught to the patient and carer, who must continue the daily regime of exercise and massage themselves (Williams, 1997). Thus lymphoedema management requires on-going motivation and commitment from the patient and carer.

Acute inflammatory episodes

Attention to the above regime will minimize infection occurrence, but the presence of stagnant, protein-rich oedema in the tissues predisposes the area to infection, which can spread diffusely through the subcutaneous and connective tissues if unchecked (Jeffs, 1993). Bacterial entry is gained through breaks in the skin. It is commonly believed that streptococcus is the causative organism. These acute inflammatory episodes are often referred to as cellulitis. The patient will experience fever, chills and malaise. The neck and head become red, inflamed and tender. Any inflammatory episode should be treated promptly with antibiotics. Streptococcal infections are sensitive to penicillin, or erythromycin for individuals allergic to penicillin (Jeffs, 1993). Jeffs recommends that patients who suffer repeated attacks of cellulitis should carry an emergency supply of broad-spectrum antibiotics to be taken at the first indication of attack. Infections which repeatedly recur may require long-term prophylactic antibiotics (Jeffs, 1993; Gillham, 1994).

Pharmacological management

Pharmacological management may sometimes be needed alongside conservative management (Hardy & Baum, 1991). Benzopyrones are used in some countries. Benzopyrones are said to increase lymphatic flow by increasing the pumping capacity, increasing capillary resistance and decreasing hyperpermeability, resulting in decreased protein loss from blood vessels. They also stimulate the proteolytic activities of macrophages, resulting in more phagocytosis of protein in the tissues (Casley-Smith et al, 1993).

Surgical management

Surgical management is only indicated if conservative management proves unsuccessful. This involves debulking or removing skin and subcutaneous tissue (Humble, 1995).

Summary

Head and neck lymphoedema is a distressing problem associated with impaired lymphatic drainage caused by surgery, radiotherapy and advanced or recurrent disease. It is a problem that has not attracted much attention in the literature. However, the evidence available suggests that it can be controlled conservatively by a skilled therapist.

Lymphoedema management is labour-intensive and time-consuming. It is much less well provided for in the UK than in other areas of the world. Many patients today are told that it is an unavoidable cost of life-saving treatment and that they will 'just have to live with it' (Gillham, 1994). If head and neck lymphoedema is to be treated, as with any other kind of lymphoedema, a significant amount of resources will be required in order to provide a service with the requisite specialist skills and time. Few lymphoedema treatment centres exist in the UK, despite the fact that more advanced cancer treatment is now leaving survivors living with significant lymphoedema. With improvements in survival in head and neck cancer due to increasingly more extensive surgery and radiotherapy, the effective and efficient management of subsequent lymphoedema requires urgent investigation by head and neck cancer centres.

Strategy for practice

• Ensure all patients undergoing neck dissection and radiotherapy to lymphatic chains are trained to self-administer MLD.

- Ensure patients understand how to look after their skin to prevent infection occurring.
- Incorporate written information on lymphoedema into information booklets.
- Research and development is needed in this area.

For more information on lymphoedema contact:

The British Lymphology Interest Group (BLIG)
PO Box 1059
Caterham
Surrey CR3 6ZU

The Lymphoedema Association of Australia
Henry Thomas Laboratory
University of Adelaide
Adelaide
SA 5005
Australia

Chapter 2.10
Altered sensory function

Introduction

The extent to which human beings can cope with their environment, whether physically, socially or emotionally, depends on the information they receive from their sensory organs. The eyes and ears are of primary importance, and the other senses of taste, smell, touch and proprioception all have a part to play (Wigmore, 1981). The senses also have a tremendous amount of importance in relation to quality of life. There is the visual enjoyment of scenery, colour and art; the appetizing smell and taste of food; the scents of flowers and perfumes; and the myriad beautiful sounds in the environment: music, voices, birdsong, wind and so on.

This chapter will focus on the sensory organs at risk of impairment in head and neck cancer. That is, olfaction, gustation, hearing and equilibrium and sight. Each section will cover an overview of the anatomy and physiology, the causes and impact of impairment, and the nursing management.

Olfaction

Function of olfaction

Unlike hearing and sight deficits, impaired olfaction receives little attention in the literature (Souder & Yoder, 1992). This may be due to the association of olfaction and taste with sensual and emotional activities, rather than intellectual activities.

Olfaction is important for monitoring the safety of the environment. Smell alerts the individual to fires, leaking gas and the presence of toxins in food that has spoilt.

Olfaction is also important as it plays a crucial role in the ability to appreciate the flavour of food. The appreciation of aromas such as cooking, flowers, soaps and perfumes all contribute to quality of life. The importance of smell is demonstrated by the major industry in fragrances, from cosmetic companies and perfumiers, to manufacturers of deodorants, room fresheners, detergents and aromatherapy products.

Anatomy and physiology
Martini, 1992a
There is a pair of olfactory organs, one on either side of the nasal septum in the upper portion of the nasal cavity below the cribriform plate of the ethmoid bone. Each olfactory organ contains mucous glands and olfactory epithelium. This epithelium contains the olfactory receptors, neurons sensitive to chemicals dissolved in the overlying mucus. It also contains supporting cells and basal (stem) cells. Beneath the basement membrane, large olfactory glands produce a pigmented mucus that covers the epithelium.

The olfactory epithelium covers the roof of each nasal cavity and extends across portions of the nasal septum and superior conchae. When air is drawn in through the nose, turbulence generates eddies that bring airborne compounds to the olfactory organs. A normal, relaxed inspiration provides a small sample of air. Sniffing repeatedly creates more extensive eddies, increasing the airflow to, and thus the stimulation of, the olfactory organs.

Once the airborne compounds have reached the olfactory neuroepithelium, water-soluble and lipid-soluble materials must dissolve it into the epithelial mucus before the olfactory receptors can be stimulated. A continual stream of mucus dissolves airborne molecules, prevents the build-up of dangerous or overpowering stimuli and keeps the area clean and moist.

The olfactory receptors are highly modified neurons. The apical portion of each receptor projects above the epithelial surface, providing a base for up to 20 cilia. The cilia are in constant motion, exposing their considerable surface area to dissolved chemical compounds in the surrounding mucus. There are about 10 to 20 million olfactory receptors altogether in an area of roughly 5 cm^2.

Axons leaving the olfactory epithelium collect into 20 or more bundles which penetrate the cribriform plate of the ethmoid to reach the olfactory bulbs of the cerebrum. Efferent fibres from nuclei elsewhere in the brain also contact the neurons of the olfactory bulb and provide a mechanism for central modification of olfactory sensitivities. Axons leaving the olfactory bulb travel along the olfactory tract to reach the olfactory cortex, the hypothalamus, and portions of the limbic system. Olfactory stimuli are the only type of sensory information that reaches the cerebral cortex without first synapsing in the thalamus. The extensive limbic and hypothalamic connections help to explain the profound emotional and behavioural responses that can be produced by certain smells.

There is a strong relationship between olfaction and behaviour which is mediated at a subcortical level, in the limbic and paralimbic structures of the brain. Olfaction is a very primitive sense and the limbic structures involved may be essential to the expression of normal behaviour, including sexual behaviour. Sensuous fragrances may have strong activating properties on the emotional and sexual centres of the brain (Zasler et al, 1992).

Olfactory receptors are the only neurons that are regularly replaced in the adult human. New receptor cells are produced by the basal membrane of the epithelium. Despite this, the number of receptors declines with age and the elderly may have difficulty detecting odours in low concentrations.

Causes of olfactory impairment

Olfactory impairment can be described as anosmia (absence of smell) and dysosmia (distortion of smell). Anosmia plays an important part in the loss of taste.

- Smoking has been shown to produce an olfactory deficit. Improvement in smell function occurs slowly after smoking has stopped, and may never completely return to normal (Frye et al, 1990). Malnutrition and vitamin B12 deficiency have also been shown to impair the sense of smell (Schiffman, 1983a).
- Some medications may cause smell deficits; chlorpheniramine maleate, levodopa, codeine, morphine, carbamazepine, amphetamines and various antimicrobial agents (Schiffman, 1983a).
- Factors that cause decrease in cell renewal, affecting the replacement of olfactory receptors, also affect smell. Thus irradiation of the olfactory gland (for example if the nasopharynx or sinuses are being treated) will cause anosmia. Cytotoxic chemotherapy can

have a similar effect (Schiffman, 1983a). Radiotherapy can cause dysosmia, with some patients reporting being able to 'smell' pungent odours during treatment, especially if it is to the nasopharynx (Sagar et al, 1991). Smells reported are commonly those of 'ozone, chlorine, bleach and celery'. The sensation usually goes as soon as the machine is switched off. In a study by Chang et al (1996), patients receiving radical radiotherapy to the nasopharynx reported 'foul odour' because of nasopharyngeal crust. Smell acuity is profoundly affected, for long periods of time, by irradiation of the olfactory epithelium (Ophir et al, 1988). Impaired olfaction was still present 6 months after irradiation in Ophir et al's study (1988); there is no data on later recovery.

- Procedures that damage the olfactory nerve, such as craniofacial surgery, cause anosmia.
- Diseases affecting the nervous system, including Korsakoff's psychosis, are associated with anosmia (Mair et al, 1986).
- Diseases that affect the flow of air over the olfactory epithelium cause anosmia. Rhinitis and nasal sinus disease are commonly implicated (Schiffman, 1983a). Laryngectomy causes a decrease in smell function as the individual breathes via the neck, having lost the function of the upper airway (Schiffman, 1983a). In one study, 95% of 63 laryngectomees reported hyposmia immediately after surgery, with 52% going on to have long-term hyposmia (Ackerstaff et al, 1994). Tatchell et al (1985) demonstrated that hyposmia was directly related to the ability of the laryngectomee to move air in through the nose; oesophageal speakers were best able to do this. Craniofacial, nasal and paranasal sinus surgery and radiotherapy can also cause anosmia due to intranasal mechanical obstruction by causing scarring and oedema (Freedman & Kern, 1979; Mott, 1992).

Helping the patient with impaired olfaction

The nurse plays a very important role in educating the patient and family about impaired olfaction.

The patient and family must take additional precautions to check gas appliances for leaks. Smoke alarms should be installed in the house and checked regularly (Souder & Yoder, 1992). Free gas checks are available from British Gas for people with disabilities, and some local fire services provide free smoke alarms to the elderly and disabled. Carbon monoxide monitors are available from British Gas and DIY stores.

Food should always be labelled with the date and discarded as soon as the expiry date is reached. When possible, a family member or friend should evaluate perishable foods such as raw meats or fish for freshness. Toxic substances such as insecticides, cleaning agents, paint thinners, petrol, etc., should be kept in labelled containers, as the individual will no longer be able to identify them by the sense of smell. Personal and household hygiene must also be carefully maintained, as odour detection to indicate a need for cleaning or washing can no longer be relied upon (Souder & Yoder, 1992).

Individuals with impaired olfaction will experience decreased sensitivity to the taste of food. Taste nerves are sensitive to sweet, sour, bitter and salt taste (see Gustation, below), but it is olfactory receptors which are responsible for carrying information about the many volatiles in food and beverages. Food flavour involves smell as much as it does taste (Murphy & Davidson, 1992). Impairment can severely impair the enjoyment of food and lead to nutritional deficits with the overuse of seasonings such as sugar and salt to compensate. High-sugar and high-fat foods may be consumed to a level associated with a higher risk of cardiac disease and obesity (Duffy et al, 1996). Coping with taste alteration is discussed in the next section.

Gustation

Function of gustation

Gustation, or tasting, provides information about the safety of material for ingestion; that is, whether it is likely to be toxic or bacteria-laden. Taste has also been implicated in 'states of need' hungers. For example, craving for salty foods develops if the body is in negative sodium balance (Schiffman, 1983b). However, gustation is much more than a survival function — it is essential for appetite, enjoyment of food and thus quality of life.

Anatomy and physiology
Martini, 1992b

The gustatory receptors are distributed over the surface of the tongue and adjacent portions of the pharynx and larynx. The receptors are clustered in individual taste buds. Each taste bud contains around 40 receptors, called gustatory cells. A typical gustatory cell survives for about 10 days before being replaced.

Tasting occurs whilst the mouth holds and manipulates food, dissolving it in salivary secretions. The taste buds are recessed into the epithelium and each gustatory cell extends microvilli (taste hairs) into the surrounding fluids through a narrow taste pore. This protects the delicate sensory cells from any damage caused by direct contact with unprocessed food.

The taste buds of the tongue are the major gustatory receptors. They are well protected by epithelial projections called papillae. There are three different types of papillae: filiform, fungiform and circumvallate. The largest number of taste buds are associated with the circumvallate papillae, which form a V near the posterior margin of the tongue.

The mechanism of gustation is similar to olfaction. Dissolved chemicals contacting the taste hairs cause stimulation of the gustatory cell. There are four primary taste sensations: sweet, salt, bitter and sour. Each taste bud shows a particular sensitivity to one of these tastes and there are regional differences in the distribution of sensitivity on the tongue. Taste receptors respond more readily to unpleasant rather than attractive stimuli. They are much more sensitive to acids (sour taste) and toxins (bitter taste) than to either sweet or salty chemicals.

Taste buds are monitored by the VIIth (facial), IXth (glossopharyngeal) and Xth (vagus) cranial nerves. The sensory afferents synapse within the nucleus solitarius of the medulla to travel on to the medial lemniscus. After another synapse in the thalamus, the information is sent to the primary sensory cortex. In assembling a conscious perception of taste, the information from the taste buds is correlated with other data. The perception of the general texture of food, together with the sensations of warmth, cold, irritation and pungency, result from stimulation of general sensory afferents in the trigeminal nerve. Information from the olfactory receptors also play a very important role, making perceptions of tastes and flavours much more sensitive than information from the taste buds alone. Visual information about the colour and appearance of food also adds to total perception.

Causes of altered taste

Altered taste can be described as ageusia (absence of taste), hypogeusia (decreased taste acuity) and dysgeusia (abnormal taste sensation).

Altered taste is a very common problem for patients who have undergone treatment for head and neck cancer. There are a number of factors that contribute to the problem.

- Old age causes hypogeusia. In childhood there are over 10,000 taste buds, but the numbers decline dramatically after 50 years of age. This, combined with loss of olfaction, means that many elderly people find their food tastes bland and unappetizing (Murphy & Davidson, 1992). As most head and neck cancer patients fall into the over-65 age group, decreased taste may already be a problem before the onslaught of various taste-altering treatments compounds this problem.
- Many drugs cause altered taste (Mott, 1992). There may be several factors causing the problem. Dysgeusia can result from the drug's metabolites presence in saliva producing bitter, metallic or unpleasant taste. As salivary function is important in taste (to put substances in solution for the taste buds), drugs that reduce salivary flow (for example antidepressants) will affect taste in this way. Some drugs alter taste by modifying the taste system directly. Chlorhexidine (Corsodyl) is thought to alter taste by binding to specific sodium receptor molecules in the taste bud. Chemotherapy agents damage frequently regenerating cells such as taste cells. Medications acting on the nervous system can affect taste; elevated taste thresholds and an aversion to alcohol occur with carbamazepine, a drug commonly used to control nerve pain in head and neck cancer (Halbreich, 1974).
- Radiotherapy to the tongue causes loss of cell replication, which is temporary, and damage to salivary flow, which is permanent. Taste alteration may be noted as early as 2 to 3 days from the beginning of irradiation, with degeneration of the taste buds occurring after 6 to 7 days (Nelson, 1998). This is manifested as dysgeusia or ageusia, depending on the area of tongue in the treatment field. Wilson et al (1991) record patients' descriptions of dysgeusia during radiotherapy: 'Everything tasted like wet cardboard ... rubber ... mush'. Patients in their study described taste changes as the most difficult problem to solve. The sense of taste does return after radiotherapy as the taste buds repair themselves. A partial improvement occurs between the 20th and 60th days after radiotherapy, and a full recovery is usually achieved after 4 months (Ripamonti et al, 1997). However, hyposalivation may also be a factor causing hypogeusia (Conger, 1973).

- Surgical procedures that damage the taste pathways in the cranial nerves (facial, glossopharyngeal and vagus nerves) can cause taste problems, but as it would be unusual to damage all these nerves, total ageusia would not be expected (Mott, 1992).
- Oral infections, such as *Candida*, can alter the sense of taste (Mott, 1992).
- Laryngectomy causes hypogeusia, and this is probably related to the hyposmia which it also causes. In one study 44% of laryngectomees reported hypogeusia immediately after surgery, with 15% finding this a long-term problem (Ackerstaff et al, 1994).

Helping the patient with altered taste

The most important effect of altered taste is on nutritional status (Murphy & Davidson, 1992). Ageusia, dysgeusia and hypogeusia can both cause and compound poor appetite and malnutrition. The patient may also use sugar and salt excessively to compensate for lack of taste in food. A nutritional assessment should be made and the patient and family should be given dietary advice. Spices, texture, temperature and visual presentation can all be used to compensate for altered taste.

Texture is a highly valued food attribute in people with hypogeusia (Duffy, 1996). Patients can be encouraged to experiment with different textures: creamy, rough, crunchy, or sticky. Increasing the amount of seasoning in food can also help; condiments such as pepper, horseradish, mustards, herbs, spices, vinegar, lemon juice and hot peppers stimulate the trigeminal nerve and thus give additional sensation (Zasler et al, 1992). Spices such as nutmeg, vanilla and cinnamon may be used to enhance the flavour of sweet foods instead of adding extra sugar. Nurses must suspend old beliefs that patients with eating difficulties due to radiotherapy and chemotherapy should eat soft, bland foods and encourage them to be much more creative.

Meals should also incorporate visual aspects in the form of colour, and presentation. The caregiver should pay close attention to the aesthetics of food presentation. Serving the meal in a friendly, caring environment can also help to stimulate the patient's appetite (Souder & Yoder, 1992).

Patients with dysgeusia can learn to avoid foods that cause unpleasant taste sensations, and can also minimize the taste sensation by eating cold, non-aromatic food.

A small but rigorous study (18 patients) seems to show that hypogeusia and ageusia caused by radiotherapy of the oral cavity can be improved by taking zinc sulphate 45 mg three times per day. The zinc sulphate slowed down the worsening and accelerated the improvement of taste acuity in a clinically and statistically relevant way (Ripamonti et al, 1997). The authors recommend that this clinical practice be used to improve supportive care for people with head and neck cancer who experience altered taste.

Despite all these measures, and because taste dysfunction may be only one of several eating difficulties, some individuals may remain anorectic. On a practical level, the nurse must encourage such patients to see food as an essential medicine to be taken at regular intervals throughout the day.

Cooking for other people can become problematic, as the patient can no longer rely on tasting the food to adjust seasoning. They may need to depend on a friend or family member to test the food, or on following recipes carefully. Conversely, preparing a meal for the affected individual becomes difficult. Preparing and enjoying family meals is important for psychological and social wellbeing. Family tensions may increase when carefully prepared meals are rejected (Stubbs, 1989), and patients may feel isolated if they can no longer enjoy the social event of a meal.

Deems et al (1991) found that 68% of 750 patients with taste and smell dysfunction reported that the disorder affected their quality of life. Specifically, 56% reported impaired daily living or psychological wellbeing, and almost half noted changes in either appetite or body weight. Food is for the soul as well as the body (Duffy, 1996). Eating is one of life's greatest pleasures, an emotional, social and sensory experience, not just a nutritional process.

Hearing and equilibrium

Function of hearing and equilibrium

The sense of hearing helps the individual function within the social environment. It is especially important for verbal communication and acts as a warning of approaching threats. Most alarm systems rely on the sense of hearing. The sense of equilibrium is essential for the body to maintain balance during even the most simple of movements.

Anatomy and physiology

Martini, 1992b

The senses of equilibrium and hearing are both provided by the receptors of the inner ear, a collection of fluid-filled chambers and tubes also known as the membranous labyrinth. The fluid is called endolymph. The inner ear is surrounded by protective bone called the bony labyrinth. Between the bony and membranous labyrinths flows a fluid similar to CSF called perilymph. The entire inner ear is contained in the temporal bone of the skull.

The bony labyrinth can be subdivided into the vestibule, the semicircular canals and the cochlea. Receptors in the vestibule and the semicircular canals provide the sense of equilibrium; those in the cochlear provide the sense of hearing.

The external ear includes the cartilaginous pinna which surrounds the external auditory meatus, the entry to the external auditory canal. Ceruminous glands lining the canal secrete a waxy material, and many small hairs prevent the entry of foreign objects. The external auditory canal ends at the tympanic membrane which divides the external ear from the middle ear. The middle ear communicates with the nasopharynx via the pharyngotympanic (Eustachian) tube and also with the mastoid sinuses via other small connections. The middle ear contains the auditory ossicles that connect the tympanic membrane with the receptor complex of the inner ear.

Sensory information on equilibrium is transmitted from the inner ear via the vestibular nerve to the vestibulocochlear nerve (eighth cranial nerve). These nerve fibres synapse on neurons within the vestibular nuclei, which integrate information from either side of the head and relay it on to the cerebellum, the cerebral cortex and the motor nuclei in the brain stem and spinal cord.

Auditory information from the cochlea is transmitted through the cochlear nerve to the vestibulocochlear nerve. These axons enter the medulla and synapse at the cochlear nucleus. This transmits information to the opposite side of the brain, at the inferior colliculus of the midbrain. This processes unconscious reflexes to auditory stimuli. From here information travels to the auditory cortex of the temporal lobe, where it reaches conscious awareness.

Causes of impaired hearing and equilibrium

- Tumours of the ear and their surgical or radiotherapeutic treatment will obviously carry a risk of hearing loss, tinnitus and disturbed equilibrium. Fortunately, this is often a unilateral problem, and the patient can adjust to coping with one ear alone. The main problem is in not being able to hear people standing or sitting on the affected side, and difficulty in locating the direction from which sounds (such as someone shouting from a distance) are coming.

- Radiotherapy to the nasopharyngeal area frequently causes long-term bilateral hearing loss (Low & Fong, 1998). This is because the ear structures are within the target area. Patients will experience soreness and crusting in the ear canal, as well as hearing loss. Post-irradiation serous otitis media was found to cause 46.9% of hearing loss in 132 patients who had undergone treatment for nasopharyngeal cancer. Persistence of hearing loss was found to be age related; there was no persistence in under-30s, whilst 37.4% of those in the over-50 age group had persistent loss (Kwong et al, 1996).

- Hearing loss can also be caused by cisplatin, a cytotoxic drug commonly used to treat head and neck cancer which has ototoxic effects. Patients in poor general medical condition are at an increased risk of hearing loss from cisplatin chemotherapy (Blakley et al, 1994).

Helping the patient with hearing loss

Human effectiveness is heavily dependent on verbal communication. Communication can become very stressful for both the individual affected and those communicating with them when hearing is impaired. Hearing loss can also be very isolating. Friends and relatives may avoid conversation with the patient, and family tensions may result from the need to increase the volume of the television and radio. The patient will experience feelings of frustration, anger and insecurity (Anon, 1994). Embarrassment and loss of confidence can be experienced in social situations, with inappropriate responses to things that are misheard, and feelings of uneasiness due to being unable to join in the general conversation (Lysons, 1978). Herth (1998) conducted a phenomenological study to explore the effects of hearing loss in adults. Integrating hearing loss was a complex and dynamic process that involved loss of feeling capable, control, independence, connectedness and belonging, dignity and self-esteem, plus fear of failure, dependency, ridicule, being slighted or avoided, being made conspicuous, new situations and people. This resulted in emotions such as grief, anger, denial, frustration, isolation, depression, loneliness and sadness. Hearing loss thus may be an important factor in altered body image to which the patient has to adjust. The nurse should encourage the patient's expression of concerns and anxieties about altered auditory skills and provide information to facilitate coping strategies.

Improving communication

All patients experiencing hearing loss should be referred to the audiology department for an assessment. An individually tailored hearing aid can help patients with conductive deafness. The nurse can check that the patient maintains and fits his or her hearing aid correctly. Some patients may be reluctant to wear a hearing aid as they regard it as a stigma which advertises their disability (Lysons, 1978).

Loss of hearing can be partly overcome by focusing more on visual communication. Eye contact, speech reading and gesture can be used to enhance understanding. The difference between facing the patient whilst speaking and turning away can be dramatic. The nurse should firstly attract the patient's attention by raising an arm or touching, then speak directly to them in good light, using appropriate gesture and facial expression. If the patient has one good ear, the nurse should stand or sit on this side while communicating with the patient. Speech should be clear and distinctive in a moderate voice (vowels carry the power of spoken English, whilst the consonants and other higher frequency sounds carry the intelligibility), letting the patient's hearing aid do the amplifying of the sound (Fotheringham, 1998). If there are any doubts about the efficacy of the hearing aid, the audiologist should be consulted. When verbal communication fails, finger writing on the palm of the hand can be used to spell out key words. Touch can also be used appropriately to overcome communication barriers and convey sympathy, friendship and comfort. It is important that the nurse teach the family these constructive methods to help.

Hearing impairment means that a person deviates from social norms and so becomes stigmatized. The person will become aware of this when people with normal hearing react with impatience, avoidance, or adopting an assumption that the deaf person must be deficient in intelligence as well as hearing (Lysons, 1978). Deafness, unlike blindness, is not a disability that makes an instinctive appeal to human sympathy. The nurse should coach patients to be assertive and disclose their hearing impairment to other people, giving hearing people instructions to help them communicate effectively; for example, asking the person in question to sit or stand on the side of their hearing ear, or to repeat something more clearly. Guessing what people have said is not an effective coping strategy and should be discouraged.

Hearing loss can present a threat to safety as hearing can warn of dangers that cannot be seen, such as oncoming traffic, shouts of warning, or footsteps approaching in the dark. The patient should be made aware of the need for extra vigilance. Technical aids such as a flashing light on the doorbell, an extra-loud doorbell, special alarm clocks, etc., can be supplied by the local social services department. BT supply specially adapted telephone systems. The nurse should always put the patient in touch with local social services for specialist help (see Chapter 1.4 for more details).

Helping the patient with disturbed equilibrium

Disturbed equilibrium is a sensory disturbance and motor impairment that causes distressing symptoms of dizziness, nausea and unsteadiness which can be extremely debilitating. In one study, 56% of patients who had undergone surgery for acoustic neuroma still had dizziness 6 months later (Parving et al, 1992). These symptoms can be helped by physical therapy with selected balance retraining exercises using graded activities (Freeman & Nairne, 1995; Gill-Body et al, 1997). The occupational therapist can provide adaptive equipment and teach alternative strategies for performing activities of daily living (Cohen, 1994). Patients often avoid movement during the early postoperative period, but this can delay the onset of recovery (Herdman et al, 1995). It is therefore important that the nurse ensures that an early referral is made to the physiotherapist and occupational therapist, and that the nursing team work with the rehabilitation team to encourage the patient to practice exercises daily. Patients will also require nursing interventions to relieve depression and anxiety. The long-term outlook is good for these patients; Black et al (1989) followed 17 patients for 4 years and found that 75% eventually recovered normal postural control.

Dizziness and nausea can also require pharmacological management. The most common pharmacological agents are antihistamines — prochlorperazine, cinnarizine, promethazine, diphenhydramine and cyclizine, and antimuscarinics — scopolamine (hyoscine) (Lucot, 1998). Their mechanism of action is poorly understood. The most common theory is that they suppress integration of sensory stimuli in the vestibular nuclei. 5-HT_3 antagonists are not effective in preventing motion sickness.

The eyes and vision

Function of the eyes and vision

Unlike many other animals, humans rely more on vision than on any other sense. It is vital for the individual to function effectively in the environment. Without vision, moving around becomes a hazardous activity. All tasks of daily living become much more difficult, and a large amount of independence may be lost. Vision is tremendously important in quality of life. It is difficult to think of many leisure activities that do not require vision for participation.

Anatomy and physiology
Martini, 1992b
The visual receptors are contained in elaborate structures, the eyes. The eyes enable us to create detailed visual images. In head and neck cancer, the effect of the disease or treatment is usually related to the loss of one eye, or altered function in the accessory structures. The anatomy and physiology of the eye itself will therefore not be described.

The accessory structures of the eye

The accessory structures of the eye include the eyelids, the superficial epithelium of the eye, and the structures associated with the production, secretion and removal of tears. The eyelids can close firmly to protect the delicate surface of the eye. Their continual blinking movements keep the surface lubricated and free from dust and debris. The upper and lower eyelids are joined at the medial canthus (near the nose) and the lateral canthus (outer edge of the eye). The eyelashes help to prevent foreign particles and insects from entering the eye. Along the inner margin of the eyelids, large sebaceous glands secrete a lipid-rich product that helps to stop the eyelids sticking together. At the medial canthus the lacrimal caruncle contains glands that produce thick secretions to lubricate the eye. The outer surface of the eye is covered by an epithelium called the conjunctiva. Goblet cells within this epithelium also provide a superficial lubricant that prevents friction.

The lacrimal gland is an almond-shaped gland that sits in a depression in the frontal bone, just inside the orbit, superior and lateral to the eyeball. The lacrimal gland provides the key ingredients and most of the volume of tears that bathe the conjunctival surfaces. Its secretions are watery, slightly alkaline, and contain lysozyme, an antibacterial enzyme. Tears mix with the other secretions on the ocular surface. The mixture provides lubrication, slows evaporation, reduces friction, removes debris, prevents infection, and provides nutrients and oxygen to the conjunctiva. The secretions accumulate at the medial canthus in the lacus lacrimalis. Two small pores drain this collection into lacrimal canals in the surface of the lacrimal bone. These end at the lacrimal sac, which drains into the nasolacrimal duct. This carries the tears to the inferior meatus of the nose.

Visual information from each eye is carried in the optic nerve (second cranial nerve) to the optic chiasm. From here about half of the fibres cross over to reach the lateral geniculate on the opposite side of the brain, whilst the other half travel to the lateral geniculate on the same side. The lateral geniculates relay information to the reflex centres in the brainstem as well as to the cerebral cortex. Each eye receives a slightly different image and the crossover that occurs at the optic chiasm ensures that the visual cortex receives a composite picture of the entire visual field. The different images are also used to provide depth perception.

Causes of impaired vision

- Impaired vision can be caused by disease process affecting the accessory structures or the eye itself; for example advanced tumours of the paranasal sinuses can cause oedema of the accessory structures which prevents opening of the eye.
- The tumour itself may grow to affect vision externally, or by invading the orbit.
- Damage to the optic nerves causes loss of vision. Damage can be

caused surgically or by the disease itself. Nasopharyngeal tumours can impair the eye movement or vision itself by affecting motor and sensory nerves. Radiotherapy may cause optic nerve neuropathy.

- Surgery for disease of the nose and sinuses can impair vision. Enuclectomy leaves the patient with monocular vision, whilst extensive surgery to the sinuses with retention of the orbit can leave the patient with dystopia (mis-alignment of the eyes), diplopia (double vision) and epiphora (abnormality of tear drainage causing water to flow on to the cheek) (Mathog et al, 1997). In a review of 58 patients who had undergone craniofacial resection with preservation of the orbit, 43% had some ocular sequelae (Andersen et al, 1996). This consisted of epiphora in 21 patients, diplopia in eight, vision loss in six and pain and enopthalmus (eye sunken into the socket) in two.
- Radiotherapy treatment to areas near the eyes has to be carefully planned to avoid damage, but sometimes low doses to the eyes cannot be avoided and there is a long-term risk of cataracts developing (Brady & Davis, 1988). Andersen et al (1996) attribute the vision loss in their six patients (cited above) to postoperative radiotherapy.
- Radiotherapy can also cause damage to the lacrimal gland causing desiccation or 'dry eye'.
- Surgery which damages the facial nerve (e.g. parotidectomy) will bring about unilateral facial droop, unilateral inability to close the eye and unilateral loss of tear production. This may lead to exposure keratitis (inflammation of the cornea) (Andersen et al, 1996).

Helping the patient with impaired vision

Patients experiencing loss of lacrimal production or eyelid function should be observed carefully for signs of keratitis, which must be treated promptly with topical antibiotics. Artificial tears/lubricants must be applied regularly. The eye may need to be taped closed, and protected with a patch, particularly when the patient is sleeping.

Visual impairment often causes the loss of self-management skills, and alternative techniques are required to accomplish tasks that could be carried out quite easily by a sighted person. It is unusual for head and neck cancer to cause total loss of vision, and patients most commonly have to contend with visual impairment such as double vision and monocular vision.

Vision plays an important part in everyday social interactions. Non-verbal cues and expressions are frequently used and without these the visually impaired person loses important sources of information. This makes interaction and communication with other people much more difficult. The individual may also experience fear and embarrassment about going out and coping in public places. Independence may be lost if the patient is unable to drive or travel alone. Personal relationships may become strained as the patient becomes more reliant on others for assistance with activities such as shopping and travel. The patient may also experience loss of confidence, low self-esteem and anxiety. Psychological reactions of shock, denial, isolation and anger are common reactions to impaired vision (Hall & Waterman, 1997). Patients will require sensitive counselling to facilitate adjustment to their loss.

An important role of the nurse is to begin the process of helping the patient learn to adjust to altered visual perception. The other senses must be used to compensate, for example feeling the wall, chair or bed, feeling stairs with the feet, hearing people approaching and so on. Nurses should do everything they can to orientate the patient to the environment (Hughes-Lamb, 1981). Basic considerations such as always placing the bedside locker and possessions in the same place so they can easily be located, and placing food and cutlery conveniently, are very important. The patient should also know what food is being served! A hospital ward or clinic can be a dangerous place for a visually impaired individual. Unnecessary furniture in the floor space, trolleys left in the walkways, bedstrippers left projecting, are all hazardous for the visually impaired.

Monocular vision and double vision cause loss of depth perception. Double vision sends especially confusing information to the brain. The best way to manage double vision is to keep the 'bad' eye covered, either by an eye patch, or a pair of spectacles with one lens made specially to prevent the eye from seeing. Moving around can be a demoralizing experience, with negotiation of furniture and stairs being particularly difficult. The patient may be inclined to wait for assistance, but daily practice with the nursing staff will help him/her to gradually adjust to the altered visual input, and so become independent. Supervised practice of tasks such as pouring a glass of water or cup of tea are vital to prevent accidents. The nurse should ensure a referral is made to the occupational therapist for help with this. It may take people as long as a year to adapt to altered visual images (Hughes-Lamb, 1981).

Jones & Diner (1992) suggest that the best way for the patient to cope with monocular vision is to move the head, instead of trying to look with the eye alone (i.e. moving the head sideways or up and down instead of glancing sideways, up or down). A hand mirror and wall mirror used together can be helpful for checking to see if makeup is blended properly, the face has been shaved evenly, or the hair is groomed correctly on the affected side. Good lighting is essential to maximize visual perception (Jones & Diner, 1992). A spotlight that can be angled to shine directly on to a page or object will help with grooming, reading or handicrafts.

Tactile examination of surfaces and objects is a must (Jones & Diner, 1992). As the patient reaches out for things, they will find that they are not exactly where they seem to be. Sliding the hand over the surface on which the object is will help to determine the exact location. On irregular surfaces, it helps to feel the surface with the hand before trying to set an object down, to locate a flat surface and avoid spills. When pouring into a glass or cup, it helps to rest the spout of the jug on the edge of the receptacle. Feeling fabrics and papers is the best way to determine their texture. If an object is being handed to a monocular individual, Jones & Diner (1992) advise that the individual keep their hand still, allowing the other person to put the object into it. This also works with hand shakes.

Driving is still possible for monocular people (Jones & Diner 1992). Although it can be frightening at first, the individual can learn to compensate for altered perception. Use of side and rear mirrors is very important and they should be adjusted to maximize range of perception. Special mirrors used by heavy goods vehicles, and for caravan towing can give a wider side and rear view and can be purchased at motor suppliers. Kerb feelers can also be purchased to give a scraping sound and alert the driver that the car is in the proper position next to the kerb.

It is recommended that patients protect their remaining eye with glasses (Jones & Diner, 1992), even if the vision in this eye does not require correction.

For people with low overall vision, magnifying lenses can be vital to allow them to read or perform handicrafts. There are many kinds of lenses available, from mirrors to help with grooming, to hand-held lenses for reading or close inspection, to floor stand models, or clip on models for sewing machines for example.

The patient may feel considerable loss of confidence and anxiety about the future if vision is impaired. It is essential that the nurse accesses such patients to the occupational therapist and specialist social services for the blind. This service will provide special equipment, such as clocks, medicine measures, electronic fluid indicators, etc., as well as advice on coping skills and benefits (see Chapter 1.4). A visual assessment by the local ophthalmology department is essential because, if vision is impaired significantly, being registered as partially sighted by an ophthalmologist ensures that the patient has access to more help. The nurse can help by ensuring that medical colleagues make this referral.

Summary

Head and neck cancer can frequently have a profound effect on sensory perception. Nurses should be aware that people with visual, auditory, olfactory or gustatory impairment are in fact suffering from sensory-perceptual deprivation. This means that their ability to function fully in their physical environment will be reduced. A sense of loss, and a feeling of threat to their future independence and quality of life will be experienced. The stress and negative impact of these disabilities can be minimized by sensitive and intelligent help from the nurse.

Strategy for practice

- Access patients with hearing and visual problems to specialist audiology and ophthalmology help, as well as social services.
- Provide information on coping strategies for all forms of altered sensory perception.
- Do not underestimate the negative effect on quality of life of altered taste and smell.
- Ensure that the patient with altered taste and smell takes measures to ensure safety, such as installing smoke alarms and careful storage of food (reading use by dates on food).

Resources

The Partially Sighted Society
Queen's Road
Doncaster
South Yorkshire DN1 2NX
Tel. 01302 323132

RNIB Talking Books Service
Mount Pleasant
Wembley
Middlesex HA0 1RR
Tel. 020 8903 6666

Royal National Institute for the Blind (RNIB)
224 Great Portland Street
London W1N 6AA
Tel. 020 7388 1266

Royal National Institute for the Deaf (RNID)
105 Gower Street
London WC1E 6AH
Tel. 020 7387 8033

Patient information books

- Jones J, Diner J (1992) A different dimension. Adapting to monocular vision. Available from Mr C Laycock, Oral Surgery Unit, West Middlesex University Hospital, Twickenham Road, Isleworth , Middlesex TW7 6AF
- What happened to your eye? Available from Changing Faces.
- A guide for blind and partially sighted people; Leaflet FB 19, The Benefits Agency. Available from social services departments.
- There is some very useful patient information about smell and taste disorders on the World Wide Web:

  http://www.blkbox.com/~rdevere/tsdc/index.html
  http://www.netdoor.com/entinfo/smellaao.html
  http://www.nih.gov/nidcd/smltaste.html
  http://www.entnet.org/smelltaste.html

Chapter 2.11
Pain

Introduction

Pain is often a problem with any type of cancer diagnosis, but the significance of pain in the head and neck region is magnified because of the importance of this area in nutrition, communication, and social and psychological interactions. Pain can be caused by oncological treatment, as well as by disease processes. It is important that this pain is managed well in order to ensure that patients tolerate their course of treatment. Chronic malignant pain is progressive, irreversible, cyclic (varying from aching to agonizing), intractable, and conveys a sense of hopelessness to the patient. It is therefore also very important that this pain is managed well. The role of the nurse is central to optimum pain management and therefore a good knowledge of pain and pain management is essential. This chapter will give a brief overview of pain and then discuss the management of head and neck cancer pain in more detail.

Pain: overview and the vital role of nursing

Pain is an incredibly complex concept consisting of a multitude of theories, mechanisms, dimensions, meanings and experiences. The experience of pain is highly individual and gives rise to a language of pain, both verbal and non-verbal. It is beyond the scope of this chapter to describe all aspects of pain in great depth, but a brief overview will be given as background information. The reader is referred to McGuire & Sheidler's (1997) excellent chapter on pain in cancer nursing. A brief summary of salient points is given below.

The six dimensions of pain

McGuire and Sheidler (1997) describe a conceptual model of cancer pain in which six dimensions of pain are defined:

- Physiological: pain associated with tumour (bone infiltration, nerve infiltration, viscera infiltration), pain associated with cancer therapy (surgery, radiotherapy, chemotherapy) and pain unrelated to cancer or its treatment.
- Sensory: the location(s), intensity (none, mild, moderate, severe, excruciating, bad, intense) and quality (tender, aching, throbbing, stabbing, shooting, sore) of pain.
- Affective: depression, anxiety, or other psychological factors associated with pain.
- Cognitive: the manner in which pain influences the individual's thought processes. The meaning that pain holds for an individual significantly affects their ability to cope with it, their perceived level of pain, and their affective state.
- Behavioural: activity levels, intake of analgesics, verbal and non-verbal communication of pain, use of pain controlling activities.
- Sociocultural: demographic, ethnic, cultural and spiritual factors.

Factors affecting pain management

Pain has a significant impact on quality of life for both patients and their families. Good pain management is an essential part of the nurse's role. Evidence shows, however, that pain is frequently not well managed due to factors involving healthcare professionals, patients and healthcare organizations. These factors include:

- lack of understanding about pain
- expectation that pain should be present
- relief of pain not viewed as a goal of treatment
- inadequate or non-existent assessment
- under-treatment with analgesics
- inadequate knowledge of analgesics and other drugs
- fears of addiction, sedation, and respiratory depression
- inadequate knowledge of other interventions for pain
- perceptual differences between patients and healthcare providers
- legal impediments.

The nurse's role

The Oncology Nursing Society's position paper on cancer pain (Spross et al, 1990) defines the nurse's role as:

1. describing the pain
2. identifying aggravating and relieving factors
3. determining the meaning of pain
4. determining its cause
5. determining the individual's definition of optimal pain relief
6. deriving nursing diagnoses
7. assisting in selecting interventions
8. evaluating the efficacy of interventions.

The nurse's emphasis should be on the individual as a whole and their response to pain. Attention is also paid to the effect on significant others and support systems.

McGuire and Sheidler (1997) assert that oncology nurses, by virtue of their prolonged contact and relationships with patients and families across a variety of settings, are best prepared to assume a leadership role in the assessment and management of pain.

Assessment of pain

Systematic nursing assessment of pain is essential. It establishes a baseline, assists in the selection of interventions, and allows evaluation of interventions. This assessment is different from the simple measurement of pain, as it includes assessment of the pain in all of the six dimensions described above. Pain assessment in the head and neck cancer patient may be particularly difficult due to impaired speech and communication (see Chapter 2.5 on altered communication).

Assessment tools are very helpful in systematic pain assessment, and there is extensive literature on instruments (see McGuire and Sheidler, 1997, Chapter 20, for a comprehensive summary of tools). Pain assessment tools have the potential to improve pain management but they are often not used effectively (Carr, 1997; MacLellan, 1997). Additionally, most of the tools used in the clinical setting tend to measure only the sensory dimension of pain. There is an urgent need to develop pain management strategies that reflect the multidimensional nature of pain (Carr, 1997). Indeed, behavioural, affec-

tive and cognitive problems amenable to treatment can go unde-
tected when pain is evaluated and treated purely as a biological
phenomenon.

Keefe et al (1985) believe that cancer of the head and neck is a
particularly appropriate form of cancer in which to apply behavioural assessment techniques. Behavioural approaches to the assessment of cancer pain help to identify specific daily activities and
events that exacerbate pain. These activities and the patient's
response to them may then be modified. They can also help to assess
the effects of pain control interventions. In order to clarify what is
meant by behavioural pain assessment, it might be helpful to
summarize Keefe et al's study of a group of 30 individuals with head
and neck cancer undergoing active radiotherapy treatment. They
describe the following pain behaviours:

- Motor pain behaviours (guarding movement, body posturing,
  grimacing, rubbing, sighing). These are all observable actions
  which communicate that pain is being experienced. Keefe at al
  (1985) report grimacing to be the most common behaviour of
  pain in patients undergoing radiotherapy treatment.
- Activities that increase pain (chewing, swallowing, movement of
  the head and neck). Patients tended to avoid such activities, especially eating; there was a strong tendency for patients to lose
  weight.
- Methods to relieve pain (heat, cold, pain medication, rest,
  massage, avoidance of activity). Patients significantly increased
  the number of pain-relieving methods used over time of treatment. The main activity was use of narcotic analgesics.
- Activity level. Patients' activity levels decreased significantly over
  the duration of their treatment. However, more time was spent
  sitting than lying down.

Behavioural Dysfunction Index scores were strongly related to
pain ratings in this study; pain-related behaviour problems are
clearly evident in head and neck cancer patients. The authors
conclude that the focus of pain assessments for this group of patients
should be broadened to consider the impact of pain on behaviour
and lifestyle.

It is also important to determine accurately the type and cause of
pain in order to identify the most effective intervention. Inaccurate

pain assessment is a major cause of misdiagnosis and inappropriate management (World Health Organization, 1990).

Causes and sites of pain in head and neck cancer

Keefe et al (1986) report that pain in head and neck cancer patients is most frequent in the jaw, mouth, neck and shoulder; 50% of their sample of 30 patients experienced pain. Patients with advanced disease experienced considerably more pain than those with early disease. Pain was localized to tumour and incision site. Patients who experienced severe pain before treatment were likely to experience pain after treatment. Other studies report pain rates of 40% to 80% in head and neck cancer (Shedd et al, 1980; Grond et al, 1993; Forbes, 1997). Vecht et al (1992) found that 64% of 25 patients had cancer-related pain, 20% therapy-related pain and 16% debility-related pain. Grond et al (1993) found that 83% of 167 head and neck cancer patients had pain caused by cancer, and 28% pain due to the effects of treatment. Seventy per cent of patients had nociceptive pain, and 25% had neuropathic pain (definitions of nociceptive and neuropathic pain are given below). The causes of head and neck cancer pain are as follows.

Tumour and metastasis

Pain is often a presenting symptom in head and neck cancer (Epstein & Stewart, 1993; Epstein & Jones, 1993); for example, denture pain may often be the first symptom of an oral lesion (Amagasa et al, 1985). Pain frequently precedes recurrent disease in head and neck cancer (Wong et al, 1998). Tumour may have a direct effect on muscles, limiting mandibular movement. It may cause bone destruction and fracture, and nerve compression or infiltration. Bone destruction is common in head and neck cancer, in the mandible, maxilla, skull base, sinuses and nasopharynx. Metastasis or direct extension of tumours into the base of skull cause specific pain syndromes. These consist of headache (frontal, vertex or occipital pain) and dysfunction of the affected cranial nerve, depending on the site of the lesion (Twycross, 1994). Pathological evidence of perineural invasion was found to occur in 44% of 100 head and neck cancer surgical cases, and 88% of 17 terminal cases (Carter et al, 1982).

Lymphoedema

Lymphoedema often causes distension of pain-sensitive structures, with sensations of 'tightness' and 'pulling'.

Infection

Infection can be secondary to tumour, surgery, chemotherapy, radiotherapy and implants. Superimposed infection of the oral mucosa during radiotherapy and chemotherapy exacerbates mucositis. Acute infection of ulcerating lesions causes pain. Fungal infections of the oral cavity are also problems associated with xerostomia, causing a 'burning' pain.

Surgery

Pain is an obvious immediate complication of surgery (Epstein & Stewart, 1993). In addition, surgery may result in damage to neural structures and may lead to persistent neuropathic pain. Pain may also develop due to the impairment of function of the jaw following resection, discontinuity of the jaw, and fibrosis of tissue leading to altered function. Neuropathic pain often occurs after surgery due to the sacrificing of sensory nerve branches, particularly during lymph node dissection (see Chapter 4.1). In Vecht et al's study (1992), 24% of patients experienced pain due to neck dissection. The auriculotemporal, transversus colli, and supraclavicular nerves are most commonly associated with pain after neck dissection.

Watt-Watson & Graydon (1995) report 65% of 44 head and neck cancer patients experiencing moderate to severe pain post-surgery. They were not given adequate analgesia and pain was often unrelieved. Patients with higher pain scores had correspondingly higher fatigue scores. The authors recommend that the common use of codeine preparations for pain relief for patients with moderate to severe pain after surgery be reviewed.

Radiotherapy

Radiotherapy-related pain results from direct damage to normal tissues due to mucosal inflammation and ulceration, epithelial thinning, mucosal atrophy and xerostomia (see Chapter 4.3). These conditions all create a severe, continuous 'burning' pain that usually begins during the second or third week of treatment. Modern techniques for delivering head and neck radiation include accelerated fractionation and hyperfractionation. Neoadjuvant and concurrent chemotherapy are also increasingly being used (see Chapter 4.4). All of these treatment modalities may cause more severe mucosal reactions. Management of these side effects is imperative, since a delay in treatment due to intolerance of side effects will reduce its efficacy and therefore reduce chances of cure (Weissman et al, 1989).

Epstein & Stewart (1993) found that all of 34 patients undergoing head and neck irradiation reported pain of increasing severity during treatment; 73% of these experienced severe pain. From the middle to the end of their treatment courses they described it as 'distressing' (50% of patients from mid-treatment to end of treatment) and 'horrible' (21% from mid-treatment, rising to 23% by the end of treatment).

Similarly, Weissman et al (1989) found that 21 patients undergoing head and neck irradiation experienced severe pain during radiotherapy treatment which they described as 'burning', 'aching', 'sharp', 'throbbing' and 'shooting'. In this study 93% of patients experienced eating disturbance due to pain (eight patients experienced greater than 2 kg weight loss), 79% noted sleep disturbance due to pain, 64% noted disturbance in energy levels due to pain. On 58% of treatment days the pain was 'always present' or 'present throughout most of the day', despite analgesics. Weissman et al conclude that pain control was poor due to:

- analgesics administered being of insufficient potency, or inadequate dosing schedule
- direct mucosal irritation by some drugs negated their analgesic effects
- topical anaesthetics are not optimal for continuous pain due to their short activity
- alcohol in drug preparations produced a burning effect.

The authors recommend more liberal use of strong opioids given 'around the clock', preferably in a transdermal delivery system. These issues will be discussed below.

Good oral hygiene is also essential to minimize mucositis. See Chapter 2.2 for more information.

Radiation fibrosis of muscles and soft tissue may occur as late effects of treatment. Osteoradionecrosis of the mandible is a most distressing late effect. The treatment of pain caused by soft tissue and bone injury due to radiotherapy includes antibiotic therapy, and wound debridement (Futran et al, 1997). Occasionally, surgery is required to remove the damaged tissue and bring in new blood supply. Hyperbaric oxygen may contribute to wound healing in some patients (Hart & Mainous, 1976; King et al, 1989). Pentoxifylline may be helpful in the healing of less severe forms of soft tissue injury (Futran et al, 1997). It produces lower blood viscosity, improved erythrocyte flexibility and increased tissue oxygenation.

Psychosocial and emotional causes of pain

Stress, anxiety and depression associated with cancer, dysfunction and disfigurement heighten perceptions of pain. They play a major part in myofascial pain. Importantly, they also modify the benefits of analgesia. Interestingly, they are also factors associated with disorder of the temporomandibular joint (Epstein & Stewart, 1993).

Types of pain in head and neck cancer

There are a great many specific pain syndromes in head and neck cancer due to the dense sensory innervation of the face and anterior skull (Vecht et al, 1992). These factors also mean that head and neck cancer pain is often difficult to treat. The types of pain can be categorized as follows (information from Melzack & Wall, 1991a; Twycross, 1994 unless otherwise stated).

Nociceptive pain

Tissue damage caused by tumour, surgery, radiotherapy, infection or chemotherapy causes the release of chemicals. These chemicals include bradykinin, histamine, peptides such as substance P and prostaglandins. These all cause local inflammation and sensitize nociceptors, causing swelling, aching, tenderness and soreness, or *nociceptive* pain. Prostaglandin is particularly important in this process. Bone pain is a specific type of nociceptive pain which is common in head and neck cancer.

Neuropathic pain

Neuropathic pain is usually present with little or no evidence of inflammation and is caused by pathological changes in the function of nerve input and processing. The result is distorted and unpleasant sensation. This includes:

- hyperalgesia (increased response to painful stimuli)
- allodynia (hypersensitivity to light stimuli; touch of fabric, changes in temperature, wind)
- paraesthesias (tingling, pins and needles)
- spontaneous stabbing or shooting pain
- dysaesthesia (a very unpleasant sensation which is hard for the patient to describe)
- causalgia (burning pain).

  There are several causes of neuropathic pain.

'Wind up'

Prolonged nociceptive pain can cause changes in the central nervous system processing of pain, and thus can lead to the development of neuropathic pain. One mechanism for this is via increased activity of the B and C nerve fibres which causes increased sensitivity of receptors in the spinal cord to stimuli. This can contribute to a phenomenon called 'wind up' whereby N-methyl-D-aspartate (NMDA) receptors in the spinal cord become more excitable to stimuli, and less responsive to opioids (Twycross, 1994).

Peripheral nerve damage

Nerve damage can be caused by treatment (surgery, chemotherapy, radiotherapy), infiltration of a nerve by cancer and compression of a nerve by tumour.

- After nerves have been cut during surgery, sprouts are formed from the severed end which can grow to form neuromas. Neuromas cause paraesthesia sensations when touched. The ends of these nerve sprouts can also become sensitized to chemicals in the tissues around them. Some develop adrenergic receptors and thus can become sensitized to sympathetic chemicals such as noradrenaline.
- Peripheral nerves damaged by tumour infiltration or compression give off abnormal afferent impulses causing nerve pain sensations. These sensations are confined to the dermatomes of the specific nerve or nerves affected (see Tables 2.11.1 and 2.11.2 and Figure 2.11.1).
- Radiotherapy can damage the Schwann cells of the myelin sheath and also the glial cells. This damage leads to abnormal afferent impulses.

Table 2.11.1: The cervical plexus (see Figure 2.11.1 for dermatomes) consists of the ventral rami of spinal nerves C1 to C5

Nerve	Distribution
Great auricular nerve	Skin and muscle of the
Lesser occipital nerve	scalp, neck, ear
Supraclavicular nerves	Shoulder
Transverse cervical nerve	Upper chest
Phrenic nerve	Diaphragm muscle
Ansa cervicalis	Extrinsic laryngeal muscles

Information from Agur (1991), Martini (1992c) and McMinn et al (1994).

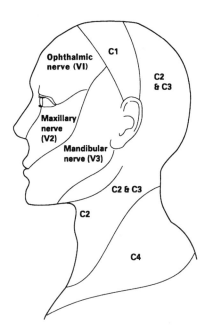

Figure 2.11.1: Dermatomes of the trigeminal nerve and cervical plexus.

Referred pain may be caused by compression of a peripheral nerve. A common example is the laryngeal tumour which compresses the vagus nerve. The vagus nerve provides sensory innervation to the external auditory meatus, and the brain misinterprets the impulses caused by this compression, perceiving them as earache. Another example is the headache caused by compression of cranial nerves in the skull base (see section on Tumour and metastasis, p. 286).

Table 2.11.2: The cranial nerves

No.	Name	Special sense function	Sensory function	Motor function	Parasympathetic function
I	Olfactory	Smell			
II	Optic	Sight			
III	Oculomotor			Orbital muscles	Ciliary muscle and pupils
IV	Trochlear			Orbital muscles	
V	Trigeminal		CN V1 ophthalmic nerve CN V2 maxillary nerve CN V3 mandibular nerve • see Figure 2.11.1 for dermatomes	Temporalis, masseter, pterygoid, tensor veli palatini, tensor tympani, mylohyoid and anterior digastric muscles	
VI	Abducens			Orbital muscles	
VII	Facial	Taste (palate and anterior tongue)	External acoustic meatus and the auricle	The muscles of expression around the eye, nose, mouth and ear, scalp, platysma, stylohyoid, posterior digastric, stapedius muscles	Glands of nose, palate, lacrimal gland, submandibular and sublingual salivary glands
VIII	Vestibulocochlear	Balance and hearing			
IX	Glossopharyngeal	Taste (posterior tongue)	Pharynx, oropharynx, auditory tube, tympanum, inner eardrum, mastoid antrum, mastoid cells, carotid sinus and body	Stylopharyngeus muscle	Parotid gland

(contd)

Table 2.11.2: (contd)

No.	Name	Special sense function	Sensory function	Motor function	Parasympathetic function
X	Vagus	Taste (epiglottis)	Outer eardrum, external acoustic meatus, back of auricle, mucous surface of lower pharynx, larynx, trachea. Also extends to lungs, oesophagus and abdomen	All smooth muscle, all laryngeal muscles, all pharyngeal muscles (except stylopharyngeus), all muscles of palate (except tensor veli palatini)	All secretory glands
XI	Accessory			Sternocleidomastoid, trapezius muscles	
XII	Hypoglossal			All the muscles of the tongue (except palatoglossus), geniohyoid, thyrohyoid, strap muscles of hyoid	

Information from Agur (1991).

Changes in processing in the central nervous system

Continuous abnormal messages from local inflammatory processes and peripheral nerve damage eventually cause changes in both the spinal cord and the brain. These changes include the activation of normally inhibited inputs (causing increased sensitivity), changes in the dorsal root ganglion cells (causing increased sensitivity), changes in the spinal cord terminals (causing inhibitory mechanisms to fail) and changes in the brain (also causing increased sensitivity). All these factors lead to chronic neuropathic pain.

Neuropathic pain may sometimes be accompanied by sympathetic dysfunction such as cutaneous vasodilatation, increased skin temperature and abnormal sweating (Twycross, 1997).

Neuropathic pain is less responsive to opioids than nociceptive pain. Mercadante et al (1997) report that patients with head and neck cancer had pain that was less responsive to opioid treatment. They surmise that this may be due to a higher incidence of neuropathic pain, as well as psychological distress due to disfigurement. Thus additional drugs and interventions must be used to treat neuropathic pain.

Sympathetically maintained pain

In this condition there is an interaction between the sympathetic and sensory nerves that results in pain similar to neuropathic pain. It can be produced by tissue or nerve injury. Malignant cervical lymph nodes can cause sympathetically mediated pain which is manifested as burning pain up the line of the carotid vessels (see Figure 2.8.1) and over the hemicranium. It may be worse lying down. The patient will dislike using a hairbrush on the affected side.

Myofascial pain

Myofascial pain is a form of cramp often associated with the presence of one or more hypersensitive trigger points within the muscle, together with muscle spasm, pain (often referred into neighbouring areas), tenderness, stiffness and reduced movement (Twycross, 1997). This type of pain is often opioid resistant. It is often associated with bone pain and anxiety is an important exacerbating factor. Injection of trigger points can be performed using normal saline or local anaesthetic (King & Jacob, 1993). The trigger point is located by palpation, with the muscle stretched, to find a taut band of muscle. Correct location is confirmed by the patient stating when he/she feels the worst pain.

Interventions for pain

Antitumour therapy

Radiotherapy, surgery and chemotherapy are all used as first-line treatment; however second-line antitumour treatment in extensively pre-treated patients gives a small chance of response (Vecht et al, 1992). Radiotherapy treats the pain of bone metastases very successfully (Needham & Hoskin, 1994). It can also be useful in pain resulting from nerve root infiltration (Abrams & Hansen, 1989). Chemotherapy can also be used to palliate symptoms.

Pharmacological therapy

Pharmacological treatment of pain is the mainstay of therapy. Because of the complex mechanisms of pain in the head and neck, a combination of drugs may be required to act on the different types of pain. Vecht et al (1992) recommend that treatment for head and neck cancer pain should be based on the type of pain; assessment of the type and cause of the pain helps to define proper therapy.

Drugs for nociceptive pain

The World Health Organization (WHO) analgesic ladder (Table 2.11.3) gives the recommended steps of treatment for nociceptive pain. Several studies show that the WHO guidelines for relief of cancer pain are very effective for individuals with head and neck cancer (Vecht et al, 1992; Grond et al, 1993; Talmi et al, 1997).

Table 2.11.3: The World Health Organization three-step analgesic ladder

Step one	Non-opioid (NSAID, paracetamol) ± adjuvant
Step two	Weak opioid (e.g. codeine, distalgesic) plus step one drug ± adjuvant
Step three	Strong opioid (e.g. morphine, fentanyl) plus step one drug ± adjuvant

WHO (1990).

Non-opioids

- *Non-steroidal anti-inflammatory drugs (NSAIDs)*, their site of action is the site of injury where they inhibit prostaglandin synthesis. They do not produce physical dependence, tolerance or addiction. NSAIDs have antiplatelet properties and therefore should be used with caution in the preoperative and perioperative period. They are also thought to act on the central nervous system. Examples are aspirin, ibuprofen, flurbiprofen, indomethacin, naproxen and diclofenac.
- *Paracetamol* is thought to act on the central nervous system.

Opioids

- Opioids are very effective analgesics that interact with the opioid receptors in the spinal cord to inhibit nociception. Drugs in this group include weak opioids (e.g. codeine, dihydrocodeine, co-proxamol and tramadol) and strong opioids (e.g. morphine, fentanyl and methadone). Morphine is very commonly used for cancer pain; it has highly effective anti-nociceptive and anti-anxiety effects and is available in short-acting, immediate release preparations and sustained-release preparations (Laurence et al, 1997a). Morphine is also the cornerstone of postoperative pain management, especially for extensive surgical procedures that cause moderate to severe pain (Carr et al, 1992). A combination of NSAID and opioid works best, as this gives combined action at the site of injury and centrally in the spinal cord.

Drugs for neuropathic pain

It is important to understand that the drugs listed above for nociceptive pain also help with neuropathic pain, but may be enhanced by the addition of drugs that reverse the abnormal processing in peripheral nerves and the central nervous system. Twycross (1997) proposes an additional ladder for neuropathic pain (Table 2.11.4).

Table 2.11.4: A four-step analgesic ladder for nerve injury pain

Step one	Tricyclic antidepressant or anticonvulsant
Step two	Tricyclic antidepressant and anticonvulsant
Step three	Class 1 cardiac anti-arrhythmic or ketamine
Step four	Spinal analgesia

From Twycross (1997).

- *Antidepressants.* This group of drugs act against changes in processing in the central nervous system (described above). They inhibit the reuptake of serotonin and noradrenaline (inhibitory chemicals), thus reducing excitability in the spinal cord. They also potentiate the effects of opioids and can thus be used in conjunction with opioids. They are useful for pain that has a continuous, dysaesthetic, burning quality. The most commonly used are the tricyclic antidepressants, particularly amitriptyline. A major disadvantage of these drugs in head and neck cancer is the exacerbation of dry mouth. Analgesic action is effected within 24 to 48 hours. Dosage is less than that used for antidepressant effect; the dose range is from 10 to 100 mg per day.
- *Anticonvulsants.* This group of drugs are useful for shooting/stabbing pains (Swerdlow & Cundill, 1981). They act against changes in processing in the central nervous system (described above) in preventing neuronal excitation by stabilizing the cell membrane and enhancing inhibitory mechanisms. Examples are sodium valproate, clonazepam, gabapentin, carbamazopine and lamotrigine.
- *Class 1 cardiac anti-arrhythmics.* These drugs are chemically related to local anaesthetics and act as cell membrane stabilizers. They should never be given to patients with heart failure and never administered with tricyclic antidepressants (Twycross, 1997). Examples are mexiletine and flecainide. A specialist pain team would normally be involved in the prescribing of these drugs.
- *Ketamine.* This is used for neuropathic pain because, as an NMDA antagonist, it reduces excitability of receptors in the spinal cord (see changes in processing in the central nervous system, above), and also enhances the action of opioids (Twycross, 1997). Thus it can be useful with an opioid. It is an effective drug for the treatment of 'wind up'. A specialist pain team would normally be involved in the prescribing of this drug. Other drugs with an NMDA antagonist effect include co-proxamol and methadone.
- *Antispasmodics.* Baclofen inhibits transmission in the spinal cord. It can be useful in myofascial pain (Laurence et al, 1997a). Diazepam can also be used as a muscle relaxant.
- *Capsaicin.* This is a substance found in chili peppers. It affects the synthesis and release of substance P and is toxic to C fibres. It is therefore useful as a topical agent in causalgic pain. A specialist pain team would normally be involved in the prescribing of this drug.

- *Corticosteroids.* These are pure anti-inflammatory agents and are very effective in the treatment of nerve compression (Twycross, 1997) and pain due to inflammation.

Adjuvants: drugs to control other symptoms and side effects of analgesics

- Adjuvant drugs should be used to manage other symptoms that may arise. For example, antibiotics to treat infection, and topical therapy such as mucosal coating agents to treat mucositis (Grond et al, 1993).
- Adjuvants such as laxatives, antacids, histamine-2 receptor antagonists, anti-emetics, anxiolytics and hypnotics should also be prescribed to ameliorate coexisting symptoms or side effects of analgesic treatment (Grond et al, 1993).

Analgesic drug administration

Analgesics should be administered on a regular, fixed-time dosing schedule. Dosing should be continually monitored and adjusted promptly to control pain and reduce side effects. It should include measures to deal with breakthrough pain (Twycross, 1997).

In Vecht et al's (1992) study of 25 patients with severe head and neck cancer pain referred to a pain clinic, good pain relief was achieved in 72% of patients using the WHO interventions. However, several successive attempts at treating the pain were usually needed, alone or in combination. Grond et al (1993) report that use of the WHO guidelines in the treatment of 167 head and neck cancer patients was very successful; severe pain was experienced during only 5% of their treatment days. They conclude that WHO guidelines are the most effective way of managing head and neck cancer pain. The most common reason for failure to control pain was failure to use the WHO guidelines, especially regarding the use of step one analgesics and coanalgesics.

For those who would like a more comprehensive overview of pharmacological therapy, Twycross 1994 is recommended reading.

Nerve blocks

Nerve blocks are used to achieve pain relief by the blocking or destruction of the nerve fibres (Melzack & Wall, 1991). Non-destructive nerve blocks involve the use of local anaesthetic. They treat pain for a short time (12–24 hours) but when steroids are also injected they can take the pressure off nerves and exert a longer effect. Destructive nerve blocks offer more prolonged relief . This can be achieved by injecting toxic agents such as alcohol or phenol, or burning the nerve fibres by passing a high-frequency current through the tip of a needle (radiofrequency electrocoagulation). Another method is to freeze the nerve (cryoanalgesia); function usually returns some time after this procedure. If the painful area is large or close to the spine, more central structures may need to be treated (King & Jacob, 1993). Because of the range of neurophysiological disturbances that contribute to pain in the head and neck, responses to nerve blocks can be very variable (Twycross, 1994).

Peripheral, paravertebral and sympathetic nerve blocks may be useful in head and neck cancer pain. Common nerve blocks for head and neck pain are: stellate ganglion blocks, trigeminal blocks, cervical plexus blocks and glossopharyngeal blocks. The indication for paravertebral blocks is intractable pain in a limited segmental area served by peripheral nerves in a patient whose life expectancy is 1 year or less (Wood, 1994). The indication for peripheral nerve block (e.g. trigeminal or glossopharyngeal) is pain in a specific area supplied by a single nerve.

Prior to the procedure, the skin is numbed using local anaesthetic. Using X-ray to visualize placement, a local anaesthetic is injected first to check correct placement, before administering the neurolytic agent. The ultimate effect of a block cannot be evaluated for 24–48 hours, by which time the local anaesthetic effect will have been replaced by the effect of the nerve destruction. If blocks are effective, the duration of pain relief varies from 2 to 4 months (paravertebral blocks) and 3 weeks to 6 months (peripheral nerve blocks) (Wood, 1994).

Side effects of nerve blocks

Several complications may occur as a result of the use of nerve blocks (Latham, 1983). Complications common to all nerve blocks in the head and neck include:

- pain at the puncture site; if this persists for more than a few days causes other than local tissue trauma should be sought, for example infection or trauma to a nerve

- bruising or haematoma at the puncture site
- haemorrhage; if a blood vessel is accidentally punctured (neural block is contraindicated in patients with prolonged clotting time)
- inadvertent injection into the cerebral subarachnoid space, leading to loss of consciousness and possible respiratory arrest
- nerve blocks will destroy both motor and sensory nerve fibres and the muscles supplied by the nerve blocked will be weakened or paralysed unless the nerve carries only sensory fibres.

Specific nerve blocks

Stellate ganglion block: Sympathetically maintained pain does not respond to analgesics, but it does respond to sympathetic nerve blocks. Sympathetic blockade is only effective for sympathetically maintained pain (Verrill, 1994). The sympathetic supply to the head, neck and arm can be interrupted at the stellate ganglion. The stellate ganglion (the combined inferior cervical and first thoracic ganglia) lies in the neck just over the neck of the first rib.

Side effects of stellate ganglion block include temporary hoarse voice, difficulty swallowing, transient arm weakness on the side treated, and Horner's syndrome (ptosis, facial flushing, blocked nose and pupil constriction on the treated side). Pneumothorax is a possible complication of stellate ganglion block (King & Jacob, 1993).

Trigeminal block: See Table 2.11.2 and Figure 2.11.1 for the distribution and functions of the trigeminal nerve. Side effects of a trigeminal block include muscle weakness (which often recovers after 3–4 days; weakness lasting beyond this is likely to be permanent), temporary loss of corneal reflex, numbness and unpleasant paraesthesia in the numbed area (Shapsay et al, 1980). Transient trismus may occur, resolving over 72 hours.

Glossopharyngeal block: See Table 2.11.2 and Figure 2.11.1 for the distribution and functions of the glossopharyngeal nerve. Side effects include possible temporary vocal cord paralysis and swallowing difficulties (Shapsay et al, 1980). There is also a possibility of late paraesthesia.

Cervical plexus block: See Figure 2.11.1 and Table 2.11.1 for the distribution of the cervical plexus. Side effects include accidental block of the phrenic nerve, causing diaphragmatic paralysis and hypoxia, blocking of the vagus nerve, block of the sympathetic chain causing

Horner's syndrome, and the recurrent laryngeal nerve causing hoarseness (Latham, 1983). Puncture of the oesophagus is also a possibility, causing dysphagia and tenderness at the puncture site. Antibiotic therapy is essential if this should occur (Latham, 1983).

Nursing care following nerve blocks

Nursing care for the patient undergoing nerve block includes preparation for the procedure, outlining the postoperative side effects to be expected. The patient should understand that it is important to lie very still during the procedure, to minimize accidental trauma to adjacent nerves and blood vessels. Postoperatively, the nurse should observe carefully for any complications, such as hypotension and haematoma, for 2 hours. If injected neurolytic agents have been used, the position of the patient is crucial and should be maintained as instructed.

Opinion is divided as to how frequently neuro-destructive techniques should be used in the head and neck. Receptors for a variety of pain stimuli (pressure, chemical, temperature) densely populate the tissues of the head and neck, and the afferents subserving these tissues pass through several cranial and peripheral nerves making efficacy of nerve blocks very variable. Grond et al (1993) recommend that they should only be used if pharmacological therapy has failed. However Boys et al (1993) propose that 'less morphine and more nerve blocks' be used in order to minimize the side effects of high opiate dosage.

Psychological interventions

Medical interventions are used to treat physiological and sensory aspects of pain, whilst non-drug methods are aimed at treating the affective, cognitive, behavioural and sociocultural dimensions of pain. The benefits of these techniques are that they increase the individual's sense of control, reduce feelings of helplessness, reduce anxiety and stress, elevate mood and raise pain thresholds. They are not intended as the main treatment of pain, but rather as adjuvant therapies (McGuire & Sheidler, 1997).

- Psychosocial care is very important, as psychological distress and sociocultural factors are probably the most important factors limiting an effective analgesic regime (Mercandante et al, 1997). Psychological responses to pain such as hopelessness, fear and anxiety can heighten the severity and behavioural impact of pain (Keefe et al, 1985). Secondary effects of pain, such as decreased eating leading to weight loss; decreased exercise; and depression, can play an important role in reducing tolerance to treatment regimes. Professional time spent exploring worries and fears is time well spent and relates directly to pain management (Twycross, 1997).

- Cognitive therapy attempts to modify thought processes through strategies such as information and education provision, distraction, imagery and calming self-statements.

- Behavioural therapy attempts to modify physiological reactions to pain, or behavioural manifestations of pain, through strategies such as relaxation techniques, biofeedback, meditation, music therapy and hypnosis. Teaching patients to alter maladaptive behavioural reactions to pain can help to control pain, but this method is often under-utilized (Keefe et al, 1985). Behavioural and cognitive methods may be used together; for example, relaxation with guided imagery. The nurse should be aware that myofascial pain and trismus may respond well to interventions to manage anxiety and to specific relaxation exercises for the jaw.

- Diversional activity is another important factor in pain control. Pain perception requires consciousness and attention. Pain is worse when it occupies a person's whole attention. Diversional activity does more than pass time: it diminishes pain (Twycross, 1997).

Stimulation techniques

Cutaneous stimulation

Cutaneous stimulation takes several forms, the exact mechanisms of which are poorly understood. They can, however, be very effective. Transcutaneous electrical nerve stimulation (TENS) acts by activating the large A fibres which inhibit the response of the dorsal horn cells to input from B and C fibres (Melzack & Wall, 1991b). Other techniques include application of menthol ointments, heat and cold and massage (Melzack & Wall, 1991). These act by changing the perception of pain, and also fall within the domain of behavioural interventions. Massage may be used very effectively alongside relaxation techniques.

Acupuncture

Acupuncture is an ancient Chinese practice that has been in continuous use for at least 2,000 years. It involves the insertion of fine needles through specific points of the skin and then twirling them for some time at a very slow rate. Pain is believed to be due to disharmony between Yin and Yang energies (Chi) which flow through the body in channels called meridians. There are 14 meridians and on these lie 361 acupuncture points. Acupuncture has been demonstrated to have significantly greater effects on pain than placebo stimulation (Melzack & Wall, 1991). There are no specific rigorous studies on the use of acupuncture in head and neck cancer, but a systematic review of 16 studies on the use of acupuncture in dental pain concluded that it is effective in relieving dental pain (Ernst & Pittler, 1998). In a small pilot study of four head and neck cancer patients undergoing radiotherapy, Hidderley and Weinel (1997) seemed to demonstrate enhanced pain relief when TENS was applied to acupuncture points related to the site of pain.

Routes of analgesic administration in head and neck cancer

The route chosen for analgesic administration should always be the simplest, which will have the least effect on the patient's quality of life.

Oral/enteral

The oral route for analgesics is the most straightforward, inexpensive and safe route of administration but may not always be possible in head and neck cancer because of swallowing difficulties. Many patients will be able to manage oral drugs in liquid or soluble form, but if oral administration is not possible, the next route to consider is via the patient's enteral feeding tube (nasogastric tube or gastrostomy tube). Again, liquid or soluble preparations of analgesics are available for this purpose (Grond et al, 1993). Some tablets may be crushed and dissolved; check with the pharmacist. Morphine is supplied in both rapid-acting and slow-release forms. Once the patient has been titrated to the appropriate dose with rapid-acting morphine, conversion to slow-release morphine will greatly reduce the disruption of 4-hourly doses and allow a good night's sleep. Slow-release morphine sulphate tablets should never be crushed; sachets of slow-release granules are readily available for dissolving in water.

Transdermal

The transdermal route is a useful option for head and neck cancer patients. Fentanyl is a potent opioid analgesic, available in the form of a transdermal patch (Durogesic). This is much easier for patients who experience difficulty instilling medication via their feeding tube, or who have poor compliance. It also simplifies medication regimes and saves nursing time. It may also be much more acceptable to patients who have a psychological dislike of 'taking tablets'. In one study, 54% of 136 patients preferred fentanyl patches to sustained-release morphine; they caused less interruption to daily activities, and the activities of family and carers (Ahmedzai & Brooks, 1997).

Transdermal fentanyl has been shown to be as effective as morphine for pain control. It was also associated with significantly less constipation and daytime drowsiness (Ahmedzai & Brooks, 1997; Donner et al, 1998). Analgesic fentanyl concentrations in the plasma can be expected within the first 6–12 hours of the first application. Plasma concentrations rise steadily for the first 5 days and once steady levels are achieved they remain relatively constant for 72 hours and can be maintained by patch replacement every 72 hours thereafter (Janssen-Cilag Limited, 1996). Some patients may require more frequent application (Donner et al, 1998). Patients converted from a morphine regimen should continue to take morphine for 12 to 24 hours after the first application. If a syringe driver is in place, fentanyl should be allowed to reach therapeutic levels before removal of the driver. Morphine withdrawal symptoms may be experienced for the first 72 hours (diarrhoea, nausea, depression, anxiety, shivering) and these can be relieved by adequate rescue doses of immediate release morphine. Table 2.11.5 shows a simple conversion guide from morphine.

Durogesic is applied by peeling off the backing film and sticking the patch to a clean, dry, undamaged, hairless area of skin. The area used should be rotated. It should not be applied under a clothing strap or tight band. A high temperature may enhance absorption of the drug. Hot baths and showers should be avoided, as should the application of heat pads over the patch. Individuals who experience difficulties with patch adherence can use adhesive tape (e.g. Microp-

Table 2.11.5: Morphine to fentanyl conversion

4-hourly morphine dose (mg)	Durogesic patch size (μg/hour)
5–20	25
25–35	50
40–50	75
55–65	100

Source Janssen-Cilag Ltd (1996).

ore) to stick down corners. Elderly and frail individuals may be more sensitive to Durogesic. Plasma concentrations continue to fall after removal and may be detectable for up to 5 days.

Transdermal fentanyl is contraindicated in patients who need rapid titration for severe uncontrolled pain. It will *not* relieve pain that has not responded to morphine (Twycross et al, 1998).

Rectal

Rectal administration is possible for many analgesics, and this route should be considered if the patient cannot take drugs orally. For example, diclofenac suppositories are particularly useful for nociceptive pain. Adjuvants such as anti-emetics can also be given rectally.

Subcutaneous infusion

Subcutaneous infusions of drugs using a syringe driver is often useful if the enteral route cannot be used, for example if nausea and vomiting are a problem, if constipation is severe, and in the case of inadequate enteral absorption of analgesia. It is useful for giving adjuvant drugs such as corticosteroids, anti-inflammatory agents, anti-emetics and hypnotics, etc., when the enteral route cannot be used.

Intravenous infusion

Intravenous administration of analgesics is the route of choice in the initial postoperative period, and for rapid titration for patients in severe pain. Patient-controlled analgesia (PCA) devices deliver analgesics usually intravenously, although subcutaneous and epidural infusions are also possible (Cowan, 1997).

Summary

Pain is a very common problem in head and neck cancer, and the nurse has a central role in its management. The accurate and detailed assessment of pain is essential if interventions are to be effective. The patient will require close and continuous monitoring. The management of pain in head and neck cancer is a challenge for the whole team, and is one of the areas where teamwork is essential. Nurses should review their current methods of pain assessment, monitoring and evaluation and establish evidence-based pain control tailored to the individual head and neck cancer patient. Despite the central role of nursing, there is relatively little nursing research in this area. Nurses working with head and neck cancer patients should make this issue a research priority.

Strategy for practice

- Ensure that your ward is using a comprehensive, validated pain assessment tool.
- Always titrate analgesia using the WHO guidelines and a regular, by-the-clock schedule.
- Refer all patients who do not respond to WHO guidelines to a specialist pain team.
- Be aware of the value of all pain control methods and incorporate these into care plans.
- More research and development is needed in this area.

The following references are highly recommended for those with a particular interest in the subject: Carroll & Bowsher, 1993; Twycross, 1994, 1997; McGuire & Sheidler, 1997.

Chapter 2.12
Fungating lesions

Introduction

Fungating wounds are caused by the infiltration and proliferation of malignant cells into and through the epidermis of the skin, or mucosa, and its supporting blood and lymph vessels. This involves the spread of malignant cells along pathways that offer minimal resistance: tissue planes, blood and lymph vessels, and in the perineural spaces. Their origin may be a local tumour, or they may be a metastatic deposit from a distant primary lesion. These tumours may grow rapidly, with a fungus- or cauliflower-like appearance (Collier, 1997). They may also ulcerate and form shallow craters. The tumour grows until capillary rupture causes it to lose its vascularity and tissue necrosis occurs (Grocott, 1995).

In the head and neck, fungating lesions are often complicated by fistula formation; orocutaneous fistulas are very distressing; constant saliva leakage is a major problem, eating and drinking becomes impossible, and speech is impaired. Skin may quickly become excoriated. Stomal recurrence can lead to distressing fungating lesions around the stoma, which compromise the airway, cause tracheoesophageal fistula with salivary leakage, and can lead to erosion of major vessels.

Thus fungating tumours in the head and neck present a major challenge to nursing care. Psychological and emotional care is the most important component of this challenge. A fungating lesion severely affects quality of life, often alienating and isolating the individual from normal life. It is a constant visible reminder of cancer. It often gives a sense of a lingering death, 'rotting' away. Patients with fungating head and neck cancer lesions represent extreme cases of distress to both carers and professionals.

The thoughts of a woman newly diagnosed with cancer are described below.

> She knows there will be a lot of pain. She knows there is itching, and a foul smell. And people find it harder and harder to look you in the eye, keep their patience with your moaning, keep from holding their noses. The bit about the smell bothers her. It picks away at the insistent image of the freshly bathed martyr, gently declining on a snowy bed — the received image of a terminal patient, spouting words of wisdom for the benefit of those left behind.

Incidence

There is no hard data on the incidence of fungating lesions in head and neck cancer. However, Thomas (1990) reports estimates of 24% of all fungating lesions seen in oncology units; these are second only to breast lesions at 62%.

Medical and surgical treatment

Palliative radiotherapy and chemotherapy can often help to reduce the size of the lesion, and prevent bleeding. Surgical excision of lymph nodes in the neck and face may sometimes be possible as a palliative measure to prevent fungation; it may give the patient several months of life without the need for wound dressings. However, ulcerating lesions may often occur in very end-stage disease, in extensively treated patients, where no further treatment options are available. Thus the mainstay of treatment is good wound care.

Management of a malignant fungating wound

Fungating wounds are invariably chronic, and are extremely complex wounds to manage as they require a range of highly individualized interventions. The primary goal of management may not include healing of the lesion, but should include minimization of complications. There are many products available to the nurse and patient, and creative use of these can do much to reduce discomfort and enhance quality of life. Wounds are dynamic and therefore care should be re-evaluated on a daily basis. Products may need to be changed as the situation changes. Every individual lesion is different, and the fixation of dressing to the face and neck is extremely problematic. Thus finding the optimum regime and dressing is often a process of trial and error for the nurse and patient.

Assessment

Careful and frequent assessment of a fungating lesion is essential. The initial assessment should include a holistic assessment of the individual and family, in order to plan wound management care with the patient and family's needs and goals as priorities. Ongoing monitoring will be on a daily basis. Assessment will include:

- location and size of the wound; it is important to keep accurate visual records to evaluate efficacy of interventions. A paper ruler and hand-drawn diagram, or photographic record, may be useful
- presence of infection, exudate (amount and colour), malodour, bleeding
- condition of surrounding skin
- effects on daily activities of living, appearance and function
- pain
- dressing fit, type and performance
- frequency of dressing changes required
- physical condition of the patient
- psychological and emotional status of the patient and family
- need for social services such as laundry service, soiled clinical waste collection, etc.

Grocott (1997) reports an assessment tool for the management of fungating wounds measuring the number of dressing changes, the amount of exudate leakage and dressing fit. Finlay et al (1996) describe a grading system to measure malodour. A suggested assessment tool, adapted from these reports, is shown in Table 2.12.1.

Table 2.12.1: A suggested wound management assessment tool

Date

Smell

0 = none

1 = present but not offensive

2 = mildly offensive

3 = moderately offensive

4 = extremely offensive

Exudate

0 = none

1 = small, not offensive

2 = small, offensive

3 = moderate, offensive

4 = large, offensive

Dressing fit

0 = dressing conformed, all edges remained attached for 24 hours

1 = dressing conformed, but edges required retaping once or twice in 24 hours

2 = dressing did not conform, edges required retaping several times in 24 hours

3 = dressing did not conform, became completely detached after several hours

4 = dressing did not conform, became completely detached within 1 hour of application

Exudate absorption

0 = no repadding required in 24 hours, no strike through

1 = no repadding required, but strike through occurred within 24 hours

2 = dressing soaked through, requires repadding twice in 24 hours

3 = dressing soaked through, leakage on to skin and clothing, requires repadding several times per day

4 = dressing sodden within an hour of application, frequent leakage on to skin and clothing

Surrounding skin condition

0 = normal, no excoriation

1 = slight redness

2 = moderate redness, signs of breakdown

3 = severe excoriation, maceration present; requires dressing

4 = severe maceration and cellulitis present

Fistula leakage

0 = no leakage in 24 hours, plugged effectively

1 = small leakage in 24 hours, absorbent dressing or occasional wiping required

2 = moderate leakage in 24 hours, absorbent dressing replaced once or twice

3 = large amount of leakage, requires several dressings per day, suction, protection for clothing

4 = uncontrolled copious leakage, constant suction required, dressing soaked within an hour, protection for clothing

---

For each section, scores of 2 or more indicate a review of wound management plan is needed — try a different dressing, seek specialist advice.

Wound management plan

Grocott has recommended that the following factors be considered when devising a wound management plan for a fungating wound:

- maintenance of optimum wound humidity to minimize pain
- non-adherent dressing to prevent trauma and thus minimize pain and bleeding at dressing changes
- facilitation of wound debridement, with the removal of excess exudate and toxic materials to prevent bacterial proliferation and control odour
- topical or systemic antimicrobials to control odour as appropriate
- restoration of body symmetry by the use of cavity dressings
- maximizing cosmetic acceptability by minimizing the use of bulky secondary dressings
- control of bleeding by use of haemostatic dressings as appropriate.

Malodour

Tissue hypoxia in a fungating wound can be a significant problem, as anaerobic organisms flourish in accessible necrotic tissue — a characteristic of the majority of fungating wounds. The malodorous volatile fatty acids that are released as a metabolic end product are responsible for the characteristic smell and profuse exudate often associated with these wound types (Collier, 1997a). Malodour can be extremely unpleasant, triggering a gagging or vomit reflex in both patients and carers (Collier, 1997b). It permeates the whole of the patient's environment, and many families find it difficult to live with the smell (Moody, 1998). The patient may be very self-conscious, with social embarrassment heightening the misery of advanced disease, and deepening the individual's sense of worthlessness and social isolation, at a time when the support of family and friends is crucial (Price, 1996). Malodorous wounds often make patients feel they are 'rotting away'.

The most common groups of anaerobes involved are *Bacteroides fragilis*, *Bacteroides prevotella*, *Fusobacterium nucleatum*, *Clostridium perfringens* and anaerobic cocci. Other pathogenic organisms that may cause malodour belong to the aerobic group of bacteria, commonly *Proteus*, *Pseudomonas spp.*, and *Klebsiella*. Most malodorous wounds contain at least two anaerobic as well as aerobic organisms (Moody, 1998).

The primary aim in control of malodour should be to kill the causative micro-organism (Moody, 1998). In order to do this, the nurse must consider the use of:

- systemic antimicrobial agents (Figure 2.12.1)
- topical antimicrobial agents (Figure 2.12.2)
- cleansing (Figure 2.12.3)
- debridement/desloughing (Figure 2.12.4).

Odour control measures should be taken until the primary aim has been achieved.

One method is the use of external deodorizers such as aromatherapy oils, which can be sprinkled on to the top of the dressing itself and around the room, diffused or sprayed into the air. These agents mask odours but some have powerful smells that, when mixed with the wound odour, can be nauseating (Haisfield-Wolfe, 1997).

- Metronidazole can be used systemically (200 mg TDS) to eliminate pathogenic anaerobes (Hampson, 1996). It can be administered orally, as a suspension via a tube feed, or as suppositories. A disadvantage of systemic treatment is the side effects experienced by many individuals. Systemic metronidazole may cause an unpleasant taste in the mouth, furred tongue, nausea, vomiting and gastrointestinal disturbance (Moody, 1998). Metronidazole is often withheld if the patient is using alcohol, yet the rationale for this intervention is not clear in the literature. It is has been reported to cause a 'disulfiram reaction' (headaches, tachycardia, emesis, facial flushing) when given concurrently with alcohol. This complication has been reported as occurring at rates varying from 10% to 25% to 100% (Alexander, 1985; Stockley, 1991; Dukes, 1993). However, a randomized, placebo-controlled trial in 10 patients with alcoholism found no evidence of an adverse reaction, except for alcohol being reported as tasting less pleasant (Gelder & Edwards, 1968). More research is needed on this issue, particularly as many head and neck patients use alcohol. Hampson (1996) suggests that is may be possible to circumvent an interaction by taking metronidazole and alcohol at different times of the day.
- Hampson (1996) suggests that metronidazole should not be prescribed blindly for malodorous wounds; culture and sensitivity of micro-organisms should be obtained in order to determine which antimicrobial agent to use.

Figure 2.12.1: Systemic antimicrobial agents.

- Metronidazole gel (Metrotop, Seton Healthcare Group) has been suggested for effective odour control, 0.8% being the most effective (Clarkem, 1992). In the majority of wounds, authors suggest effect will be noted between 2 and 7 days (Newman et al, 1989; Finlay et al, 1996). Finlay et al (1996) also report improvements in cellulitis and pain with metronidazole gel. However, there is a distinct lack of good randomized controlled trials to prove this. Metronidazole gel should be applied generously directly to the cleansed wound surface. The wound should then be covered with a secondary dressing. Small cavity wounds can be filled with metronidazole gel and covered with a secondary dressing. In larger cavities, a cavity dressing can be generously smeared with metronidazole gel before being inserted.
- Flamazine is an agent containing 1% silver sulphadiazine which has a broad spectrum of action against Gram-negative and Gram-positive organisms, fungi and yeasts. It has to be used with an occlusive dressing to prevent oxidation and cannot be used during radiotherapy (Bale, 1997).
- Iodine (Inadine and Iodoflex) controls bacteria on the wound surface. It should not be used on large wounds, or individuals with thyroid disease or iodine allergy (Bale, 1997).
- Non-conventional treatments reported in the literature include live yogurt and buttermilk (Welch, 1982), baking soda (Foltz, 1980), icing sugar (Sims & Fitzgerald, 1985), honey (Thomas, 1990). However, reports on the efficacy of these agents is entirely anecdotal. Sugar paste (icing sugar and lubricating gel) or honey can be useful for fungating lesions in the oral cavity, where use of metronidazole gel would be unpleasant.

Figure 2.12.2: Topical agents.

Topical antiseptics (Eusol, Milton, povidone iodine, chlorhexidine, cetrimide, hydrogen peroxide) have all been used in an attempt to control odour in lesions. However, there is now a body of evidence to show that these agents are inactivated by body fluids, blood, pus and slough. They have also been found to damage new tissue and suppress normal lymphocytic response, thus impairing wound healing (Ivetic & Lyne, 1990). The optimum wound cleansing agent is therefore normal saline (Collier, 1997b; Tonge, 1997).

Figure 2.12.3: Cleansing agents.

Debridement is the process of removing dead tissue from a wound. Necrotic tissue acts as a medium for bacterial proliferation. Its removal will also reduce wound odour.

- Hydrocolloids/hydrogels (Duoderm, Comfeel, Granugel, Purilon Gel, Intrasite Gel, Aquacel). These dressings will promote debridement by autolysis (natural degradation of devitalized tissue). Autolysis depends on the phagocytic activity of neutrophils and macrophages to ingest debris and on enzymes released by these cells to help digest necrotic tissue. Devitalized tissue eventually separates from viable tissue. This may take several days. Initially, there may be an increase in exudate. However, as slough is removed, the volume of exudate will diminish.

  Cells and enzymes require a moist environment in order to function; hydrocolloids and hydrogels provide this environment, helping to rehydrate and soften necrotic tissue and promote autolysis. These products also have a capacity to absorb fluid and debris. Another advantage is that a hydrocolloid does not require a secondary dressing, and can be cosmetically pleasing as it conforms to the body's contours and is 'skin coloured'. It is waterproof and so the individual can bathe or shower with it in situ.

- Irrigation. Wounds can be cleared of debris using saline or water under pressure, e.g. syringes, spray canisters, shower head. Care must be taken not to exert too much pressure and cause bleeding (Flannagan, 1997).

- Surgical and sharp debridement. Extensive debridement of necrotic, crusted lesions, particularly those which are inaccessible such as those in the nasopharynx, may require surgical intervention in theatre. An experienced nurse can debride necrotic tissue at dressing changes, using sterile scissors, or a surgical blade.

Figure 2.12.4: Debriding agents.

Another option is the use of charcoal-impregnated dressings, which absorb gases and filter odours from the wound (Figure 2.12.5).

Infection

Nearly 100% of wounds will be colonized by some organism. However, the presence of bacteria or slough alone may not be of any clinical significance (Collier, 1997b). The clinical signs of infection are pyrexia, raised white cell count, inflammation, localized erythema, heat or pain. Infection is often indicated by the presence of cellulitis in the surrounding skin (Cutting, 1997). Odour is also a factor, as noted above.

It is important to eliminate infection as it may result in additional discomfort and odour. It may also progress to systemic infection.

- Activated charcoal incorporated into dressings helps to control odour (Lyofoam C, Actisorb Plus, Kaltocarb).
- Alginate sheets and cavity dressings (Melgisorb, Sorbsan, Kaltostat, Kaltostat Fortex) — Melgisorb has the highest absorbency in g/dressing (British Pharmacopoeia, 1995). Alginates should be trimmed to the shape of the wound to prevent maceration and excoriation of the surrounding skin (Seymour, 1997).
- Mesalt (Molnlycke) is a dressing ideal for heavily exuding wounds, designed to cleanse the wound by absorbing infected exudate. It is impregnated with sodium chloride and creates a hypertonic environment, pulling exudate from the wound and also removing bacteria and necrotic material.
- Hydrocolloid sheets and gels, thin hydrocolloids have low absorbency, normal hydrocolloids and hydrogels have moderate absorbency (Duoderm, Comfeel, Aquacel).
- Foam/hydrocellular dressings, sheet dressings (Allevyn, Mepilex, Lyofoam, Lyofoam Extra) have moderate to high absorbency whilst Tielle and Spyrosorb have a light to moderate absorbency. Cavity foams (Cavicare, Allevyn cavity dressing) have moderate to high absorbency.
- Low-adherent dressings, Mepitel (a silicone dressing which is very useful for protecting very delicate, sensitive tissue), Tricotex, Tegapore, Release, Melolin.
- Semi-permeable film membranes, a less obtrusive way of securing dressings (Tegaderm, Opsite, Epiview).
- Protective barrier films for surrounding skin (Clinishield, 3M Cavilon).

Figure 2.12.5: Dressing materials.

Observation of the wound appearance can often help to identify infection before the classic signs appear (Cutting, 1997):

- red, raw, tender, friable tissue that bleeds easily
- discoloration of the tissue; a dull, dark red hue signifies infection with anaerobes (*Bacteroides fragilis* or anaerobic streptococci). Pseudomonal infections may cause a green or blue appearance
- pocketing in the wound due to islands of infection
- change in odour; infections due to Gram-negative bacilli usually result in a distinctive and slightly unpleasant smell. Infections by anaerobic bacteria produce the characteristic 'acrid or putrid' smell.

Management of infection includes systemic antimicrobials (Figure 2.12.1), topical antimicrobials (Figure 2.12.2), wound cleansing (Figure 2.12.3) and effective management of exudate (Figure 2.12.5).

Exudate

Exudate is a fluid produced by wounds and plays an essential part in wound healing as it provides nutrients for cells, a transport medium for white blood cells, and a moist environment for wound healing. It is normally pale yellow in colour, and is discoloured by contaminants such as infected and necrotic tissue. Tumour microvasculature is hyperpermeable to fibrinogen and plasma colloid, and many tumours also secrete a vascular permeability factor that increases permeability and accounts for the large amounts of exudate which some wounds secrete (Haisfield-Wolfe, 1997). Exudate becomes more viscous and malodorous in infected wounds, due to the activity of bacterial enzymes (proteases). Stagnant exudate also causes wound odour. By-products of anaerobic organisms such as bacteroides present in infected exudate include acetic, propionic, lactic and succinic acid (Collier, 1997a). These quickly result in maceration and damage of the skin surrounding the lesion.

Management of wound exudate is an essential part of wound care in the fungating lesion. Firstly, the underlying causes of exudate generation (infection and necrotic tissue) should be addressed and treated, as this will lead to diminished exudate. During this time an appropriate dressing to deal with exudate should be selected.

When selecting a dressing it is necessary to take into account the lesion, its depth, shape, size, location, presence of infection and necrotic material and amount of exudate present. For a heavily exuding wound, select a dressing with high absorbency; but monitor exudate levels carefully, and change to a lower absorbency as soon as exudate levels reduce. A mixture of different dressing types is often required. Use primary and secondary dressings together to increase absorbency. For example, an alginate with a hydrocolloid to secure, or a cavity dressing with an absorbent foam to secure. Skin protection of the surrounding skin is very important; use a skin barrier (Figure 2.12.5).

Infected and necrotic wounds should be managed with a debriding and antimicrobial agent plus an exudate absorber. For example, an alginate with metronidazole gel, secured by Allevyn and a semipermeable film.

Haemorrhage

Surface haemorrhage is a common problem. The fragile structure of tumour capillaries may predispose the tissue to bleeding (Grocott, 1995). Platelets are absent from the tumour stroma and their function is suppressed by tumour cells (Haisfield-Wolfe, 1997). The tumour may erode a local blood vessel. Light bleeding can be controlled with local pressure and haemostatic dressings (e.g. alginates), heavier bleeding may require ligation or cauterization (Haisfield-Wolfe & Rund, 1997). Non-adherent dressings should always be used to prevent trauma at dressing changes causing bleeding. Mepitel is useful for fragile and sensitive wounds. It is laid over the wound surface to prevent trauma. Topical agents and exudate absorbers can be applied over it (Williams, 1995).

Pain

An effective analgesic regime should be established (see Chapter 2.11). Non-adherent dressings will minimize pain at dressing changes, as will careful attention to the wound dynamics, and changing dressings to match the amount of exudate; dressings designed to manage heavy exudate will adhere to lightly exudating wounds. Sensitive wounds can be protected by a silicone-coated dressing such as Mepitel, which prevents adherence of secondary dressings, yet allows the application of topical agents (Williams, 1995). It can be safely left in situ during radiotherapy treatment without adverse effects (Adamietz et al, 1995). Wound cleansing should minimize trauma; for example, irrigation may be employed instead of swabbing.

Disfigurement

Fungating wounds in the head and neck are almost always disfiguring. The patient and significant others may feel repulsion, shame and embarrassment. The nurse must provide a positive role model in accepting the person as an individual, avoiding any negative feedback (verbal or non-verbal) on appearance. Management should aim to conceal the disfigurement in the most cosmetically pleasing way possible. Chapters 3.2 and 3.3 deal with the psychosocial issues associated with disfigurement.

Dressing fixation

It is very difficult to achieve good dressing fixation on fungating wounds on the head or neck area. Frequent retaping or repadding may be required. Presence of fistulae may also mean that frequent changes are required.

Suggested methods of fixation are use of semi-permeable film dressings (Figure 2.12.5), Hypafix, Surgifix elasticated net, Netelast, and cotton tubular bandage.

There are reports in the literature of creative approaches to dressing fixation for fungating head and neck lesions. Grocott (1992) describes the use of a latex wound dressing support device for a patient with a fungating neck lesion. A mould was made of the anatomical area, using a technique often used to make beam direction masks in radiotherapy centres. Using the mould, an appliance of foam latex was prepared, and fixed to the skin over the dressing, using surgical glue. A batch of similar appliances can be made so that a fresh one can be applied at each dressing change. The patient in this case study found the appliance to be comfortable and flexible, with fewer dressing changes needed.

Banks and Jones (1993) describe the management of a fungating nasal carcinoma with a combination of several different wound care products. The cavity was packed with an Allevyn cavity dressing, after metronidazole gel had been applied, plus Kaltostat to bleeding areas. Over this was placed a piece of Melolin trimmed to a triangular shape, secured with a semi-permeable film dressing (Opsite).

Lesions in the mouth

Lesions in the mouth or nasal cavity are particularly difficult to manage because of their inaccessibility and the impracticality of applying topical agents and dressings. Meticulous oral hygiene (see Chapter 2.2) is the mainstay of care; it may be required as frequently as once an hour. Systemic antimicrobial therapy is often the only option for eliminating bacterial contamination. Nasal lesions may cause unpleasant discharge of exudate into the pharynx, or may erode through the hard palate, and cause the discharge of unpleasant exudate directly into the mouth. This can often be managed by packing the cavity with an absorbent dressing and topical agent, and correcting the defect with a specially made maxillofacial prosthesis (obturator).

Lesions in/adjacent to the laryngostome

Tumour lesions at the site of the individual's laryngostome are highly problematic. They often compromise the airway, and the application of dressings is very difficult without compromising it further. Such tumour lesions often erode through the posterior tracheal wall, causing a tracheoesophageal fistula. They are also very close to major blood vessels (the innominate and right common carotid arteries). The primary aim of management is to protect the airway; patients are often terrified by the thought they may 'choke to death'. A rigid laryngectomy tube should be inserted to prevent tumour growth into the airway. A cuffed tracheostomy tube may be necessary to protect the airway from a leaking fistula. See Chapter 2.1 for more information on airway management. Dressings need to be carefully shaped, trimmed and fixed to avoid compromising the airway. Management of haemorrhage is discussed in Chapter 2.8.

Fistulae

Leakage of saliva and oral contents is an extremely distressing consequence of orocutaneous, pharyngocutaneous and tracheoesophageal fistulas. Some suggestions for management include:

- plugging the fistula — for tracheoesophageal fistulas it is sometimes possible to use a device such as a tracheoesophageal valve or tampon; orocutaneous fistulas can sometimes benefit from a specially made maxillofacial prosthesis. Fistulae can be plugged to some extent by cavity dressings, such as alginate ribbons
- containing the leakage using a high-absorbency dressing
- containing the leakage using a wound drainage or ostomy bag
- minimizing leakage by avoiding oral intake completely, providing nutrition via a nasogastric or gastrostomy feed
- protecting the surrounding skin from excoriation by using a skin barrier.

Chambers and Worral (1994) describe the use of a silastic foam dressing (now replaced by Cavicare) to occlude a large orocutaneous defect in the floor of mouth. They made an acrylic shield from a mould of the patient's mandible and neck area and this was used to mould the silastic dressing to shape. The shield was then used to keep the dressing in place, by fixing it in place with orthodontic head gear.

Case examples

The following case examples demonstrate the creative approaches possible to deal with difficult problems.

Case one: Derek

Derek was a 56-year-old salesman with a fungating nasal carcinoma, eroding backwards into his face, leaving a large cavity right back to the nasopharynx. He had been treated both surgically (including a radical maxillectomy) and with radiotherapy. He had a prosthesis wired into his remaining maxilla to correct the maxillectomy defect. The aim of our wound management was to contain the exudate that dripped down into his throat, minimize the reflux of drinks and food into the cavity and thus out over his face, and to make his appearance as cosmetically acceptable as possible.

First, crusting and necrotic tissue was debrided using a surgical blade and forceps. Kaltostat was applied to bleeding areas. The wound cavity was lined with clingfilm which had been lightly smeared with Vaseline, then Cavicare mixture (2 pots were needed) was poured in. The clingfilm prevented the Cavicare from running down Derek's throat (we found that the clingfilm stuck to the Cavicare unless smeared with Vaseline). Derek had a nose prosthesis that had been made by the maxillofacial prosthetics technician. This was secured by elastic straps behind his ears. He did not like wearing it. The inside of this was smeared with Vaseline in preparation, and as soon as the Cavicare had been poured in, the prosthesis was placed over the cavity. The Cavicare then foamed up to fill the prosthesis, and set inside it. The whole dressing was then lifted out, and separated from the prosthesis and clingfilm. It was then reinserted, trimmed around the edges, and fixed with strips of semi-permeable film dressing (Tegaderm).

The Cavicare absorbed any exudate and mostly prevented reflux of food or fluid; any that did get through was absorbed into the dressing. An additional benefit was that it was nose-shaped. Derek was highly pleased with this dressing and felt able to walk around the hospital and grounds whilst it was in place. It was changed daily. Cavicare can be cleaned and re-used, but it was so soiled with food debris that we made a new one each day. The whole procedure took approximately 30 minutes once we had practised a few times.

Case two: David

David was a 52-year-old engineer with recurrent squamous cell cancer in his trachea, after extensive surgery (pharyngolaryngectomy and glossectomy), radical radiotherapy and palliative chemotherapy. He was married with a young family and wanted to spend as much time as possible at home with them. The recurrence was a small area at the back of his laryngostome, which had eroded through the tracheal wall, causing a tracheoesophageal fistula that constantly leaked saliva and prevented David from eating and drinking. David had a gastrostomy tube inserted to maintain his nutrition, and a cuffed tracheostomy tube to prevent aspiration problems. The fistula was very small, and we managed to insert a 16 French Blomsinger duckbill tracheoesophageal valve which successfully stopped the leak. This was attached to a thread and safety pinned to his collar in case it fell out. David was able to dispense with his cuffed tracheostomy tube and return to normal eating and drinking for 2 weeks. However, the fistula continued to enlarge as the tumour grew and was too large for a 20 French valve after a few months. It also became malodorous. David was treated with systemic metronidazole 200 mg TDS and returned to his cuffed tracheostomy tube and nil by mouth status. Clinishield skin barrier was applied to the skin around the stoma to prevent excoriation. A portable suction pump was supplied but David mostly managed his leakage by frequently wiping with soft tissues (Kleenex Ultrabalm).

Case three: Kevin

Kevin was a 68-year-old man with recurrent squamous cell cancer in the trachea after laryngectomy. The tumour had ulcerated in his laryngostome, causing a huge tracheoesophageal fistula. A cuffed tracheostomy tube was inserted to protect Kevin's airway, but he did not like wearing it. He was expectorating offensive green sputum. He did not want a gastrostomy or nasogastric tube inserted. His main goal was to get out of hospital, back to the caravan where he lived, and to have a last ride on his beloved motorbike.

Kevin was given antibiotic treatment for his chest infection, but we were concerned that it would soon recur due to his frequent removal of his cuffed tube, which he said made him cough and felt uncomfortable. The fistula was so large that three fingers could easily be inserted into it. We therefore tried inserting two super absorbency tampons to plug the leakage. These expanded to plug the oesophagus extremely well. Kevin was so relieved to be free of the copious leakage of saliva that he agreed to have a nasogastric tube passed through the fistula into his stomach for feeding. This was secured to his neck using semi-permeable film membrane. The tampons required changing every 3–4 hours, with suction at the ready as they were pulled out. Kevin easily learnt to do this himself, with the aid of a mirror.

The district nurse visited Kevin in hospital to learn about the dressing technique, and how to re-insert the feeding tube when necessary. She arranged for a supply of tampons from the local chemist. Kevin was discharged home to his caravan with a portable suction pump and feeding pump (fortunately, the caravan had mains electricity). He was able to have several 'last' rides on his motorbike before deteriorating and dying in his local hospice.

Summary

Management of a malignant fungating wound in the head and neck is time consuming, complex and often only partially successful. There is no perfect management or dressing. Nurses need to be highly creative in their approach to such wounds, and make full use of all the wound care products available. The need for systematic research and development in the area of fungating wound management has been highlighted by several authors (Grocott, 1995). It should be a research priority in head and neck cancer care.

Strategy for practice

- Use systematic assessment tools for fungating lesions.
- Use evidence-based wound care interventions.
- Fungating wounds require continuous review and refinement of care as they are constantly changing.
- Research and development is needed in this area.

For those who would like to read more widely in this area, the following publications are recommended: Grocott P (1995) The palliative management of fungating malignant wounds: preparatory work. Chapter 12 in Richardson A, Wilson-Barnett J (eds) *Nursing Research in Cancer Care*. London: Scutari Press, RCN and Morison M et al (1997) *Nursing Management of Chronic Wounds*, 2nd edn. London: Mosby.

Section Three
Quality of life, psychological, social and emotional management

Chapter 3.1
Quality of life in head and neck cancer

'As we move towards evidence-based care, it is important to acknowledge that there is a good deal of other evidence to suggest that methods and achievements of medicine are frequently overrated and under researched ... there is evidence that medicine itself can be a significant barrier in the attempt to achieve health' (Milligan, 1998).

Introduction

George had become increasingly depressed over the 18 months after his laryngopharyngectomy, thyroidectomy, bilateral neck dissection and postoperative radiotherapy. His jejunal graft was kinked, so that he could only swallow tiny amounts of food. He had a feeding gastrostomy. His neck felt so tight that it was a constant source of discomfort. He had severe trismus that prevented him opening his mouth. He had to walk around with his head facing down because of the tight scar tissue. He could not use the tracheoesophageal valve that had been inserted for speech. He could not use electronic speaking aids because of his trismus and facial and submental lymphoedema. He had progressively lost hope that he would ever improve. His social life was ruined as he could see no point in going out if he couldn't enjoy the large meals he used to love. His relationship with his partner was strained due to the communication difficulty, loss of sexual activity and loss of social life. He felt totally miserable. Every day he had to force himself to get up and face another day. Today he decided it was not worth bothering. He laid in bed with his eyes closed and said 'I just don't want to wake up. I would rather be dead than face a lifetime of this misery'.

Joseph had undergone a total laryngectomy, bilateral neck dissection and postoperative radiotherapy a year earlier. He had severe submental lymphoedema, swallowing problems, and breathing problems due to excessive mucus. Even light activity made him breathless because his trachea had become very narrow and stenosed due to a postoperative wound infection. Joseph felt acutely self-conscious about his appearance and his frequent coughing and therefore would not go out socially. His relationship with his wife was strained; they had no sexual or social activity and she felt exhausted because she had to do all the household tasks that Joseph used to do, as well as her own. He told his doctor: 'I wish I had never had this operation'. His doctor replied, 'But you would not be here now if you had not had it'. Joseph replied, 'Exactly; I really don't want to be alive now'.

The concept of quality of life is extremely important in head and neck cancer. Radical surgery and radiotherapy may give individuals a high chance of cure, but the cost of this cure may be more than the survivor can bear. Radical treatment is also given in head and neck cancer for 'palliative' reasons: to prevent an unpleasant death from airway obstruction, bleeding or fungating tumour. However, the common assumption that death from distant metastases is preferable to death from local symptoms is not evidence-based, and must be balanced against the distress that surgery and radiotherapy inflict in the name of palliation. Patients' objectives for treatment may be unrealistic and differ from their perceptions of actual treatment outcome, even when, in a technical sense, treatment is successful. Thus the definition of success can often differ widely between patients and their doctors (Hodder et al, 1997), and the nurse has to help the patient come to terms with, and cope with, the gap between the quality of life they used to enjoy and the quality of life that is their new reality.

Strauss (1989) suggests that fear of death affects decision-making for both the patient and the clinician when head and neck cancer is diagnosed, and may allow therapeutic activism to proceed to an extreme degree. He says that 'it is an unusual patient who can question the wisdom of active treatment because this involves a challenge to professional norms'. Strauss also noted that patients regarded their surgeon in heroic terms, with a sense of awe. The author concludes that patients are initially grateful for the chance to survive, but as the long-term impact of the surgery on their function, relationships, social life and wellbeing becomes apparent, they often reappraise, and then regret, their initial decision.

Factors that patients use to measure success are not only medical but also social, economic and cultural. A cured patient who is permanently disabled or is experiencing symptoms or other medical morbidity is not the same as a cured patient who is working full-time, earning his or her pre-diagnosis income, and requiring only modest ongoing involvement within the healthcare system (Harrison et al, 1997). The traditional outcome measures of treatment efficacy, such as tumour recurrence and survival time, are often meaningless to the patient. What matters is the ability to return to pre-illness function and psychosocial wellbeing (Deleyiannis et al, 1997). Quality of life issues are of great importance to patients when deciding treatment options. Clinicians need to integrate quality of life issues into descriptions of treatment options, side effects and expected outcomes (Terrell et al, 1997).

Nurses, who are often acutely aware of the patients' disease experience, and what their disability actually means to their life and personhood, are in a position to act as an advocate for the patient, and future patients, by ensuring that the surgeon and oncologist are aware of the quality of life implications of their therapeutic interventions. Quality of life may sometimes even present conflicts of beliefs between professionals, and between patients and professionals. These difficulties lie in the different priorities each individual has; the nurse's priorities are to enhance quality of life and act as the patient's advocate, whilst the doctor's priority is to cure the disease, and the patients priority is to lead as normal a life as possible.

The need to measure quality of life

Measuring the many dimensions of quality of life is the only way in which clinicians can obtain a quantitative evaluation of the true outcomes of their interventions. Quantitative data about quality of life can help nurses who are coaching patients in the diagnostic phase, facilitating decision-making; it can provide important additional information to be used in the decision-making process, especially when two treatment modalities are known to be equivalent in terms of survival, or where the aims of treatment are palliative rather than curative. Decisions about treatment for head and neck cancer inevitably involve trade-offs between length of survival and quality of life, and there may be differences between individual patients regarding the extent they wish to trade quality of life for length of survival (Morris, 1991). Here, data can help nurses act as the patient's advocate, for example in presenting their decisions to forego survival if they feel they cannot cope with the impact of treatment.

Comprehensive assessment of the impact of head and neck cancer — the disease, its therapy, and rehabilitation — goes beyond traditional biomedical outcomes such as survival and disease progression to include patient wellbeing. Quality of life assessment has been used increasingly over the last decade to provide vital treatment-related information (Gotay & Moore, 1992). Quality of life assessment is particularly important in head and neck cancer because the disease and its treatment have such a profound impact on quality of life, and also because advances in treatment may produce survival results that are equivalent between two groups (e.g. concurrent chemoradiation versus surgery). In this situation, quality of life may be the measure that indicates the best outcomes.

The large multidisciplinary team approach to care involves many different professionals. Quality of life outcomes are of concern to all these professionals. While each professional can identify the effect that his/her interventions have in a specific area, it is the patient who can evaluate the total impact of treatment as a whole (Gotay & Moore, 1992). Thus, incorporating quality of life assessment in clinical research allows professionals to understand and appreciate the outcome of their therapeutic regimens more fully and to use this information to make modifications.

Quality of life information can be used to help when giving patients an overview of their treatment and its side effects, when setting a timetable for recovery, and to help patients decide on treatment options. Quality of life measurement can also provide a focus for rehabilitation programmes and help to identify those individuals who are unlikely to cope with the consequences of diagnosis and treatment, so that they can be given additional support. It can also help to identify specific time periods during the patient's 'cancer journey' when additional interventions are most needed; for example the diagnostic phase, post-surgery and during radiotherapy.

Measuring quality of life

Quality of life is a difficult concept to define and measure because it is multidimensional. In order to assess quality of life, it has to be broken down into its component parts (or 'domains'). Aaronson et al (1988) suggest that the minimum four aspects that should be considered are: physical symptoms, social functioning, psychological distress and functional status. Morton (1995b) adds that it incorporates other life experiences such as economic/financial, occupational and domestic/family domains. Morton suggests that the following domains be considered in a quality of life questionnaire:

- physical functioning
- symptoms (disease- and treatment-specific)
- emotional functioning
- role functioning
- social functioning
- coping ability
- financial impact
- health status
- sexuality
- global index.

The EORTC (European Organization for Research into the Treatment of Cancer) core questionnaire, for example, has been designed to fulfil these criteria for cancer patients. It is a 30-item core questionnaire that incorporates domains relevant for cancer patients: five functioning scales (physical, role, cognitive, emotional and social), a global quality of life scale, three symptom scales (fatigue, pain, emesis) and six single-item symptom measures. This core instrument is designed to be supplemented by questionnaire modules assessing quality of life aspects relevant to specific cancer sites (Bjordal et al, 1994a).

Glikich et al (1997) demonstrated that, for patients with head and neck cancer, a general tool alone is not sensitive enough to give a precise picture of the problems they experience, especially when comparing treatment modalities. They recommended that a head and neck specific tool is used to supplement a general cancer questionnaire.

The criteria for a good head and neck quality of life tool

Statistical criteria

Prior to the introduction and use of a questionnaire in clinical practice, the statistical criteria of *acceptability*, *validity*, *reliability* and *responsiveness* must be satisfied (Hassan & Weymuller, 1993).

- Acceptability refers to the patient preference for a questionnaire; for example the ease and speed with which it can be completed.

Practicality refers to both patient and clinician preference. Patients prefer shorter, concise questionnaires, whilst health professionals prefer scales that receive good patient response rates and also achieve clinical significance. They should also be cost effective.

- Reliability is a measure of random error. It can be assessed by repeated applications of the same test (test–retest reliability) or by analysing the internal consistency (scale reliability), which is a measure of the relationships between a set of indicators for the same underlying variable. As the test–retest reliability can be difficult to measure for a set of variables that fluctuates, internal consistency is often used to determine the reliability of quality of life instruments.

- Validity is the extent to which the result of a method measures the underlying construct in question. It is connected to the degree of systematic measurement error or bias. There are three basic types of validity: criterion, content and construct validity. As there is no golden standard for measuring cancer patients' quality of life, indirect approaches must be used, such as interview-based ratings, or analysis of the psychometric properties of the given instrument (how particular instruments relate to each other and their consistency with prior expectations or theory). This is construct validity (Bjordal & Kaasa, 1992).

- Responsiveness and sensitivity refer to the ability of the question-naire to detect clinical changes that occur after therapeutic inter-ventions. Thus responsiveness is proportional to the change in scores on a particular questionnaire during treatment. Ideally, a clinically responsive questionnaire can detect small changes in quality of life. The measurement should also be sensitive enough to differentiate between stages of disease, extent of treatment and changes over time (Baker, 1995).

Who should score quality of life — the clinician or the patient?

Slevin et al (1988) demonstrated clearly that clinicians cannot adequately rate patients' quality of life. They also demonstrated that healthcare professionals had a wide variability in the scores they produced, even for the objective Karnofsky scale. Hodder et al (1997) also found that clinician-rated scales are likely to under-estimate the extent of the problems. They found that surgeons attached widely differing weights of importance to various compo-nents of outcome, and propose that this may affect their treatment decisions. D'Antonio et al (1996) similarly found that physicians consistently underrated their patients' emotional wellbeing when asked to score it for them.

Gotay and Moore (1992) note that as head and neck cancers frequently affect the patient's ability to verbalize, self-administered questionnaires may be more appropriate than interviews.

Patient self-rating is therefore the methodology of choice in quality of life assessment.

Recommendations for head and neck quality of life tools

Several authors (Maguire & Selby, 1989; Terrell et al, 1997; D'Antonio et al, 1998) recommend that an assessment tool should be completed by the patient, easy and quick to complete and score, valid and reliable, and able to reflect changes over time. A head and neck module should be suitable for patients before, during and after treatment, receiving combinations of radiotherapy, chemotherapy and surgery. It should measure all the important disease specific symptoms that affect the patient's functional status and wellbeing. It should also be adaptable to cross-cultural settings.

Several authors have presented proposals for head and neck cancer specific quality of life assessment tools. Table 3.1.1 (p. 333) gives a summary of some of these instruments.

Quality of life studies and their findings

Table 3.1.2 (p. 340) gives a comprehensive overview of quality of life studies in head and neck cancer over this decade. The findings relevant to nursing practice are summarized briefly.

Summary

Quality of life measurement has several important implications for nursing practice in head and neck cancer:

- It can help patients and clinicians make treatment decisions.
- It can help to give patients an overview of their treatment, side effects and recovery trajectory.
- It can help to identify areas for practice development.
- It can help to identify the individual patient's needs for additional supportive interventions.

- It can help to evaluate therapeutic interventions.
- It can give an accurate picture of the patient's overall benefit from the whole service.

There is now enough data from quality of life studies to suggest that head and neck cancer service providers should be routinely incorporating the use of a validated instrument by all their patients.

Table 3.1.1: An overview of head and neck quality of life assessment tools developed during the 1990s

Tool	Items covered	Scoring system	Ability to meet criteria
Performance status scale for head and neck cancer patients (PSS-HN) (List et al, 1990) Developed as there was a need for a tool more specific than Karnofsky. Developed in consultation with otolaryngology, surgical and speech and swallowing experts	Eating in public Understandability of speech Normalcy of diet	Patients are rated in each item through use of an unstructured interview. Scores range from 0 (worst function) to 100 (best function) Clinician-rated	Correlation statistics, one way analyses of variance, t-tests, Kappa statistics and Kruskal–Wallis statistics were used. High levels of inter-rater reliability were found, and significant correlations between the items. The PSS-HN was more sensitive to specific head and neck patient problems than Karnofsky. On tests for validity, reliability and sensitivity, it performed well. It can be easily administered with no training to screen patients for difficulties and expedites appropriate interventions
University of Washington QOL head and neck questionnaire (UW QOL) (Hassan et al, 1993) Method of development is not described	Pain Disfigurement Activity Recreation/entertainment Employment Chewing Swallowing Speech Shoulder disability	Each category is assigned 100 points. Best function scores 100, worst function scores 0. The total possible score is 900 points	The UW QOL demonstrated a high level of acceptability. Correlation coefficients showed that the UW QOL correlated significantly with the SIP and the Karnofsky. A statistically significant reliability was demonstrated. It was more responsive to head and neck cancer than the SIP or Karnofsky

(contd)

Table 3.1.1: (contd)

Tool	Items covered	Scoring system	Ability to meet criteria
The Head and Neck Radiotherapy Questionnaire (HNRQ) (Browman et al, 1993b) Developed by literature review, consultation with oncologists, radiation technologists, nurses and patients	Pain/soreness in mouth Dryness of skin Difficulty swallowing Energy levels Emotional wellbeing Nausea Itching skin Sleep Dry mouth Fatigue Pain/soreness in throat Upset stomach Sticky saliva Taste Appetite Self-esteem Swallowing Hoarseness	Each domain is covered by three questions. There are seven possible responses on a Likert scale. The worst toxicity gives the lowest score; the final score is expressed as the mean of the 22 questions Clinician-rated	The HNRQ demonstrated significant sensitivity to change, using analyses of variance. It correlated well with WHO stomatitis and skin scales, ECOG performance status and Karnofsky, using product-moment correlation coefficients. Inter-rater reliability or patient acceptability was not tested
European Organization for Research and Treatment of Cancer (EORTC) Head and Neck Module (EORTC QLQ-H&N37)	Pain in the mouth, jaw, throat Soreness in the mouth Problems swallowing liquids, pureed food, solid food	Each item has four response categories; 1 (best function) to 4 (worst function). Use of painkillers, supplements, feeding tube and weight gain/loss are scored as yes	The module content has been extensively researched and pretested across Europe and therefore has a high level of content validity. It is designed for use with

(Bjordal et al, 1994a)

Developed from literature search (MEDLINE and CANCERLIT, medical textbooks), structured interviews with clinicians and nurses, structured interviews with patients

Choking when swallowing
Problems with teeth, dry mouth, sticky saliva
Problems opening the mouth
Change of sense of taste and smell
Coughing, hoarseness
Feeling ill
Bothered by appearance
Trouble in eating in front of others
Enjoyment of meals
Talking to other people and telephone
Carrying out normal work
Practising hobbies or leisure time activities
Contact with family and friends
Going out in public
Physical contact with family or friends
Sexual interest and enjoyment
Use of painkillers, nutritional supplements, feeding tube
Weight loss and weight gain

(2) or no (1). Thus higher scores represent worse function

Patient-rated

the EORTC QLQ-C30. It is now being field tested. There is no statistical data on acceptability, reliability, validity and sensitivity at the time of writing

(contd)

Table 3.1.1: (contd)

Tool	Items covered	Scoring system	Ability to meet criteria
Functional Status in Head and Neck Cancer — Self Report (FSH&N-SR) (Baker, 1995) Developed from patient interviews	Shoulder/upper body mobility Chewing Swallowing Drooling Taste Dry mouth Eating in public Speech Breathing Appearance Pain Fatigue Overall QOL	Five statements about each item are rank ordered with 'no problem' scored 5, and those statements associated with greatest dysfunction scored 1. Scores range from 15 (worst function) to 75 (best function) Patient-rated	*t*-Tests, analysis of variance, multiple comparison tests of significance, Pearson correlation, Cronbach's alpha showed the FSH&N-SR is a sensitive, reliable and valid tool to reflect functional status after multimodality treatment. It is an excellent screening tool for the identification of symptom management and rehabilitation needs
Functional Assessment of Cancer Therapy — Head and Neck Scale (FACT-HN) (List et al, 1996a; D'Antonio et al, 1996) Development not described	Eating food I like Dry mouth Breathing Voice Eating as much as I want Self-conscious Swallow Smoking Alcohol use	Each item is rated on a 0 to 4 Likert type scale, with an extra item on overall effect on QOL rated 0 to 10. High scores represent better QOL Patient-rated Designed for use with the	Kruskal–Wallis one-way analysis of variance, Mann–Whitney nonparametric analyses, and Spearman correlation coefficients suggested a high degree of sensitivity and correlation between the FACT-HN and the UW QOL. There was a lower degree of correlation with the PSS-HN

	Communication Eating solid food Global QOL	FACT-G, a 28-question general cancer questionnaire	The FACT-HN had a low internal consistency coefficient, particularly on the emotional wellbeing subscale
Multiattribute utility assessment of outcomes of treatment for head and neck cancer (Hodder et al, 1997) Developed by interviews with patients, consultant maxillofacial surgeons, a Delphi panel (head and neck oncologist, four maxillofacial surgeons, head and neck counsellor, researcher)	Social function Pain Physical appearance Swallowing Speech Nausea Donor-site problems Shoulder function	Eight domains, each domain has a score between 0 (worst health) and 100 (best health) Clinician-rated	Acceptability, reliability, sensitivity, validity not tested as yet
Head and Neck Survey (H&NS) (Gliklich et al, 1997) Developed by an expert panel	Eating (normalcy of diet) Eating (in public) Swallowing (aspiration) Swallowing (sticking in throat) Speech; intelligibility and in a noisy room Social anxiety related to appearance Appearance and self-esteem Pain	Each item has five response categories assigned a score of 0 (worst) to 100 (best). A total score is calculated based on the cumulative score of the nine questions Patient-rated	Cronbach's alpha and Multiple t-tests showed the H&NS was highly correlated to the UW QOL and PSS-HN, which are also head and neck specific. It was only moderately correlated to the SF-36, which is a general health measure. The SF-36 failed to measure eating, speech and appearance domains adequately

(contd)

Table 3.1.1: (contd)

Tool	Items covered	Scoring system	Ability to meet criteria
Head and Neck Quality of Life Questionnaire (HNQOL) (Terrell et al, 1997) Developed by a literature review, interviews with healthcare workers, patient surveys, consultation with head and neck oncologists and surgeons	Speaking to others and phone Voice Chewing Dryness while eating Taste Swallowing Difficulty opening mouth Embarrassment about condition Concerns about appearance Emotional problems Financial worries Concern about the future Frustration Pain in neck/shoulder Pain/burning in mouth Frequency of pain medication use General physical problems	Responses as five choices are rated as 0 (worst score) to 100 (best score) Patient-rated	Principle factor analysis varimax rotation, Cronbach's alpha, Pearson product correlations, intraclass correlations, and paired *t*-tests were performed. The HNQOL showed reliability, validity and sensitivity. Acceptability not discussed. The authors believe that the multiple domains of which it consists are an advantage over the UW QOL, FACT and EORTC composite scores for three reasons. 1. It more accurately reflects the multidimensional nature of the patient's functional status and wellbeing. 2. It allows for breakdown of the patient's QOL for analysis. 3. It has a larger potential range of responses for each domain. They believe its Pain domain is more comprehensive as it includes shoulder pain

Instrument	Items	Scoring	Comments
Head and Neck Quality of Life Radiation Therapy Instrument (QOL-RTI/H&N) (Trotti et al, 1998) Developed from a review of current tools and panel of health professionals. The authors felt that existing tools did not adequately address radiation side effects	Pain in mouth Pain in throat Amount of saliva Quality of saliva Mucus in mouth or throat Taste Appearance Speech intelligibility Coughing Chewing Eating (normalcy of diet) Eating (in public) Swallowing (food and liquids)	Each item is rated on a 0–10 Likert scale. The scores are summed and averaged to yield a single score Patient-rated	Cronbach's alpha demonstrated satisfactory internal consistency. Test–retest reliability was demonstrated. Designed for use with the general quality of life-radiation therapy instrument (QOL-RTI) There was satisfactory correlation with the FACT/H&N; the QOL-RTI/H&N seemed to demonstrate superior sensitivity. The authors say that patient compliance was good, therefore acceptability was high. The authors say that this tool is more accurate than others in measuring radiation side effects

Please note that copyright for these QOL instruments is retained by the author of each instrument and permission to use any of the instruments must be obtained directly from the author of that instrument.

Abbreviations: ECOG = Eastern Co-operative Oncology Group Performance Status (Oken et al, 1982); Karnofsky = Karnofsky Performance Status Scale (Karnofsky & Burchenall, 1949); QOL = quality of life; SF-36 = Medical Outcomes Study Short-Form 36-Item Health Survey (Ware & Sherbourne, 1992); SIP = Sickness Impact Profile (Bergner & Bobbitt, 1981); WHO = World Health Organization.

Table 3.1.2: An overview of recent quality of life studies and their main findings

Author Aim	Tools	Sample size	Treatment modalities and cancer sites	Disease stages	Statistical tests	QOL Findings
Rathmell et al (1991) Aim: to find a series of questions which identify specific QOL issues for head and neck cancer patients	Own QOL questionnaire (PR) Structured interview and Hospital Anxiety and Depression score for 11 patients	96	Surgery and postop radiotherapy, radiotherapy alone, surgery alone: Larynx/ hypopharynx 45 Oral cavity/ oropharynx 37 Sinuses/nose 6 Salivary glands 5 Ear 3	Not reported	Proportions only	QOL improved with time after treatment in both groups, but more rapidly in the radiotherapy alone group. Surgery patients had more problems with eating. More than half the surgery patients reported problems with arm morbidity due to neck dissection and forearm flap Conclusion: radical surgery should only be used if it gives significant survival benefits
Jones et al (1992) Aim: to evaluate tool	EORTC QLQ-C30 (PR) Own H and N module (PR)	48	Surgical only: Laryngectomy 15 Craniofacial 11 PLO 5 Hemiglossectomy 4 Tonsillectomy 3 Thyroidectomy 2 Recurrence 8	Not reported	Mean values Wilcoxon Rank Sum Test	Laryngectomy patients reported best QOL but had speech difficulties and hyposmia. Craniofacial patients reported next best QOL but reported headaches, altered vision (usually blurred), fatigue, pain, anxiety, hyposmia. PLO patients reported worse overall QOL with eating problems, fatigue, speech difficulties, isolation, hyposmia, sexual problems, anxiety and depression

Study / Aim	Tool	Number	Sample		Statistics	Results
						Hemiglossectomy patients reported speech and eating difficulties. Recurrence patients reported worst QOL with eating, speech, sexual difficulties, hyposmia and hypogeusia, anxiety. High levels of fatigue in PLO and craniofacial patients. Conclusion: the EORTC QLQ is a sensitive tool and information collected will enhance our understanding of patients' difficulties, facilitating improved rehabilitation and better QOL
Bjordal & Kaasa (1992) Aim: to evaluate tool	EORTC QLQ-C30 (PR) Own H and N module (PR) General Health Questionnaire (GHQ-20) (PR)	126	Radiotherapy: Oral cavity 33% Pharynx 19% Larynx 19% Skin 18% Salivary gland, sinuses, thyroid, cervical nodes 18%	Not reported	Mean values Cronbach's alpha coefficient Pearson correlation coefficients One-way analysis of variance	High levels of fatigue reported. Work, family and social activities suffered. Sore mouth, swallowing problems, salivation and mucus production was worst from halfway through to follow-up after radiotherapy. Taste change and dry mouth were worst at follow up after radiotherapy, as was fatigue and social functioning. Conclusion: patient compliance was high in completing the QLQ. The QLQ showed reliability, validity and sensitivity, with some problems which will be modified in future QLQs

(contd)

Table 3.1.2: (contd)

Author Aim	Tools	Sample size	Treatment modalities and cancer sites	Disease stages	Statistical tests	QOL Findings
Harrison et al (1994) Aim: to compare QOL and functional outcome in base of tongue treated by surgery and primary radiotherapy	Performance status scale	40	Primary radiotherapy, surgery and postop radiotherapy: base of tongue	I/II 26 III/IV 14	Mean values t-tests estimated residual variance F-test	Much better functional outcome for radiotherapy group for eating in public, normalcy of diet and speech understandability. Conclusion: performance status is better after radiotherapy for base of tongue tumours. When both radiotherapy and surgery have similar survival outcomes, QOL measurement is an important factor when deciding on the optimal treatment strategy
Bjordal et al (1994b) Aim: to compare QOL in patients treated by conventional and hypofractionated radiotherapy	EORTC QLQ-C30 Head and neck cancer module General Health Questionnaire	204	Primary, postop and preop radiotherapy: Oral cavity 44 Pharynx 14 Larynx 102 Nose/sinus 12 Other 32	I 97 II 39 III 31 IV 34 NS 3	Cronbach's alpha Pearson correlation coefficients Multiple regression	Both groups reported high levels of symptoms, especially dry mouth, mucus production, fatigue and swallowing. Patients who also underwent major surgery had most symptoms. Emotional function was significantly influenced by the extent of surgery. The patients receiving the hypofractionated regime reported better QOL than the conventional group

	n	Treatment and site	Stage	Statistics	Conclusion
Morton (1995) Aim: to evaluate tool — Own Life Satisfaction self-reported questionnaire (PR)	130	Radiotherapy, surgery and combined modality: Glottic 39, Oral/oropharynx 31, Nasopharynx 8, Hypopharynx 29, Other 23	I 25, II 21, III 25, IV 41, NS 18	2-way paired t-tests Pearson chi-square	Conclusion: functional and emotional outcomes are important parameters. QOL measurements are an easy and valid way of assessing treatment effects. They can be used to identify patients in need of support and rehabilitation and thus improve their QOL
Bjordal et al (1995) Aim: to assess QOL 1–6 years after treatment, to compare clinician ratings and patient self ratings — Spitzer QOL index (CR) EORTC QLQ-C30 (PR) General Health Questionnaire (GHQ-20) (PR) Karnofsky Performance Status (CR)	50	Surgery, chemotherapy and radiotherapy: Oral 22, Parotid 9, Pharynx 14, Other 5	I 14, II 12, III 8, IV 12, NS 4	Descriptive; Multivariate analyses not performed due to small sample size	Life satisfaction improves with time after successful treatment. The principal determinants are pain, dysphagia, and speech difficulty Conclusion: it is important that attention is paid to pain, communications skills, swallowing problems—improvements will improve QOL
					Patients reported high frequency of treatment-related side effects and psychological distress; including fatigue, sleep disturbance, dry mouth, mucus production, taste and swallowing problems. Clinicians rated these symptoms significantly lower than the patients. 72% of smokers continued to smoke

(contd)

Table 3.1.2: (contd)

Author Aim	Tools	Sample size	Treatment modalities and cancer sites	Disease stages	Statistical tests	QOL Findings
						Conclusion: a stop smoking programme may benefit patients; patient self-reported questionnaires could be used as a tool for better communication of problems
De Boer et al (1995) Aim: to describe the rehabilitation outcomes of three different treatment groups	Cancer Locus of Control (PR) Self-esteem Scale (PR) Uncertainty Scale (PR) Rotterdam Symptom Checklist (PR) Head and Neck Self-efficacy Scale (PR)	110	Primary radiotherapy for T1 larynx 66 Total laryngectomy ± neck dissection and radiotherapy 32 Commando procedure ± radiotherapy 12	Not stated	Student's t-test Multiple regression analysis	T1 larynx patients experience a considerable number of physical complaints (fatigue, mucus, speech and swallowing problems) between 2 and 6 years after treatment. Laryngectomy and commando procedure patients experience severe psychosocial distress; the laryngectomees with communication problems, commando patients with eating and disfigurement problems. Laryngectomy patients particularly have difficulty with self-esteem and self-efficacy Conclusion: open discussion of illness in the family, social support and adequate information for both

Author (year) / Aim	Measures	N	Treatment	Stage	Analysis	Results / Conclusion
						patient and partner from the specialist are the most important predictors of positive rehabilitation outcomes
Long et al (1996) Aim: to measure QOL and function in patients after major surgery and examine their relationship to physical and psychosocial variables	FACT-G (PR) FACT-HNS (PR) UW-QOL (PR) PSS-HN (CR) Disfigurement and dysfunction scales	50	Major surgery for stage III/IV, recurrence, disease unresponsive to radiotherapy: Larynx 22 Oral cavity 17 Pharynx 7 Other 4	III and IV	Analysis of variance Duncan's multiple range testing	Larynx patients scored better for QOL and eating than oral and pharyngeal patients. Higher disfigurement ratings and pain were related to worse QOL scores. Married patients had significantly better scores and less pain, patients living alone had worse scores Conclusion: social support is an important variable and should be considered when planning discharge
Moore et al (1996) Aim: to determine quality of life functional outcome after primary radiotherapy for base of tongue cancer	PSS-HN (CR)	49	Radiotherapy: base of tongue	I 8 II 21 III 16 IV 4	Inter-rater agreement Mean scores	Eating in public scores were worse as T stage increased. Speech intelligibility declined with T stage. All patients had difficulty swallowing solid and dry foods. Hot spicy foods, and citrus fruit and juice were avoided. Difficulty was related to tumour stage Conclusion: patients and families should be educated extensively regarding treatment effects on eating and speech

(contd)

Table 3.1.2: (contd)

Author Aim	Tools	Sample size	Treatment modalities and cancer sites	Disease stages	Statistical tests	QOL Findings
List et al (1996b) Aim: to evaluate QOL and performance outcome in laryngeal cancer patients over time	PSS-HN (CR) FACT-HN (PR) Karnofsky performance status rating scale (CR)	21	Total and partial laryngectomy, radiotherapy alone	I 8 II 3 III 6 IV 4	Freidman's test Kruskal-Wallis test Analysis of variance Spearman correlation coefficients Median scores	Total laryngectomy patients fared worst performance-wise and took longest to improve; 40% still had significant problems at 6 months. Partial laryngectomy patients were mostly returned to normal at 6 months; eating recovered slowest. Radiotherapy patients experienced most problems at the time of treatment completion (6 weeks), but had little overall dysfunction Conclusion: clinicians can use this information to inform and prepare patients, and as a yardstick against which to evaluate individual patients
McDonough et al (1996) Aim: to compare QOL	UW QOL (PR) Social Avoidance and Distress Scale	24	Neoadjuvant chemotherapy + radiotherapy alone, Neoadjuvant chemotherapy +	III and IV	Correlation coefficients Means Standard deviations	As QOL decreased, social distress and avoidance increased. There was a significant and sharp decline in QOL for the group undergoing surgery compared with the non-

in patients treated by chemotherapy + radiotherapy with patients treated with chemotherapy + surgery + radiotherapy			surgery + radiotherapy Sites not reported			surgical group, and their scores continued to be the lowest. Both groups' QOL scores worsened mid-radiation. Scores started to improve 1 month post-radiation. At all time points, the surgical group reported higher levels of social avoidance, but these improved over time Conclusion: 1. organ preservation treatment gives better QOL, 2. social avoidance and distress peak after surgery and during radio-therapy and increased levels of support should be given at these times
Chaturvedi et al (1996) Aim: to identify the concerns and coping mechanisms used by patients with oral cancer	50	Coping and concerns inventory Hospital Anxiety and Depression Scale	Oral/oropharyngeal cancer 25 Laryngeal cancer 25	Not reported	Chi-square test Fisher's exact test	Commonest concerns (> 50% of patients) were about the future, finances, physical problems, communication, emotional difficulties and inability to do things. The commonest coping mechanisms were helplessness and fatalism. Resolution of concerns was noted in less than 40% of patients. There was a high percentage of patients suffering from significant anxiety and depression amongst those with moderate/severe concerns and those using helplessness and fatalism

(contd)

Table 3.1.2: (contd)

Author Aim	Tools	Sample size	Treatment modalities and cancer sites	Disease stages	Statistical tests	QOL Findings
						Conclusion: patients with head and neck cancer have numerous concerns and often use negative coping strategies. They need counselling in order to explore their concerns and assist in selection of more effective coping mechanisms
Harrison et al (1997) Aim: to evaluate QOL in patients treated with primary radiotherapy to base of tongue	Memorial Symptoms Assessment Scale (MSAS) (PR) Functional Assessment of Cancer Therapy (FACT) (PR) PSS-HN (CR)	36	External beam radiotherapy + brachytherapy boost: base of tongue	I 11 II 14 III 10 IV 1	Mean values Standard deviations Percentages	Most prevalent problems: dry mouth, difficulty swallowing, fatigue, pain. Psychological distress and physical, emotional and social wellbeing scores were relatively good. 72% could eat in public, 86% had understandable speech, however, only 35% had normal diet. The majority of patients were able to return to work Conclusion: QOL measurement is vital to select optimal therapy. It will also help to give a perspective of the economic cost of cancer treatment. A cured patient who is permanently disabled is not the same as a cured patient who is earning his or her prediagnosis income

| Deleyiannis et al (1997)

Aim: to compare QOL in surgery versus radiotherapy for oropharyngeal cancer | UW QOL (PR) | 13 | Surgery + postop radiotherapy 6
Radiotherapy + chemotherapy 7: oropharynx | All patients III or IV | Mean values
Wilcoxon matched-pairs signed-ranks test
2-way t-tests | Both surgery and radiotherapy patients reported worse chewing (67%). Both groups reported worse swallowing (surgery 67%, radiotherapy 71%). After 1 year, two surgery patients still required gastrostomy. 83% of the surgery group felt their appearance was worse, against 33% of the radiotherapy group. Speech was worse in 67% of the surgery group and 43% of the radiotherapy group. 67% of the surgery group felt pain was better, 29% of the radiotherapy group felt the same. 50% of patients said they were as active as they used to be

Conclusion: different treatments for oropharyngeal cancer may have similar outcomes. Careful attention to QOL outcomes will help to identify best treatment. This information will enable patients to participate actively in decisions |

(contd)

Table 3.1.2: (contd)

Author Aim	Tools	Sample size	Treatment modalities and cancer sites	Disease stages	Statistical tests	QOL Findings
List et al (1997) Aim: to evaluate post treatment QOL in patients treated with intensive chemoradio-therapy for organ preservation	Semi-structured patient interview (CR) PSS-HN (CR) McMaster University Head and Neck Radiotherapy Questionnaire (PR) FACT - Head and Neck (FACT-H&N) (PR) Centre for Epidemiological Studies Depression Scale (CES-D) (PR)	47	Neoadjuvant + concomitant radiotherapy 32 Concomitant alone 15 Larynx 15 Oropharynx 14 Oral cavity 6 Nasopharynx 4 Hypopharynx 3 Other 5	II 4 III 14 IV 29	Mean values standard deviations frequencies chi-square t-tests	Greatest functional impairment was eating difficulty, but 79% of patients would still eat in public places. Speech outcomes were good. Overall, reasonably good quality of life. 23% were depressed. The most frequent and troublesome symptom was dry mouth (77%). Sticky saliva, swallowing, chewing and hypogeusia were also troublesome to 25–33% of patients. Ability to eat post-treatment was not related to ability to eat pre-treatment. Patients who had salvage surgery were functioning more poorly. Depression and poor overall QOL were associated with alcohol use pre-diagnosis. Residual pain had the most impact in all domains. Shoulder pain and mobility should be included in assessments Conclusion: decreased QOL and depression appear to be associated with overall number and severity of symptoms. Strategies to reduce

Study / Aim	Instruments (n)	Treatment	Stage / Data	Statistics	Results
					overall symptoms, or help patients cope with them, may have a positive impact on QOL
Ruhl et al (1997) Aim: to determine survival rate and QOL after total glossectomy	FACT (PR) EORTC QLQ-C30 (PR) PSS-HN (PR) 13 additional disease-specific questions' (PR) 7	Glossectomy with or without total laryngectomy	Data not given	Descriptive only	The most significant problems were eating and shoulder/neck function. Six patients needed gastrostomies. Only one patient found eating enjoyable. Speech was severely impaired. However, the authors report that all patients scored well for overall QOL and wellbeing. Only 7 patients out of 35 approached agreed to enter this study, therefore selection bias is a major flaw Conclusion: QOL is more than function alone and adaptation is possible with good family support and access to a skilled rehabilitation team
Hodder et al (1997) Aim: to examine QOL before, during and after treatment	EORTC QLQ-C30 and head and neck module (H&N-21) (PR) HAD scale Karnofsky performance status 44	Surgery, radiotherapy, chemotherapy: Larynx 11 Tongue 9 Mouth 8 Tonsil 5 Parotid 6 Other 5	I 12 II 5 III 7 IV 18 NS 2	Fisher's nonparametric permutation test Repeated measures analysis of variance Mean values	HAD scores revealed a high level of distress, particularly at diagnosis. Distress continued long after treatment completion. All symptoms worsened during treatment, were worst at 2–3 months and started to improve at 6 months. Swallowing was still a problem at month 12.

(contd)

Table 3.1.2: (contd)

Author Aim	Tools	Sample size	Treatment modalities and cancer sites	Disease stages	Statistical tests	QOL Findings
						Dry mouth and altered taste were still significant problems at month 12. Overall QOL dipped significantly during treatment, picked up by month 12, but was still 10 points lower than pre-treatment
						Conclusion: as symptoms are worst at the end of treatment, when many patients have been discharged, this is a period when special support should be considered. Patients may also benefit from psychiatric evaluation and treatment
Languis (1997) Aim: to describe the possibility of using three standardized instruments to assess QOL in oral cancer	Sickness Impact Profile (PR) Karnofsky Performance Status (CR) Health Index (PR)	57	Oral surgery (post op radiotherapy not reported or allowed for in analysis)	Not reported	Cronbach's alpha Friedman 2-way analysis of variance Mann–Whitney U-test Kruskal–Wallis 1-way analysis of variance	Weight loss was still significant 12 months post-surgery. Psychosocial and general wellbeing measurements were still worse at 12 months than pre-treatment. Performance status was correlated to psychosocial, functional and wellbeing parameters. The more extensive the surgery, the worse the patients did

					Spearman correlation coefficients Student's t-test Pearson product correlation coefficient	Conclusion: standardized QOL instruments may help in the assessment and evaluation processes of nursing care
Murry et al (1998) Aim: to assess QOL in patients undergoing concurrent chemoradiation	Head and Neck Radiotherapy Questionnaire (HNRQ) (PR) Swallowing Questionnaire (SQ) (PR)	37	Concurrent arterial chemotherapy and radiotherapy: Hypopharynx Larynx Oropharynx	III and IV	Analysis of variance Mean scores Pearson product correlations	During the 7-week treatment QOL and swallowing declined for all groups and was worst at the end of treatment. The hypopharynx group had the worst scores. By 6 months, the hypopharynx group QOL was better than pretreatment levels, but the larynx and oropharynx QOL was worse than pre-treatment. The oropharynx group had significant swallowing problems. Psychosocial domain scores improved before physical scores

Conclusion: the need for support services to aid psychosocial recovery should be considered when treating head and neck cancer |

(contd)

Table 3.1.2: (contd)

Author Aim	Tools	Sample size	Treatment modalities and cancer sites	Disease stages	Statistical tests	QOL Findings
Rogers et al (1998) Aim: to report the SF-36 in oral and oropharyngeal patients, to relate the SF-36 outcomes to variables, to correlate the SF-36 to the UW QOL	Medical outcomes short-form health survey (SF-36) UW QOL	48	Oral and oropharyngeal surgery; 48% had postop radiotherapy	I/II 30 III/IV 18	Mean values Wilcoxon's matched pairs tests Spearman correlation coefficients Cronbach's alpha	Scores in all domains deteriorated considerably by 3 months. A steady improvement occurred from month 3 onwards. Patients with oropharyngeal sites, stages 3 and 4 and postopradiotherapy performed worst. Poor physical and psychosocial functioning was shown to continue throughout the 12 months post-surgery Conclusion: there is a need for continued physical and psychological support throughout the first year. QOL tools could be used to identify individual problems and offer specific interventions
Hammerlid et al (1998)	EORTC QLQ-C30 Head and neck module	48	Radiotherapy, chemotherapy, surgery:	I 6 II 10 III 8	Cronbach's alpha Fisher's non-parametric	51% of the sample were clinically malnourished. This was most common before treatment and in

Study/Aim	Measures	n	Sample/Treatment	Stage	Statistics	Results
Aim: to study QOL in relation to malnutrition			Larynx 11 Sinuses 10 Oral 8 Tongue 8 Other 11	IV 16 NS 8	permutation test Fisher's exact test	recurrent disease. Only 35% of the malnourished group were alive after 2 years, compared with 64% in the well-nourished group. The malnourished patients scored worse for symptoms, QOL, physical function and role function but these differences were not significant. Stage of disease did not affect nutrition or QOL. Better QOL scores were related to survival Conclusion: individual personalities and abilities to cope may be strong factors in survival
D'Antonio et al (1998) Aim: to explore the relationship between QOL and depression	Disfigurement and dysfunction scale (CR) PSS-HN (CR) Emotional well-being rating (EWB) (CR) Beck Depression	50	Surgery, chemotherapy, radiotherapy: Larynx 22 Oral cavity 17 Pharynx 7 Other 4	I 6 II 7 III 15 IV 17 NS 5	Spearman correlation coefficients	22% of the sample demonstrated moderate to severe depression. QOL was significantly inversely related to depression. FACT and UW QOL measures correlated with the BDI. There was no relationship between the clinician-rated EWB and the patient's rating on the FACT EWB or the BDI

(contd)

Table 3.1.2: (contd)

Author Aim	Tools	Sample size	Treatment modalities and cancer sites	Disease stages	Statistical tests	QOL Findings
	Inventory (BDI) (PR) FACT-G (PR) FACT-HNS (PR) UW-QOL (PR)					Conclusion: physician estimates of EWB are inaccurate and tools such as FACT and UW QOL can help to identify distress more accurately. Studies to evaluate the effect of treating depression are needed

Abbreviations: CR = clinician-rated; PLO = pharyngolaryngo-oesophagectomy; PR = patient-rated; QLQ = quality of life questionnaire; QOL = quality of life.

Chapter 3.2
Psychosocial and emotional effects of head and neck cancer

Introduction

Head and neck cancer is so very obvious. The face is the only part of the body that cannot be covered by clothing. The consequences of this visibility can be devastating. The head and neck is a visible, prominent area that serves as the primary medium for communication, animation of intellect and emotion and representation of self (Dropkin, 1989). This is aptly demonstrated by the remarks of one woman with extensive facial cancer, sitting in a radiotherapy waiting room. She commented on the unfairness of her cancer: 'Everyone in this waiting room has cancer. But I am the only one who cannot hide it. My cancer is visible to the whole world'. Head and neck cancer and its treatment also have a profound impact on the most basic of human functions, including the ability to speak, eat, breathe and socialize normally. Thus head and neck cancer affects body image, self-esteem and normal functioning, and carries a high psychological and social morbidity.

The four main psychological responses to cancer stress are: uncertainty, negative feelings (depression, loneliness, anxiety), loss of control and threatened self-esteem (Mesters et al, 1997). Patients strive for a reduction in uncertainty and negative feelings, try to regain control of the situation, and want to restore self-esteem. Most of the studies on head and neck cancer cite problems with reduced self-esteem, social isolation, fear of rejection and abandonment, overall distress, a feeling of being handicapped and even suicidal tendencies (Gamba et al, 1992).

Drettner and Ahlbom (1983) found that survivors with a good prognosis reported better quality of life than healthy controls (although they had more eating difficulties). The authors propose that survivors may have an enhanced appreciation of life. Gotay and Moore (1992) find this encouraging and suggest that, with the proper support, head and neck cancer patients may have the chance to return to normal, or even enhanced, levels of wellbeing.

This chapter will examine the literature on the psychosocial effects of head and neck cancer in order to provide a basis for psychosocial and emotional care. The reader may find it useful to revise the section on stress, appraisal and coping in Chapter 1.2 before reading on.

Body image and concepts of self

It is helpful to understand concepts underlying altered body image.

Altered body image

Price defines altered body image as 'a state of personal distress, defined by the patient, which indicates that the body no longer supports self-esteem, and which is dysfunctional to individuals, limiting their social engagement with others. Altered body image exists when coping strategies (individual and social) to deal with changes in body reality, ideal or presentation, are overwhelmed by injury, disease, disability or social stigma' (Price, 1995). Body image is dynamic, changing throughout life. Individuals are able to accommodate these changes with the help of others who affirm their self worth and attraction in other ways. However, the ability to sustain a satisfactory body image may be overwhelmed by a sudden and overwhelming change in body circumstances. Price (1998) lists the following as potent threats to body image for people with cancer:

- pain and fatigue — especially if these are associated with a poor prognosis and are persistent in nature
- loss of physical control — through incontinence, lost neurological ability, sensory or motor control
- cancer or treatment that affects the face or sexual organs — which are imbued with special significance as the means of defining our sexual identity.
- conditions which demand that a prosthesis is utilized which may be hidden under normal circumstances, but which may become starkly apparent at other times

- the breaching of body boundaries — with catheters and tubes
- alopecia.

Many individuals with head and neck cancer will experience at least one of these harms, losses and threats. Some individuals may experience all of them. In head and neck cancer, these threats may be experienced in a very visible way, for example, loss of physical control of part of the face or mouth, the wearing of a facial prosthesis, the placement of a nasogastric tube.

The reader is referred to texts by Price (1990) and Salter (1988) for more information on body image and altered body image.

Stigmatization

People who are visibly or audibly different may feel stigmatized. Goffman (1963) defines stigma as 'the situation of an individual who is disqualified from full social acceptance: a person who has a failing or handicap is reduced in the mind of society as a tainted person'. Goffman also notes that people make assumptions about certain disabilities. For example, a person who cannot speak is often also assumed to be deaf, and impaired intelligence is assumed to go hand in hand with a physical disability.

Self-efficacy

Perceived self-efficacy is defined as a judgement as to how well one can execute a course of action required to deal with a prospective situation. Perceived self-efficacy may prove to be a powerful predicator of adjustment to specific stressful events such as the sequelae of cancer (Cunningham et al, 1991).

Self-esteem

Self-esteem has been described as 'the golden key which unlocks our potential'. It 'acts as the heart of our psychological selves' and 'is just as critical to our survival as its physical counterpart' (Lindenfield, 1995). Self-belief is the cornerstone of self-esteem: if a person believes he or she is worthless, ugly and incapable, then his or her feelings and behaviour will reflect these thoughts and his or her whole experience will be one of depression and negativity. However, if thoughts are positive, feelings and behaviour will correspond, enabling people to present themselves positively.

Disfigurement and dysfunction in head and neck cancer

Facial cancer

Head and neck surgery can result in a permanent, visible mutilation to the face which is difficult to disguise (Koster & Bergsma, 1990). Physical attractiveness has tremendous importance attached to it by society. Rumsey (1997) points out that even mythology, legends and fairy tales promote the idea that beauty is of paramount importance. Although there is no evidence to suggest a relationship between facial appearance and personality, there is a popular notion that character can be influenced by appearance. Contemporary society reinforces this concept; the cosmetic and fashion industries spend millions of pounds promoting the message that beauty is all-important. Numerous reports in the literature consistently note society's real aversion to visible deformity, particularly of the face (Dropkin et al, 1983).

The importance of the face as a specialized area of both verbal and non-verbal communication, and as a point of initial focus in an encounter, is well known (Argyle, 1972). Physical attractiveness is often gauged initially by the characteristics of the head and neck. Therefore a person with a facial abnormality may suffer from negative stereotyping as well as from disruption of normal interaction processes (Rumsey et al, 1982). This negative stereotyping may be the cause of avoidance behaviour in the general public, who were shown to stand further away from a person with facial disfigurement. Rumsey et al (1982) propose that this behaviour may be due to uncomfortable feelings, uncertainty about how to behave, and a natural desire to avoid victims of misfortune or blemish in case it may 'be caught or spread'. However, initial feelings of aversion to disfigurement are often modified by sympathy and curiosity in adults. Children, however, are less inhibited and more commonly voice their curiosity and disapproval, often in a very cruel way (Bull & Rumsey, 1988).

Harris (1997) explains that visible 'differentness' is a highly individual concept, which is derived both from self-comparison with 'normal' appearances and from others' expressed reactions to one's appearance. A perceived abnormality causes selfconsciousness, which can be defined as 'the distress and dysfunction arising from an awareness of one's own abnormality of appearance'. Grossly disfigured and aesthetically disfigured people can suffer the same degree of psychological distress and be equally dysfunctional emotionally and behaviourally. Harris (1997) describes factors that make up aesthetic dimensions of appearance (see Table 3.2.1).

Table 3.2.1: Aesthetic dimensions of appearance

Gross disfigurement	Presence	Partial or complete absence of a feature: nose, eye, teeth, hair
↑	Size	Abnormalities of height, weight
	Shape	Deformity
	Symmetry	Facial palsy, mandibulectomy, radical neck dissection
	Proportion	Disproportion of a feature
	Straightness	Crooked nose
	Tidiness	Irregular scars, lax skin
	Firmness	Flabby skin
↓	Smoothness	Uneven skin, scarring, tumour
Aesthetic disfigurement	Colour	Discoloration, radiotherapy reaction, telangectasia

Adapted from Harris (1977).

Rumsey (1997) also comments on the way language reflects negative attitudes towards those who deviate from the perceived norm: " 'abnormality', 'disfigurement', 'impairment', 'disability', 'flawed', or 'different'. All these words convey a sense that something is 'wrong' about the way a person looks". To be healthy and to have normal, unmarred looks are central ideas in nearly everyone's self-image.

The most common problems associated with facial disfigurement are those concerned with social interaction (Rumsey & Bull, 1986). People with facial disfigurement report staring, rude remarks, curiosity, disgust, horror and pity from strangers. They also report difficulty in making friends, problems obtaining jobs and problems with their sexual attractiveness. As a consequence, psychological problems such as anxiety, low self-esteem, depression, aggression, increased sensitivity and irritability may ensue (Fiegenbaum, 1981). Facial cancer patients have to learn to accept their new facial appearance, as well as learn to face reactions from those in their environment that they have never dealt with before. They may experience feelings of shame and inferiority. Communication with others is often hindered by poor speech. For this reason patients may avoid social contact and restrict themselves to a close circle of friends and relatives (Koster & Bergsma, 1990).

However, numerous studies show that many people are willing to engage in positive forms of social interaction with the disfigured (Rumsey & Bull, 1986). The non-verbal avoidance noted might be rooted in less negative reasons than the uncompromising sort of rejection and revulsion that is experienced by disfigured people. Initial negative behaviour may be due to the uncertainty as to how to behave, and consequent feelings of embarrassment. People with facial disfigurement may become preoccupied with their appearance, and find it difficult to realize that other people may also be experiencing problems with the social interaction.

Another factor is the disruption of the normal pattern of communication that some facial disfigurements cause. For example, a facial palsy restricts the movement of the face, which means that it loses its normal signalling pattern. If this normal pattern is disrupted, members of the public become unsure about how to behave (Robinson et al, 1996).

In a study by Rumsey et al (1986) an actor carried out interviews both with and without a port wine stain, and using both high levels of social skills and low levels of social skills. Interviewees were more affected by the interviewer's level of social skill than by the presence or absence of disfigurement. Rumsey et al postulate that training disfigured people to tackle communication problems could improve their social interaction by counteracting the stigma of a facial disfigurement. Robinson et al (1996) proved this to be the case. Social interaction workshops significantly decreased anxiety levels in 64 disfigured participants, as well as decreasing social avoidance and distress scores.

Whilst it may seem unfair that the whole onus of improving social interaction should lie on the disfigured person, the enormity of the task of educating the whole of the general public makes this the most realistic approach to improving quality of life for the patient with head and neck cancer.

Gamba et al (1992) examined the psychosocial adjustment of 66 patients after head and neck surgery. They divided the patients into those with extensive disfigurement and those with minor disfigurement. Patients in the extensive disfigurement group reported much more distress in relation to self image, with responses such as 'I look like a monster', and 'I hardly recognize myself'. Relationships with family were not as badly affected, although one-third of extensively disfigured patients described partners as 'somewhat ashamed'. Seventy-four per cent of the extensively disfigured group were described as having 'worsened sexuality'. Thirty-six per cent of the extensively disfigured group reported that friends no longer visited them and 50% of all patients said that real friends were relatively few. However, 'real friends' were important and were credited with boosting morale and encouraging socialization. The impact of treatment was compared over the time elapsed since surgery. From the first 6 months to 2 years, 22% of patients felt that postoperative effects were 'too harsh'. This increased to 44% from 2 to 4 years, then dropped to 29% after 4 years. In the extensively disfigured group, 30% of patients did not demonstrate any reduction in distress, even after several years. Gamba et al (1992) found that this situation was most common in patients who reported a change in self-image that led them to 'no longer recognize themselves'. They conclude that head and neck cancer patients need a rehabilitation programme offering psychosocial support in order to cope with disfigurement, and that 'such a programme should provide support not only after surgery but before it, where help should involve all the family and not just the patient alone'.

Laryngectomy

Laryngectomy may not be classed as disfigurement, but nevertheless it does constitute a visible, as well as audible, difference that often alarms or frightens others (Depondt & Gehanno, 1995). The person who has had a laryngectomy must make major psychological and social adjustments. Not only does the person have to adjust to life as a cancer patient, but he or she must breathe through a stoma in his/her neck (Stam et al, 1991). The lower respiratory tract is now in direct contact with the atmosphere and because air is no longer warmed and moistened, patients experience excessive sputum production and coughing.

The civilizing process trains people to regard certain bodily functions as unpleasant (Lawler, 1991). Excretions, softness, wetness and sliminess are seen as 'dirty', as is a 'cavity, or cleft or hole'. Thus the patient may feel repulsion of the stoma and mucus and fear rejection by family and friends, as well as in any other social interactions they may have. In her personal account of her father's laryngectomy when she was a child, Weber (1993) says 'his stoma did not bother me, and it was common to see him cough through his neck, though I never became used to the excessive secretions produced ... I warned new friends that my dad had a hole in his neck. ... I did not want my friends to be frightened by a stoma that many people see as revolting'.

Ulbricht (1986) says: 'We never know when we will experience irritants in the air which cause coughing and mucus discharge. This discharge is the problem. If not checked in time, it runs down the chest. If that area is not covered, the mucus is visible'.

Loss of the larynx means that the patient has to learn alaryngeal speech. Most individuals are able to learn functional speech, but the sound of the new voice has a noticeably unusual quality. Laryngectomees have to find the courage to learn to communicate in a new way (Lehmann & Krebs, 1991). In order to live with alaryngeal speech and non-verbal communication, they need relatives, co-workers, friends, neighbours, people on the street, on the telephone, in the shops, who are willing to accept this new method of communication. Unfortunately, many people react negatively to oesophageal or electronic speech, particularly on the telephone, which patients report as being embarrassing and upsetting.

Stam et al (1991) studied the psychosocial impact of laryngectomy on 51 patients. They found that the major factor that predicted successful speech rehabilitation was the extent of preoperative information and counselling from professionals and laryngectomee visitors. Richardson et al (1989) had similar findings. Another factor was gender; men were more likely to achieve oesophageal speech than women. Writers and gesturers had spent significantly longer periods of time in hospital postoperatively. The authors suggest that women may fail to develop oesophageal speech because they are embarrassed about the deep, throaty character of the voice. Shanks (1979) also reports that laryngectomized women are concerned about loss of femininity as a result of their new voice.

Ulbricht (1986) describes her personal experience of laryngectomy:

> After the first day or two, the patient becomes aware of the fact that she cannot make any vocal sounds. Following major surgery, every patient cries. When a laryngectomee cries, there may be floods of tears, but there is complete silence. The body shakes with sobs, but there is no sound. When this fact is realized it can be shattering.

Dhooper (1985) reports that many laryngectomees experience anger and frustration over loss of their speech, whilst others tend to withdraw. One patient is quoted as saying:

> I had lost the power of speech, that marvellous gift that separates men from the animals. Gone. Totally gone. I felt my head turn toward the wall. It was a feeling I experienced off and on for days, weeks, and months. Turn to the wall, away from life, toward blankness and death. The void of the wall, with its blank face expressionless and empty like an idiot's mind or a blind man's sockets, held comfort. Hi ya, wall. Meet Mute.

Preoperative information from professionals and particularly laryngectomee visitors, also strongly predicted long-term adjustment, measured by distress and quality of life scores (Shanks, 1979; Richardson et al, 1989; Stam et al, 1991). The authors conclude that preoperative counselling is crucial to later psychological adjustment. Because support from family and friends is also very important, they recommend that they are included in the preoperative counselling. Preoperative preparation is discussed in Chapter 1.2. Length of time in hospital postoperatively was also a significant predictor of distress and quality of life; longer stays were related to higher levels of distress.

Richardson et al (1989) found that support from speech therapists and from other laryngectomees was important for successful speech rehabilitation. Peer support provides an opportunity for social comparison as other laryngectomees model skills and provide feedback for improvement. Professional and peer support was also an important predictor of physical–psychosocial dysfunction, which underscores the importance of sources of support that are specific for the disease and develop only during treatment. Although these sources of support may be transitory, they play a crucial role in the major adjustment that takes place after surgery. The provision of peer support is discussed in Chapter 1.4.

Devins et al (1994) hypothesized that psychosocial wellbeing and distress after laryngectomy were influenced by 'illness intrusiveness'. Illness intrusiveness relates to illness interfering with or preventing the individual's participation in valued activities and interests. They also hypothesized that illness intrusiveness may be exacerbated by the individual's level of perceived stigma. They studied 51 laryngectomees and found that perceived stigma correlated significantly with illness intrusiveness. Perceived stigma and illness intrusiveness were significantly related to decreased life happiness and increased depressive symptoms. When both perceived stigma and illness intrusiveness were present, depressive symptoms rose much more rapidly. They also report that laryngectomy had the most detrimental effect in life domains of work, self-expression/self-improvement, active recreation and financial situation. Illness intrusiveness was reported less in social and interpersonal life domains, but when it was present in these domains, especially the relationship with the partner, it was an important determinant of unhappiness and depression. Intrusiveness into these domains was importantly related to perceived stigma and psychosocial outcomes.

Lehmann & Krebs (1991) report loss of job, having to change job, or having to reduce working hours as a common occurrence in 332 laryngectomees questioned. Thus laryngectomy has a significant financial impact on many people. One-third of the patients in this study reported financial problems. Dhooper (1985) cites a study by King et al (unfortunately with no reference details). This study compared laryngectomees with a group of amputees matched by age and sex. They found that twice as many amputees as laryngectomees were able to work, and concluded that the loss of the larynx was more than twice as disabling as the loss of a limb.

Jay et al (1991) questioned 65 laryngectomees and found 45% reported they felt less socially acceptable. Fifty-eight per cent found their outdoor and social activity reduced. However, 91% of patients felt that their disabilities were a fair price to pay for the treatment of cancer.

Scaling disfigurement and dysfunction

Dropkin and Scott (1983) and Dropkin (1989) have shown that the severity of disfigurement and dysfunction caused by surgery can be scaled according to others' perception, and that this scaling gives a prediction of the relative degree to which a patient will have problems with postoperative adjustment. One hundred female registered nurses were asked to judge the relative severity of disfigurement and dysfunction for 11 routinely performed head and neck procedures. Correlation in the nurses judgements were high. The ratings are shown in Tables 3.2.2 and 3.2.3. The authors note that procedures rated as most severe involved the centre of the face, or that region providing the greatest audio-visual stimuli in interaction with others. In a study of 10 patients, Dropkin (1979) demonstrated a relationship between social interaction and disfigurement in the immediate postoperative period; the more severely disfigured patients spent less time outside their room than the less severely disfigured. She also found that patients who demonstrated a low need for social approval on psychometric testing coped with disfigurement better, being more compliant with self-care and resocialization activities. Thus, coping with disfigurement depends on a variety of factors, and patients with less severe disfigurement but a high need for social approval may require just as much support. Clarke argues that the value of scaling disfigurement is questionable, as evidence shows that 'minor' disfigurements are as likely to cause distress as more severe ones (Clarke, 1998).

Table 3.2.2: Rating of disfigurement severity for head and neck surgery (Dropkin et al, 1983)

Rating (Low = 1, Severe = 11)	Surgical procedure
1	Radical neck dissection
2	Cheek resection with forehead flap repair
3	Total parotidectomy with facial nerve sacrifice
4	Total laryngectomy
5	Bilateral radical neck dissection
6	Orbital exenteration
7	Hemimandibulectomy and radical neck dissection
8	Nasal amputation
9	Anterior partial mandibulectomy
10	Segmental mandibulectomy and radical neck dissection
11	Orbital exenteration and radical maxillectomy

Table 3.2.3: Rating of dysfunction severity for head and neck surgery (Dropkin et al, 1983)

Rating (Low = 1, Severe = 8)	Dysfunction
1	Loss of smell
2	Unilateral hearing loss
3	Impaired mastication
4	Impaired speech
5	Unilateral vision loss
6	Impaired control of salivary secretions
7	Impaired deglutition
8	Aphonia

Negative coping strategies and poor social skills

The traditional approach to defining those at risk of poor psychosocial functioning after head and neck cancer is that the more severe the disfigurement, the greater the risk for psychological distress. However, this is not supported by research evidence. Evidence rather points to inadequate social support networks, negative beliefs, negative coping strategies and poor social skills (Changing Faces, 1996).

Negative beliefs include wide-ranging negativity such as 'because I am unattractive I will never be able to form friendships', and can be associated with depression. Negative coping strategies and behaviour commonly constitute avoidance. Social anxiety is such that the individual completely removes him/herself from social situations. This can be manifested as agoraphobia. Partial avoidance is also a negative coping strategy, where the individual minimizes the risk of social anxiety by only going to places where people are familiar, or going out only with family or friends. Negative coping strategies also include alcohol use and aggression. Poor social skills such as stooping to hide the face, hiding the face with hair, and poor eye contact are behaviours that actually draw attention to the individual and result in negative reactions from other people.

Chaturvedi et al (1996) report a study of 50 Indian head and neck cancer patients which examined coping mechanisms. They found that many patients used negative coping strategies such as helplessness and fatalism. They recommend that professionals explore patients' concerns and assist them in finding more effective coping mechanisms.

Loss and grief in head and neck cancer

Loss is an integral part of life. Death is not the only loss a human might experience, yet it is often the only loss that is validated as a legitimate grief experience. Patients with head and neck cancer experience a variety of losses as a consequence of their illness, the most obvious being the loss of the larynx for the laryngectomee. Less obvious are the loss of the ability to eat, loss of an attractive facial appearance, loss of normal hearing and vision, loss of previous social roles and leisure activities, and loss of a certain future, to name but a few. Humphrey and Zimpher (1996) assert that any event involving change is a loss that necessitate the process of grief and transition. A loss event requires that some part of the individual be left behind and grieved before the process of transition and rebuilding can occur.

Loss of people or objects which are personally important or loved is stressful and gives rise to emotional and physiological disturbance. It is generally accepted that the physiological effects of stress are similar whatever the cause of the stress might be. Murray Parkes (1972) postulates that the psychological effects of different causes of stress may also be similar, and that the reaction to the loss of a body part may be very similar to the reaction to other loss, such as bereavement.

The reaction to both bereavement and amputation can best be regarded as a process of realization, of making real inside the self-events which have already occurred in reality outside (Murray Parkes, 1972). This is a painful, unhappy period during which the individual moves through a succession of phases.

- Shock and numbness: occurs in the first few hours or days. During this time there is a strong tendency to deny the reality of the loss: 'I can't believe this has happened/it's not there'.
- Anxiety and distress ('pangs of grief') follows the shock and numbness. Separation anxiety is the principal emotion to arise after any major loss for which the individual is not fully prepared, and grief (the pain and suffering of loss) is the means by which the individual meets a loss that has occurred. This will be evoked by any reminder of the loss. Patients may make conscious attempts to avoid reminders and redirect their thoughts away from the loss.
- Depression and apathy follow as anxiety and distress diminish. The patient begins to give up hope of getting back what they have lost. Grieving occurs with inability to think about the future. Murray Parkes defines acute grief as pining for the lost object, searching and crying out for it. This may be manifested in an urge to recover the lost object; for example widows were shown to scan the environment for the person, misperceive strangers as the lost partner, return to places associated with the person and trea-sure objects that belonged to them.
- Reorganization and redirection gradually occur with appetites and interests slowly returning as adjustment to the loss takes place.

Humphrey and Zimpher (1996) explain that the work of bereave-ment is not linear, but cyclical in nature, with many painful returns to the start process once more. The process involves trial and error, change and frustrating returns to earlier experiences of grief.

Murray Parkes found that amputees had an internal sense of loss, or 'sense of mutilation', which correlated with the sense of loss that widows experienced. He found that amputees 'pined' for their lost limb in much the same way as widows pined for their lost partner. However, the amputees did not seem to have the same urge to search for their lost limb. More often their pining was for the loss of parts of their life that had occurred as a result of their loss of limb, for example separation from their home and family whilst in hospital, the inability to return to work or their usual leisure activities. If a laryngectomee's reaction to their loss of voice is compared, the same process can be seen to occur. However, many laryngectomees can be seen to 'search' for their lost voice; for example the hope that the insertion of a tracheoesophageal valve will restore them to normality, or, more recently, that a laryngeal transplant will be possible. Similarly, patients who have lost their ability to eat normally constantly search for a way to improve their eating, refusing to believe that they will not be able to eat again, and grieving for the losses this has imposed in their daily life; not being able to eat with the family, or socialize with their friends in the same way.

In amputees, the sense of mutilation seemed to reflect a sense of being vulnerable, laid open and helpless in a potentially hostile world. Patients feel insecure, helpless, damaged and spoiled. Widows also demonstrate these feelings. Other similarities can be seen in dreams; in a typical bereavement dream, the dead person is back again alive and well. Many of my patients have told me that when they dream, they are eating and talking normally. This again, is a typical psychological reaction to loss.

Murray Parkes hypothesizes that both widows and amputees seem to describe the existence of a wound or gap in the self, rather than actual pining for the part of the self that has been lost. He theorizes that the concept of 'working models of the world' which Bowlby (1969) has described may help to explain this phenomenon. Working models are built up from our experience of the world and constitute cognitive maps and action programmes by which we recognize sensory input and initiate motor activities. Important people, functions and body parts are components of these working models. When one of them is lost, the model tends to remain unchanged but it no longer works properly. The widow who lays the table for two, and the amputee who tries to stand on an absent leg are making use of 'models' that no longer work. Only after repeated painful disappointments do they give up their old models and acquire new ones.

Until a new working model has been created, the patient will not be able to function in an effective way. He/she will be aware of a discrepancy between him/herself and the environment. The ability to control, predict and plan life is reduced and a feeling of vulnerability, helplessness and emptiness ensues. Murray Parkes believes this accounts for the sense of mutilation and emptiness.

The modification of the old working model and creation of a new one involves both unlearning and learning and during the course of this the individual will experience anxiety, frustration and depression before the new model is developed to a point where a satisfying adjustment is made. McGarry (1993) describes the use of hypnosis to accelerate the learning process by providing a subconscious blueprint of the post-amputation body.

The nurse can help by supporting and coaching the patient through this painful process, putting the patient in touch with people who can provide a good role model, and facilitating hope for the future. The nurse must also be aware that the process can become blocked and distorted in some individuals and recognize when a referral for specialist psychological help is needed.

Eating, nasogastric and gastrostomy feeding

Although eating problems are reported in most studies, the psychosocial effects of these problems have not been fully explored in any studies. Eating is one of life's most basic and satisfying pleasures, as well as a very social activity. Patients in the King's Fund report on head and neck cancer care report that one of their most severe problems is the impairment in eating and drinking. They describe the complete loss of enjoyment of food and the willpower required to make themselves eat. Many people felt embarrassed when eating and avoided eating out. Some people coped by sitting facing a corner. A patient describes the effects on socializing: 'I get embarrassed because I can't eat properly ... I will not go out into new company because I am ashamed of the way I look and it's just finished our social life together'. Another patient says 'Eating is a major part of everybody's social life ... That's what the doctors and nurses don't ever think of. What on earth goes on when we go out to eat' (Edwards, 1997).

The loss of the ability to eat can be most devastating. Alongside this, the addition to the body of a nasogastric or gastrostomy feeding tube causes difficulties with altered body image. There is no literature on the psychosocial effects of nasogastric tubes, but the following vignette demonstrates the difficulties that can occur.

> Jane was a 42-year-old woman who had a very shy 9-year-old son, Sean. She had had surgery and radiotherapy for advanced oral cancer. Her husband Tom had an illness phobia and found her disfigurement disturbing. Jane's recurrent oral cancer made eating very difficult. She had therefore had a nasogastric tube placed to maintain nutrition. She was determined to carry on a normal home life, and to continue to perform her usual role in the household of taking her son to school, and driving her husband to the pub for his evening out. However, Sean did not want his friends to see his mother with a tube protruding out of her nose, and refused to go to school with her. Tom similarly refused to be seen with Jane. Jane had been reluctant to have a gastrostomy because she felt that, although her head was 'a mess' the rest of her body was still attractive, and a gastrostomy would spoil this. However, because of the reactions of her family, she had a gastrostomy placed and experienced an extension of her already damaged body image.

Rickman (1998) looked at the psychosocial effects of gastrostomy feeding on a sample of patients that included people with head and neck cancer. Patients reported a wide range of effects. The enjoyment of eating meals in restaurants with partners was lost and exclusion from the daily routine of family meals and festive occasions was experienced. Patients reported being unable to go on holiday because it was 'antisocial', and also because of the large amount of equipment that was required. The enjoyment of food was desperately missed. One head and neck cancer patient resented the hospital staff recommending a gastrostomy 'just in case', because to him it was a constant physical reminder of cancer and illness. Physical intimacy was curtailed because the gastrostomy sticks out, and clothing had to be selected carefully. The gastrostomy was described as being very limiting. One patient described it as 'being like a dog on a lead. I'm stuck in this chair joined to that'.

Anxiety and depression in head and neck cancer

One of the most common manifestations of psychosocial distress is depression. Fear of isolation and rejection, and concerns about the

reactions of others, occur because of the great psychological investment in the head and neck area. Social interaction and emotional
expression depend on it, especially the eyes. It is therefore not
surprising that many patients experience anxiety and depression.
Patients particularly at risk are those with poor adaptive and coping
skills preoperatively (Breitbart & Holland, 1988), personality characteristics of individuals with chronic alcohol abuse problems and nicotine dependence. Also at risk are those with poor social support
(often another characteristic of a person with alcohol problems). List
et al (1997) found a positive correlation between depression post-
treatment and alcohol use pre-treatment in patients undergoing
chemotherapy and radiotherapy.

Anxiety disorders seen in patients with head and neck cancers can
be considered in two major categories (Breitbart & Holland, 1988):

- anxiety related to illness that constitutes severe distress exceeding
  the expected level of anxiety associated with responding to severe
  stress
- pre-existing anxiety such as generalized anxiety, panic disorder
  and phobias, which can constitute major complications for treatment and rehabilitation.

Anxiety was present in 50% of head and neck cancer patients
studied by Breitbart and Holland (1988), often in combination with
depression.

Studies show depression occurring in 25% to 40% of head and
neck cancer patients; the incidence in the general population is 6%
(Baile et al, 1992; Bjordal & Kaasa, 1995). Breitbart & Holland
(1988) believe that depression is a greater risk for head and neck
cancer patients than for other cancer patients due to the response to
mutilating surgery, and because individuals with an alcohol history
are at increased risk of depression and suicide (Kennedy & Faugier,
1989). Smoking is also strongly linked to depression, with depression
being a prominent symptom of quitting for highly nicotine-depen-
dent patients (Benowitz, 1997). Head and neck cancer patients are at
increased risk of suicide compared to other cancer patients; the
larynx and tongue are the most common cancer sites of people who
committed suicide (Farberow et al, 1971; Henderson & Ord, 1997).

Rapoport et al (1993), in a study of 55 head and neck cancer
survivors, report that although coping with physical problems

improved over the years (range after treatment was 0 to 21 years), there was an 'astounding' deterioration in psychosocial and emotional state. Patients reported more fears, less intimacy with the family, more anxiety and anger. They describe this as a 'massive deterioration with time'. They surmise that this could be 'patient burnout' caused by the chronic stress of having cancer and coping with health difficulties. Bjordal and Kaasa (1995) performed a follow-up study of 204 patients treated by radical radiotherapy between 7 and 11 years previously. They report 'worrying' levels of psychological distress, especially in patients with impaired cognitive function, social function, or pain.

However, it may be wrong to assume that anxiety and depression is entirely attributable to head and neck treatment as many patients have pre-existing anxiety and depression (Baile et al, 1992). Several investigators have shown that head and neck cancer patients have significant depression before the results of their biopsies are known (Davies et al, 1986; Baile et al, 1993). Baile et al report that 43% of 63 patients assessed before biopsy results were known had significant levels of anxiety and depression. They found that depression was associated most with being single and reporting high stress levels (Baile et al, 1992).

Cancer physical sequelae such as pain and discomfort, interference with vital functions and nutritional deficits have also been associated with depression (Westin et al, 1988). Twenty-three per cent of patients in List et al's (1997) study demonstrated significant levels of depression, which also appeared to be associated with the overall number and severity of symptoms, particularly pain. Hammerlid et al (1997) found that Hospital Anxiety and Depression scores (Zigmond & Snaith, 1983) revealed high levels of distress in head and neck cancer patients, especially during and after radiotherapy. They recommend psychiatric evaluation and treatment for patients undergoing radiotherapy. Several other studies show that radiotherapy is the most distressing time in the patient's cancer experience; these are outlined in Chapter 3.1. This evidence clearly shows that radiotherapy outpatient departments should be organized so that specialist cancer nurses are available to give a high level of support to patients undergoing treatment for head and neck cancer.

Bunston et al (1995) found strong correlations between locus of control, emotional distress and hope in 98 head and neck cancer patients. The more emotional distress patients experienced, the less hope they had for the future. Gamba et al (1992) propose that it could be useful to study the patient's self-concept as a possible diagnostic parameter to identify high-risk subjects of psychosocial maladjustment.

Studies (again outlined in Chapter 3.1) consistently show that clinicians are not good at identifying depression in head and neck cancer patients. The nurse should therefore be alert to the risk and signs and symptoms of anxiety and depression, in order to access the patient to early specialist treatment and help. Easily administered screening tests such as the Hospital Anxiety and Depression Scale (Zigmond & Snaith, 1983) can be very helpful alongside good listening skills, and should be incorporated into the initial and ongoing patient assessments. D'Antonio et al (1998) recommend that future studies on the management of psychosocial problems in head and neck cancer should consider the effect of the treatment of depression on quality of life.

Fatigue

The many quality of life studies now done on head and neck cancer patients consistently show post-treatment fatigue to be a major problem (see Chapter 3.1). Jones et al (1991) found that fatigue was a very common problem after head and neck surgery, particularly craniofacial procedures and laryngopharyngoesophagectomy. In a study of 98 head and neck cancer patients, fatigue was a factor that influenced hope. Fatigue depleted physical and emotional functioning, resulting in a greater number of concerns (Bunston et al, 1995). Patients in the King's Fund report on head and neck cancer care also described fatigue as a major problem (Edwards, 1997).

Fatigue is a common symptom of radiotherapy. It presents during treatment and can last for several months afterwards (Faithfull, 1998). Fatigue can be a very distressing symptom and has been described as both mental and physical exhaustion. Knowledge about fatigue is inconclusive, as is knowledge about interventions to manage fatigue. As patients can find this a particularly worrying and debilitating symptom, which raises concerns about the success of treatment and continued presence of cancer, it is important that they are informed and prepared for it by nurses (Faithfull, 1998).

Sexuality

There is now good evidence to show that sexual dysfunction is common in head and neck cancer patients (Monga et al, 1997; Siston et al, 1997). Many patients discover the disruption in their sexual relationship only after the acute crisis of diagnosis and treatment has passed (Shell, 1995). Human sexuality is much more than a biological process; it is an expression of our psychological, emotional and sociocultural being. Psychosexual problems are well recognized for breast cancer, gynaecology and ostomy patients, but a review of the literature shows this issue seems to be inadequately addressed in head and neck cancer, although head and neck cancer can have a dramatic effect on sexuality. Body image, of which facial appearance is a component, is one of the most important entities in the concept of sexuality (Metcalfe & Fischman, 1985). The high degree of visibility of head and neck cancer and its treatment, as well as alterations in function caused by surgery and the placement of feeding tubes and tracheostomy tubes, may have a major negative impact on sexuality and sexual relationships. Libido-robbing fatigue can also contribute to the problem (Shell, 1995).

Sexual responses are often affected by a laryngectomy because the patient may feel unattractive, the loud stoma breathing can be irritating to both the patient and partner, and coughing and mucus may also be off putting (Weber & Reimer, 1993). In a study of 625 women following laryngectomy, Gardner (1966) found that 23% felt less feminine, 35% felt less attractive and 66% were afraid that their ability to display affection would be impaired. Single women were more likely to feel unattractive and unwanted. Jay et al (1991) found that 48% of 65 patients questioned in their study thought that laryngectomy had adversely affected their sexual activity. They did not explore whether gender had any bearing on this result, or in what way sexual activity had been affected. In a very limited study on sexual behaviour after laryngectomy, Meyers et al (1980) found that 33% of 48 laryngectomees felt that their operation had changed their sexual relationship with their partner, and wished that their doctor had discussed these effects. Mathieson et al (1992) found that the strongest predictor of quality of life in a group of 30 laryngectomees and their spouses was satisfaction with their present sexual relationship and the laryngectomy's effect on the relationship in general. These studies all suggest that significant sexual readjustment takes place after laryngectomy, and psychosexual counselling may be important for some patients.

Ulbricht (1986) describes how laryngectomy affected her sexuality:

> The first look in the mirror is devastating. The stoma is located at the base of the neck. It is open and obvious. If there has been additional neck surgery, that side of the neck is sunken and forever will have a 'scrawny' appearance. A man can place a piece of gauze over the stoma, put on a shirt and tie and go about his business. A woman, because most dresses are open at the neckline, must devise attractive measures to cover the stoma. Until this problem is solved, she may find herself a prisoner in her own home. Once covered the stoma is not forgotten. It is especially difficult for a woman to accept this permanent disfigurement. The neck is a sensitive, sensuous area of the body and important in lovemaking. After surgery some women cannot imagine any man wanting to stroke or kiss her mutilated neck.

She goes on to say: 'Everything about a laryngectomy is unfeminine. The most obvious is the sound of the new voice'.

Oral and maxillofacial surgery may cause sexual problems. Physical attractiveness is important in sexual relationships and oral stimulation is an essential part of this (Koster & Bergsma, 1990).

Metcalfe and Fischman (1985) report patients' experiences of sexual relationships:

> A gentleman with a history of chronic alcohol abuse had been impotent for sometime prior to diagnosis and had been meeting his wife's sexual needs through oral-genital sex. A hemiglossectomy and radical neck dissection made it difficult for him to extend his tongue. Thus, he was no longer able to use this technique to satisfy his wife. A second patient, when asked what prevented him from resuming sexual activity, stated 'I don't fool around anymore. What's the point? If I can't have it all, I don't want any part of it; besides, I can't even kiss anyone due to the shape of my mouth'. One woman said: 'If I were free to date, I don't think any man would look twice at me because of my face being the way it is. It has even kept me from going out to dinner'. Another lady was angry that her nasogastric tube interfered with her ability to kiss her husband. She felt that her facial disfigurement repulsed her husband. A gentleman who had undergone a hemimandibulectomy had not been able to have an erection since his surgery two years ago, and had abruptly ended his relationship with his girlfriend because he wasn't even able to kiss her because of his feeding tube.

Gamba et al (1992) reported that patients with extensive disfigurement reported worsening of sexual function compared to patients with minor disfigurement; worsened relationship with partner (27% versus 0%), and reduced sexuality (75% versus 39%). They conclude that disfigurement acts as a physical barrier between the patient and partner. However, the questions asked about sexuality in this study were not validated.

Monga et al (1997) describe a comprehensive study using validated tools to explore sexual functioning in 55 head and neck cancer patients following radiotherapy with or without surgery. They found that the majority of patients in their sample were experiencing problems with sexual functioning. Problems were identified in all areas of sexual functioning.

- Fantasy: 25% of patients were unable to fantasize about any aspect of sex.
- Arousal: 58% reported problems with arousal. Only 42% (23) were participating in sexual intercourse and of these only 13 were able to achieve a full erection.
- Behaviour: 42% were involved in sexual intercourse at least once per month. Thirty per cent practiced masturbation once per month (five of these could not achieve erection). Forty per cent engaged in casual kissing and petting and 31% engaged in foreplay.
- Orgasm: 58% of patients were dissatisfied with their ability to achieve orgasm. Problems were also reported in orgasm intensity, duration and control.
- Drive/satisfaction: 85% of patients reported moderate to high interest in sex, but only 58% were satisfied with their partner, and 51% considered that the quality of their sexual functioning was poor.

The most commonly reported cause of sexual problems was fear of failure (27%). Other reasons included an unwilling partner (22%), and no available partner (20%). Thirteen per cent reported that their partners were afraid of engaging in sexual activities. Patients with an external locus of control had significantly worse sexual functioning. There was no correlation between performance status and sexual functioning. Interestingly, there was no relationship between old age and sexual functioning. In fact, younger patients appeared to have poorer sexual functioning. Patients with extensive disfigurement had a trend towards poorer sexual functioning, but there was no significant difference in sexual interest, quality of functioning, or satisfaction with partner.

Siston et al (1997) studied 36 patients who had completed concomitant chemotherapy and radiation therapy for head and neck cancer. Well-validated tools for measuring sexuality and partner relationships were used. More than three-quarters of the patients rated their sex lives as important, and half reported problems. Half reported a decrease in sexual activity since diagnosis, 17 had difficulty with arousal, 15 reported a lack of sexual interest and 13 were unable to relax and enjoy sex. Thirteen of 28 men had difficulty achieving an erection. The effect of treatment that was most commonly reported to interfere with sexual activity was dry mouth. A summary of the data is shown in Table 3.2.4.

Five men who had not received cisplatin were less likely to report problems with achieving erection than the 23 who did. No relationship was found between past alcohol use and sexual functioning. The authors conclude that sexual function is a significant problem for head and neck cancer patients and that healthcare providers need to become more comfortable about assessing and discussing these problems.

Table 3.2.4: Perceived problems in sexual function after chemoradiotherapy for head and neck cancer (Siston et al, 1997)

Problems reported	Number of patients (n = 36)	Percentage
Somewhat or very much of a problem		
Dry mouth	20	55
Difficulty becoming aroused	17	46
Decrease in sexual activity	16	44
Lack of sexual interest	15	41
Inability to relax	13	36
Fatigue	10	28
Lack of kissing	10	28
Lack of affection	9	25
Mouth or throat pain	7	19
Pain during sex	6	16
Occurs rarely or never		
Sexual intercourse with partner	20	55
Kissing partner	8	23
Holding hands with partner	7	20

The following vignettes demonstrate how sexuality is frequently affected:

Jim had a total glossectomy with subtotal laryngectomy for cancer at the base of his tongue when he was 65 years old. He also had a dental clearance prior to postoperative radiotherapy. He said that the operation has 'ruined' his sex life. He cannot 'chat up' women any more, take them out to dinner, nibble their ears, nor kiss properly due to the loss of his tongue.

Patrick was a divorcee who had a total laryngectomy at the age of 62 years. Prior to his laryngectomy he enjoyed a very active sex life with several 'lady friends' as well as a woman with whom he had had a 4-year relationship. He felt very emasculated and unattractive post-surgery, perceiving that he would never be able to 'chat up' and seduce women again, or indulge in pillow talk. He thought his stoma would be a huge turn off. Two days after discharge from hospital he angrily told his girlfriend that 'it was over for ever'. He cut off all contact with his female friends.

Maureen was an attractive 49-year-old who had had a parotidectomy and right radical neck dissection. She previously enjoyed a very physical relationship with her husband. She now said that her husband was afraid to touch her in case he hurt her, and their old 'rough and tumble' games were over. Her lips 'sagged' on one side, so her mouth was the wrong shape to kiss. The worst problem, she said, was the altered sensation in the skin of her neck; it felt 'like rubber' and whenever her husband touched it during lovemaking she 'froze'.

Thus the nurse *must* address sexual concerns with the patient and partner in the same way as all other needs are addressed. However, nurses, along with other healthcare professionals, tend to shy away from discussions about patients' sexual concerns because of discomfort with their own sexuality or beliefs or a lack of sexual knowledge (Shell, 1995). Nurses must be comfortable with their own sexuality and sexual knowledge level whilst maintaining an awareness of personal sexual attitudes (Fisher, 1983). They must also be able to use the same sexual 'language' as the patient in order to facilitate a comfortable discussion.

With assistance, the client and partner should be able to identify aspects of sexuality that may be threatened by head and neck cancer, and identify ways of maintaining sexual identity (Metcalfe & Fischman, 1985). Metcalfe and Fischman recommend that a baseline sexual history should be obtained at the time of initial assessment, with a reassessment at each visit. Beyond gathering information, this also serves to reassure the client and partner that their sexual concerns are important and worthy of discussion.

For example, the nurse might say: 'A lot of people find that having this operation affects their sex life — how much of a problem has it been for you?'. This sort of question may make the patient more at ease, knowing that 'a lot of people' have sexual problems, and that the nurse is at ease discussing sexual issues. Alternatively, especially for older people for whom the word 'sex' is embarrassing, the question could be phrased 'What effect has all this treatment had on your physical relationship/love life?'.

Thus the patient and partner are given permission to raise the subject at any time during their treatment. The nurse has a responsibility to know the side effects on sexual functioning of any therapy the patient is receiving, and should provide this information to the patient and partner. Information about alternative methods of sexual expression should be provided. The nurse should also recognize when the expertise of a sexual counsellor is required and make an appropriate referral.

Summary

This chapter has examined the profound effects that head and neck cancer and its treatment can have on the patient and family. Laryngectomy and disfigurement can cause individuals to become stigmatized, and can lead to social anxiety and the use of negative coping strategies, with negative effects on self-efficacy and self-esteem. Anxiety and depression are common problems in this group of patients. They may be pre-existing conditions, or caused by the trauma of cancer and its treatment. Fatigue and sexual problems are also commonly reported. The nurse working with this group of patients must develop skills in assessing and managing these problems. Strategies for how this might be achieved are discussed in Chapter 3.3. Patients must have access to professionals who are skilled in dealing with psychosocial problems and can provide psychological interventions to help. Nurses will need clinical supervision so that they can work effectively with their patients, and must also be able to recognize when to refer patients on to specialist services. For those who are interested in reading further on this subject, Edwards 1997 is highly recommended.

Strategy for practice

- Be aware of the theoretical concepts that help to explain patients' behaviour and feelings.
- Be aware that the psychological and emotional effects of *disfigurement* can often be more disabling than the physical effects.

- Be aware that the psychological and emotional effects of *laryngectomy* can often be more disabling than the physical effects.
- Monitor patients for anxiety and depression regularly using validated tools.
- Be aware of the huge sense of loss and grief that patients may experience.
- Always give information on the side effects of therapies on sexual functioning and address the patient's sexual concerns openly.

Chapter 3.3
Improving psychosocial outcomes: coping strategies for the patient and family

To survive (cancer) is to learn to live, because the skills and attributes of survivorship are not innate, they are learned.

Bushkin, 1995

Introduction

The last two chapters have focused on the problems experienced by people with head and neck cancer. This chapter will focus on evidence-based practice to help patients and families to overcome problems. There are many ways in which nurses can help people cope with the psychosocial effects of head and neck cancer. Facilitation of a feeling of control is a crucial factor. The more patients report feeling in control of their environment and their cancer, the more they report feeling hopeful for the future (Bunston et al, 1995). In a busy healthcare environment, concentration on the patient's physical survival, wound healing, functional losses and adjustment to new physical self-care skills are the priority for nurses, but attention must also be given to psychological and emotional issues, as well as coaching the patient and family in the interpersonal skills needed to deal with the new social experiences that follow from discharge from hospital. An additional consideration is that psychosocial care is often not documented comprehensively by nurses, and this may be another reason that it is often overlooked. This chapter will examine how these issues can be addressed.

Facilitating initial postoperative recovery

The primary behavioural manifestations of the coping process post-operatively are self-care and resocialization (Dropkin & Scott, 1983).

Self-care relates to activities of daily living such as personal hygiene and grooming, and tasks specifically associated with surgery (mouth care, stoma care, care of prosthesis). This requires the patient to look in the mirror and use coping strategies related to the confrontation of altered body image. Resocialization includes ambulatory activity and social interaction with others. Confrontation is integral to face-to-face encounters and requires the patient to deal with others' reactions to their alteration in appearance. The patient's ability to accommodate the reactions of other people to his or her appearance plays a major role in the success of rehabilitation. Walking out of the room in the early postoperative period can help to begin the process of resocialization with controlled exposure to other people on the ward. Patients with severe disfigurement, and patients who require a high degree of social approval, may find the first walks out of their room very difficult and it may be helpful for the nurse to accompany them until they gain confidence (Dropkin, 1979). The early postoperative period is critical to rehabilitation.

Developing confidence in performing new skills

Patients have many new skills to learn after head and neck surgery. These skills can be a source of great anxiety for both the patient and carers. For example, many laryngectomy patients and their carers are very anxious about managing their airway when first discharged from hospital. A key component of nursing these patients is to help them develop their stoma care themselves. Monitoring the growth of their skills in a concrete way, with patient and family participation, can improve their confidence and challenge negative thoughts about choking or asphyxiating. Using a confidence rating scale (see Table 3.3.1) can help the patient to see progress, and also to more accurately identify where their concerns lie. Similar scales can be devised for patients learning to care for an obturator, prosthesis, tracheostomy or feeding tube.

Confrontation and reintegration of body image

Breitbart & Holland (1988) recommend that early confrontation is encouraged on the ward. The patient should not be allowed to avoid looking in the mirror, despite the difficulty in doing so, and should also be assisted to socialize with staff, family and patients. Patients who refuse to look at their face are often those who make a poorer

Table 3.3.1: Confidence in caring for laryngostome

Date :
Postoperative day:
Confidence Scale: 0 10 20 30 40 50 60 70 80 90 100 %

	No confidence	Very confident
Activity		Confidence rating

Removing button
Cleaning mucus from stoma
Using humidification to loosen crusts and mucus plugs
Coughing to dislodge crusts and mucus plugs
Using forceps to remove plugs
Cleaning button
Inserting clean button
Applying heat/moisture exchanger
Overall feelings of confidence

Adapted from White (1998).

adjustment and who may be less able to cooperate in their rehabilitation. Dropkin (1988) proposes that postoperative days 4 to 6 can be considered pivotal in terms of acceptance of the defect; specific change points in the performance of self-care tasks were observed to occur at this time. The performance of self-care tasks usually preceded social affiliative behaviours. Careful attention to the patient's performance of self-care tasks within this specific time frame can facilitate achievement of expected outcomes at discharge. This should be documented to facilitate observation (see Table 3.3.2).

Patients who delay performing tasks should be reviewed on day 7 to ascertain if more intensive nursing assistance is needed to facilitate adjustment. Dropkin recommends that interventions should include: reiteration that the surgery was necessary to remove the cancer and emphasizing that the alteration does not change the person (that is, encouraging a more positive reappraisal of the situation). An additional intervention would be for the nurse to use sensitive counselling to explore the patient's cognitive and affective processes in relation to their altered body image and following this up by helping the patient to use problem-solving skills to facilitate more positive coping.

Table 3.3.2: Documentation of postoperative self-care and resocialization activities days 1 to 7

Name:

Activity observed	Post-op day	Signed
Self-care tasks performed independently (using mirror):
Personal hygiene (strip wash, bath, shower)
Oral hygiene
Brushing/combing hair
Shaving/makeup
Tracheostomy care (cleaning stoma, changing tubes, suction etc.)

Resocialization activities:
Up and around in room
Up and around the ward
Up and around outside the ward (dayroom, walks outside)
Interaction with family (eye contact and conversation)
Interaction with staff (eye contact and conversation)
Interaction with other patients

If activities have not been performed by day 7, review need for extra psychological and emotional support.

Adapted from Dropkin (1988).

While facial disfigurement is assumed to be the worst aspect of head and neck cancer, Baker (1992) found that dysfunction (swallowing, shoulder function, taste, speech, chewing, smell, drooling, hearing, vision) rather than disfigurement was rated worse by patients as giving poor rehabilitation outcomes. Swallowing problems, taste and shoulder immobility were most frequently reported as problematic. Interventions to limit physical dysfunction, such as exercise regimens to increase shoulder and jaw functioning, should be one of the nursing priorities to improve quality of life.

Languis et al (1993) studied 29 patients with head and neck cancer and had similar findings; most frequently reported problems were eating problems (throat irritation, mouth pain, chewing difficulty, mouth dryness, taste and smell), and these were compounded by radiotherapy. This highlights the need for the nurse to work as part of a rehabilitation team with the dietitian, physiotherapist, occupational therapist and speech therapist.

Inability to cope with disfigurement and dysfunction at discharge can result in non-compliance with care, leading to infection and breathing problems, malnutrition, pathological obsession with or denial of the defect, depression and social isolation (Dropkin, 1988). Psychological distress and poor social support in head and neck cancer patients reduces compliance with medical care and advice (i.e. alcohol use, smoking, dietary advice, taking medicines and attending follow up) (McDonough et al, 1996). Patients who are discharged with coping problems will thus require a higher level of input from the community nursing team and clinical nurse specialist.

Psychological coping strategies

After head and neck surgery, the patient has many new skills to learn. Nurses may tend to concentrate on helping the patient with survival, wound healing, functional losses and adjustment to new physical self-care skills, but attention should also be given to coaching the patient and family in how to deal with psychological and emotional issues, as well as teaching the interpersonal skills to deal with social situations on discharge from hospital. In a study of wellbeing and coping of 42 oral and pharyngeal cancer patients, support given by healthcare professionals was perceived as the most insufficient with regard to psychosocial problems such as decreased social life, dribbling, worry, fatigue, and inability to do things as before. These psychosocial problems were significantly less well supported than practical surgical and radiotherapy problems (Languis & Lind, 1995). This is backed up by overwhelming evidence from the King's Fund report on head and neck cancer care that patients consistently felt psychosocial issues had not been addressed by healthcare professionals (Edwards, 1997).

Rehearsing

The head and neck unit is a specialized area where both staff and other patients are familiar with the problems of head and neck cancer. Outside the hospital it is a different story; the public are not used to dealing with cancer or disfigurement. Participating in social events and returning to work can be very challenging for patients. First encounters with the public are often particularly problematic (Robinson et al, 1996). The patient should be taught how to deal with other people's reactions, questions, staring, embarrassment and discomfort as early as possible, as repeated negative experiences are likely to lead to avoidance behaviour. Price (1998) recommends rehearsing with the patient different levels of verbal accounts that may be given to people outside hospital. By planning the handling of social encounters, people with cancer sense a greater degree of control over events.

Clarke (1998) points out that everyone who looks different will inevitably be asked about their face and suggests that patients are prompted as follows: 'Have you thought what you might say if anyone asks you why you have stitches/what you have had done?', as this is a good way of discovering how prepared someone is for the fact that other people will be curious about their appearance. The nurse can use a situation such as doing dressings to do this and it leads easily into a discussion of what and how much the patient might want to say.

Changing Faces produces an excellent range of booklets which are ideal for nurses to use with patients for this purpose (see Table 3.3.3). These booklets have been shown to be very helpful and effective in promoting behaviour change (Clarke, 1998) and should be an essential part of ward stock.

Clarke (1998) recommends that, as a minimum standard, every person with a facial disfigurement and their family should be offered access to written information, as well as details of relevant support groups such as Changing Faces. They should also be able to answer the question 'what happened to your face?'.

Table 3.3.3: Changing Faces resources for managing disfigurement

---

Booklets
When cancer changes the way you look
When facial paralysis affects the way you look
Everybody's staring at me
What happened to your eye?
Making your face work for you
Making the change
Video
REACHOUT

These are just a few of the resources available from Changing Faces. Contact the organization for more information:
1 & 2 Junction Mews, London W2 1PN
Tel.: 020 7706 4232
Fax: 020 7706 4234
E-mail: info@faces.demon.co.uk

Graded exposure

In addition to rehearsing, social encounters can be made less intimidating by being broken down into stages — a technique called graded exposure (White, 1998). Progress can be monitored using documentation to provide feedback for the nurse and patient (see Table 3.3.4). Each step should be repeated until the patient feels confident enough to progress to the next stage. The family can be involved in planning this programme.

Advance planning

White (1998) proposes a coping strategy called 'advance planning' for patients who have undergone stoma surgery. This technique can usefully be applied in head and neck cancer. It is useful for patients who become preoccupied with the possibility of problems developing in future situations. The patient can be asked to think of various worst-case scenarios. The details of these scenarios are written down, and then the patient is helped to generate solutions to the potential problems. It is important to help the patient write down specific problems. Rather than writing 'Everybody will think I'm a freak if I go out of the house', the patient would describe specific details such as 'If I go out to the shop, people might stare or laugh at me and I will feel embarrassed and have a panic attack'. From these

Table 3.3.4: A progress form for resuming social activity

Date:

Confidence Scale : 0 10 20 30 40 50 60 70 80 90 100 %

	No confidence	Very confident	
Step	Activity	Confidence rating	Date
1	Go to corner shop with relative/friend		
2	Go to corner shop alone		
3	Go to local pub/social club with relative/friend		
4	Go to local pub/social club alone		
5	Go to supermarket with relative/friend		
6	Go to supermarket alone		

Adapted from White (1998).

details, a practical plan can be made, and the patient can rehearse what they will do, think and say. In this way, patients are helped to appraise potential problems in a more positive way, and their confidence will gradually develop.

The following vignette demonstrates how these techniques can be used:

> Richard was experiencing severe anxiety about his stoma and breathing since discharge from hospital after a laryngectomy. This was displayed in panic attacks and frequent returns to the hospital with anxiety about his stoma care. He had no confidence in his district nurses. The clinical nurse specialist and district nurse visited Richard together at home to discuss his concerns. He was asked to rate his confidence in managing his airway and stoma. He scored himself as 0% confident. He was asked to detail the specific problems he was experiencing. The list was as follows:
> - Dry crusts and mucus built up and caused him to feel as though he would 'choke to death'.
> - He was coughing up blood in his mucus and was frightened of bleeding to death (he had had a postoperative bleed which had necessitated a return to theatre).
> - The skin around his stoma felt very tight and he was frightened his stoma would close and choke him.
> - He found it very difficult to insert his button.
>
> The effects of airway dehydration due to loss of the function of the upper airway were explained; this was causing the crusts, mucus plugs and bleeding. Richard was taught how to deal with all the identified difficult aspects of his airway management and stoma care, and the appropriate equipment provided to help with this (Kaz Therasteam, Trachi-naze, Tilley's forceps, yellow paraffin to lubricate button for insertion). He was taught to massage the scar tissue around his stoma in order to reduce the feeling of tightness. After the first visit, his confidence rating had increased to 50%. The district nurse continued to reinforce this programme and after 2 weeks Richard scored 100% confidence. He felt much more in control. The frequent visits to the hospital stopped completely.

Facilitating coping during radiotherapy

As the quality of life studies at the beginning of Chapter 3.1 clearly demonstrate, the lowest point in the patient's treatment experience is radiotherapy. Firstly, the patient has to have a beam direction mask individually made, which often causes much anxiety, and secondly, there are unpleasant side effects that affect wellbeing, including fatigue, decreased energy, inability to carry out daily activities, eating and swallowing problems, skin and oral problems, pain, taste changes, decreased concentration, sleep disturbances, decreased sexual desire, negative mood and anxiety, inability to carry out usual family, work and social roles (Woodtli & Ort, 1991). This period is very difficult for all patients and can be particularly difficult for people who have already undergone surgery, as the following vignettes demonstrates.

> Joe was very pleased that he had recovered well from his hemiglossectomy and neck dissection. He said that he knew the worst was now over, and he only had a month of outpatient radiotherapy as an extra measure just to make sure the cancer was well and truly gone. He was self employed and not insured for illness, so he intended to go back to work, as his treatment only took 10 minutes per day. The nurse warned him that the radiotherapy would cause extreme soreness and tiredness, but he could not believe anything could be worse than undergoing major surgery. However, 12 days into his treatment, Joe felt otherwise. His mouth and lips were excruciatingly sore so that even a sip of water burned intensely. His mouth was bone dry and sticky mucus in his throat stopped him from swallowing and nauseated him. Everything tasted like cardboard. He had to be admitted to hospital for nasogastric feeding. He felt like he had gone right back to square one. After another 5 days, his red skin began to blister and weep, and he felt incredibly tired. It was 2 months before Joe felt well enough to go back to work, and even then fatigue prevented him from working a normal, full day. Joe said that the radiotherapy was 10 times worse than the operation; 'sheer hell' were the exact words he used.
>
> Another patient commented: 'First you have the operation, which you are asleep for. When you wake up, the worst part is over. You just get better every day. Then they give you this shit [radiotherapy]. You start off feeling OK, but every day you get worse. They squash your face into a mask every day and by the end you are much more poorly than you have ever been before. It's barbaric'.

Krouse et al (1989) also found that postoperative radiation therapy had a major adverse effect. They studied 45 patients who had undergone surgery and found that those who underwent postoperative radiotherapy did significantly worse, with a delay in returning to work and social activities and additional physical complications. Their improvement after radiotherapy was slow.

One of the trained visitors in our buddy scheme explained: 'You can tell them (new patients) about the surgery and about what the radiotherapy entails, but you can't tell them how awful the radiotherapy will be; they have to find that out for themselves'.

Mask phobia

One of the essential parts of radiotherapy treatment is the beam direction mask. This mask has to fit 'skin tight' in order to ensure absolute accuracy in direction of the beam. Many patients find wearing the mask an extremely unpleasant experience, and some individuals develop a phobia towards it. This phenomenon has not been documented in the literature, but seems to be equivalent to the anticipatory nausea or needle phobia phenomenena described in patients undergoing intensive chemotherapy. Mayou and Smith (1997) describe the occurrence of post-traumatic stress disorder (PTSD) in patients undergoing profoundly unpleasant medical treatments, and it seems plausible that PTSD can occur as a result of the experience of a beam direction mask. This manifests as a phobic anxiety and is often accompanied by panic. If it is not managed sensitively and effectively, it may result in the patient being unable to undergo radiotherapy, as it cannot be safely given without a mask.

Preparing the patient for the beam direction mask is discussed in Chapter 1.2, and is important in prevention of problems. For patients who experience difficulties nurses can use simple neurolinguistic programming techniques to help patients overcome mask phobia:

- Teaching mental rehearsal (Rushworth, 1994); patients are asked to imagine they are directing a film of themselves going through the mask fitting feeling calm, relaxed and in control. They are instructed to find a trigger to start this behaviour; for example, walking into the treatment area. The patient 'runs through' the film in his/her head several times until they are happy with it. Next time they go for a mask fitting the situation will seem familiar and the brain will automatically go into the routine.
- The phobia cure — anchoring (Rushworth, 1994); take the patient away from the problem situation to a neutral area. Ask them about what causes their panic attack. The reply will usually be something like 'it's when they clip the mask down over my head'. Ask the patient to imagine this now, and note their non-verbal reactions (physical tensing, change in colour). This is Anchor A. Now ask the patient to imagine a pleasant memory (a positive resource state), opposite to the one being felt about the mask. The ideal feeling is a feeling of being in control. For example, 'imagine a time when you felt really confident about yourself ... remember where you were, who was there ... I'd like you to be there now, remember what you saw, what you heard'. Watch the patient closely and when they can be seen to be reliving the memory mentally (smiling, facial flushing), squeeze their shoulder firmly. This is Anchor B. If you cannot achieve a positive resource

state with this question, try others such as imagining being in an open space, a favourite place, etc. Once this has been done, ask the patient to imagine the mask being clipped down again, and as you do, squeeze the shoulder firmly. You have now anchored the positive resource state on to the negative one. This has the effect of cancelling out the phobia; the patient will no longer display the phobic non-verbal reactions. Now ask the patient how they feel about wearing the mask. Although the patient may not feel ecstatic about it, they will usually say something like, 'Well I'll just have to put up with it'. Incredible as it may sound this technique actually works astoundingly well in practice.

- Relaxation techniques and guided imagery can also be used, but need to be practised by the patient several times prior to the mask fitting. They cannot be taught to patients in the grip of a panic attack.

Clare Rushworth's excellent book *Making a Difference in Cancer Care* has more information on these techniques and is strongly recommended for anyone interested in them.

Coping with side effects

As most radiotherapy is given on an outpatient basis, patients and families have to manage side effects and symptoms in the home setting. The symptom distress experienced by patients engenders marked disruption of daily activities and a considerable self-care burden, leading to appraisals of the illness situation as stressful (Oberst et al, 1991). Fatigue is a significant problem, often aggravated by the daily travelling back and forth for treatment, sometimes over considerable distances. Studies demonstrate that patients need a strong family support system to cope effectively with radiotherapy and that patients without this resource needed additional nursing support during treatment (Hanucharurnkul, 1989; Oberst et al, 1991).

Thus during radiotherapy, more than at any other time, the patient requires intensive psychological support. Coping skills can be enhanced by good preparation pre-radiotherapy and this has been discussed in Chapter 1.2.

Johnson et al (1997) have clearly demonstrated that nursing care based on self-regulation theory enables patients undergoing radiotherapy to cope significantly better than those who do not benefit from such interventions. Self-regulation theory describes a coping process that people use when undergoing stressful health-related events. The theory provides guidance on how nurses can increase patients' ability and confidence when it comes to coping with and managing their experience. A mental image (cognitive representation) shapes the patient's expectations of an experience, and nurses can influence this mental image by providing concrete and objective information directed at helping the patient to manage side effects and reduce disruption to normal life activities. Concrete objective data include:

- physical sensations (what is felt, seen, heard, tasted, smelled)
- temporal features (sequence and duration of events)
- environmental features (people and settings involved)
- causes of the sensations.

A study group of 110 patients was given structured theory-based interventions by staff nurses who made specific appointment schedules for four interventions with each patient before, during and after treatment. Each appointment contained specific interventions to help the patient cope at that particular stage of treatment. A control group of 116 patients received the usual unstructured care, with no specific appointments, and no structured theory-based interventions. The study group experienced an impressive 31–60% decrease in disruption of normal life activities. They also demonstrated more positive moods on psychometric testing.

Weintraub and Hagopian (1990) studied 56 patients undergoing radiotherapy. Patients were assigned to a weekly consultation with a physician, a weekly general health information session from a non specialist nurse, and a weekly consultation with a specialist cancer nurse to discuss side effects and self-care strategies. The findings suggest that a weekly consultation with a specialist cancer nurse significantly reduces anxiety levels and thus has a positive impact on patient anxiety at a time when anxiety is known to interfere with wellbeing. Hinds et al (1995) found that many patients felt that active participation helped them to cope. This included being involved and in control of one's care, being a partner in care, and having the information to help oneself; all things which nursing care from an appropriately skilled cancer nurse can provide.

Wells (1998) also found that patients undergoing head and neck irradiation experience a high level of emotional and physical trauma and therefore need a correspondingly high level of support. She recommends patients be given information, symptom support and practical advice by a designated nurse or radiographer who provides continuity of care. This support needs to continue into the first month after treatment, as patients continue to experience significant difficulties during this time. An integrated rehabilitative approach to follow-up care is needed which incorporates telephone contact, practical support and liaison with the local multidisciplinary team.

Thus, evidence shows that to facilitate coping during radiotherapy, patients undergoing head and neck irradiation need:

- regular consultations with a specialist cancer nurse
- good family support
- good information provision.

Nurses need to be dynamic and creative in order to provide this care. For example, services and protocols can be designed so that patients and their family have an initial consultation with and assessment by a cancer nurse within their first week of treatment in a nurse-led clinic. This session includes the provision of information on mouth and skin care, and referral on to other professionals to help with specific eating, social and psychological problems. A referral is made to the community nursing team so that the patient also gains support at home. From this point onwards the patient is seen in a nurse-led head and neck clinic weekly, and a dietitian forms part of the team. Support from the nursing team and dietitian continues after treatment as this is the time when reactions are at their peak (Wells, 1998); the patient is reviewed in the nurse-led clinic weekly until the radiotherapy reaction has subsided, after 3 to 4 weeks. Psychological support is one of the most important functions of this service.

Physical coping strategies

Maxillofacial prosthetics

The main aim of maxillofacial prosthetics is the restoration of form and function of a missing or defective part of the maxilla, mandible or face (Jani & Schaaf, 1978). Dentures are the most common prosthetic and often one of the most important concerns for patients after surgery and radiotherapy; rehabilitation goals become centred on 'when I get my new teeth' in the patient's mind. Properly prepared and fitted palatal prostheses will usually effect near normal speech, swallowing and masticatory functions after mid-face surgery (Mathog et al, 1997). However, extensive surgery may make retention of the prostheses a difficult problem for many patients. Jani & Schaaf (1978) report 50% of patients not wearing their prosthesis due to problems with retention, discomfort and irritation. Modern techniques to implant osseointegrated rods for fixation of dental prostheses has improved, but not completely resolved, this problem (Funk et al, 1998). Nurses can ensure that referrals are made to the prosthetics department, and liaise with the prosthetics team to resolve any problems.

Demonstrating the overwhelming importance of the obturator to the patient is this quote from a patient in the King's Fund report on head and neck cancer care:

> I don't think the medical profession really realize what it really entails for a person trying to use an obturator. They don't realize that you can't talk without it, you can't eat without it, you can't drink without it. They do not realize the great immense fear. You live with the fear that it is going to break or fall out, you're going to drop it and I keep it by my bed at night so it's the biggest pot of gold I could find. (Edwards, 1997)

Limiting damage

Limiting damage to physical appearance and function is also important. This includes good wound and skin care, good oral and dental care, pain management, speech therapy, nutritional support and physiotherapy.

Cosmetic camouflage

Cosmetic camouflage can be very helpful in disguising discoloration of the skin, caused by scar tissue and radiotherapy. It cannot, however, cover changes in skin smoothness and texture due to surgery and more prominent scarring. There are several different manufacturers of cosmetic camouflage products, who are often willing to provide training sessions for nurses. Provision of cosmetic camouflage by the local nursing team can help to enhance continuity of care, and avoids the need for long journeys to, and waits to be seen at, a busy cosmetic camouflage clinic. The British Red Cross also provides a cosmetic camouflage service.

Look Good, Feel Better

This is a service provided in cancer centres by the cosmetic industry. It was established by the Estee Lauder Foundation and is funded by several of the well-known high street cosmetic companies. The project provides sessions for women undergoing cancer treatment. Beauty therapists from local department stores are recruited to the sessions to treat women to a makeup session, which includes the provision of a gift box of high-quality cosmetics. The sessions are usually run on a monthly basis.

Heat/moisture exchangers

The use of heat/moisture exchangers by the laryngectomee can significantly reduce mucus production (see Chapter 2.1), as well as prevent the unexpected expellation of mucus on to a bystander.

Clothing and hair

A well-groomed appearance can mitigate the effects of disfigurement. Attractive clothes and a good hair style will also make the individual feel more confident. Use of scarves, necklaces, romet covers, cravats etc. disguises the laryngectomy stoma, as well as any mucus that escapes. Wigs can be used to disguise alopecia, or hair shaved off for craniofacial surgery.

Group training and therapy

Fiegenbaum (1981) provided training programmes (10 weekly sessions) to improve social skills for head and neck cancer patients. Significant improvements were found in social skills and reduction of anxiety levels in the study group compared to a control group.

Sanchez-Salazar and Stark (1972) describe the use of a group interaction therapy programme for laryngectomees and families who displayed an inability to cope post-surgery. This was facilitated by the speech therapist and social worker and consisted of 1 hour per week for 10 weeks. They do not report any evaluation of the programme.

Cunningham et al (1991) studied 320 patients undergoing a 6-week psychoeducational programme to enhance a sense of control over mental/emotional states. It comprised teaching standard coping skills, relaxation, positive mental imagery, cognitive restructuring, goal setting and general issues of lifestyle change. A control group underwent six sessions of supportive discussion alone. Both groups' affective states improved, but the study sample showed twice as much improvement as the control group. This was strongly correlated with improvements in sleep patterns, energy, pain and interpersonal communication. They conclude that cognitive control (which is teachable) appears to be an important determinant of affective state in cancer patients.

Robinson et al (1996) studied 64 facially disfigured people undergoing social skills training workshops (provided by Changing Faces). The workshops significantly decreased anxiety, social avoidance and distress, and participants reported more confidence with strangers and new people. They conclude that social interaction skills training should be provided alongside surgical interventions.

Social support

Social support mitigates the negative psychosocial consequences of head and neck cancer (Mesters et al, 1997). The social support of family members is particularly important. Many studies on aspects of rehabilitation in head and neck cancer have shown that family support is a crucial factor for positive outcomes (Baker, 1992; Edwards, 1997).

Social support can be defined as a construct with several elements: informational (information that one is loved, cared for); emotional (agreement with feelings); instrumental (financial, physical); affirmation (sense of belonging); appraisal (support with feedback to patient) (Bottomley & Jones, 1997).

In a study of 51 laryngectomees, Stam et al (1991) found that satisfaction with social support was a significant predictor of distress and quality of life as well as successful speech rehabilitation. Changes in relationships with friends was a significant predictor of distress. Byrne et al (1993) also found that depression in laryngectomees was most common in those who were socially isolated, with poor professional and peer support. Richardson et al (1989) found that the quality of support from the spouse correlated most highly with depression, dysfunction and communication. They concluded that the level of support from family and friends after laryngectomy significantly influences the level of physical–psychosocial dysfunction that laryngectomees experience. This type of support encourages laryngectomees to reappraise themselves after surgery in a positive way that facilitates re-entry into social situations.

A study of 133 head and neck cancer patients (Mesters et al, 1997) found that patients who could openly discuss their illness and problems with their family experienced lower levels of anxiety, less intense feelings of fear, less loneliness, less depression and less loss of control than patients who felt unable to discuss problems with their family. More openness was associated with fewer psychological complaints as well as fewer physiological complaints. De Boer et al (1995) had similar findings. In Stam et al's study (1991), patients reported that the degree to which family and friends no longer listened to them affected quality of life.

Reasons for families being reluctant to discuss problems and emotions openly are various. Many families assume that it is important to be optimistic around a cancer patient and that the patient should avoid thinking about negative aspects. Families may be afraid of cancer and inclined to avoid discussing the topic for this reason. The patient may avoid discussions in order to avoid worrying their family. This can result in tense family relationships (Mesters et al, 1997). Nurses should therefore strive to facilitate open family discussions with the patient and give extra help to those families who have difficulty communicating.

The more speech ability was rated as inadequate (by a speech therapist) the less open discussion in the family seemed to be as time progressed. The authors propose that as time progressed, the frustration resulting from psychological problems associated with speech difficulty led to withdrawal and social isolation of the patient, even from family members. This means that nurses should pay particular attention to the psychological and emotional support of the patient with severe speech impairment and his/her family.

In summary, patients are better able to cope with radical changes in their appearance and function when they have a supportive group of relatives and friends who are appropriately briefed about the patients concerns and needs. Price (1998) suggests that if there are one or more key people who have a wide range of connections with others, they can become ambassadors for the patient — providing previously agreed accounts of a patient's new image to others outside the hospital before discharge. This limits the patient's problems of dealing with awkward social encounters and questions.

Patients with limited social support should be considered as at risk for coping difficulties, and will need additional monitoring by the primary healthcare team and in the outpatient clinic. Daycare facilities may be a good way of rehabilitating the isolated patient, and support groups may be particularly helpful for these individuals.

Concerns of significant others

Relatives often feel powerless to help patients during the acute treatment stage of cancer, and it is important that nurses acknowledge their expertise in understanding the patient and the circumstances at home.

Mah and Johnston (1993) found that there were five major categories of concerns reported by families of individuals with head and neck cancer:

- the effects and effectiveness of treatment
- interpersonal relationships
- care received by the patient in hospital
- caring for the patient on discharge
- social concerns such as ability to return to previous activities and lifestyle.

Relatives may appreciate being invited to discuss the patient's preferred ways of coping and to anticipate the role that they will play on discharge (Price, 1998). Caregiver strain and burden are common amongst family members. Caregivers are expected to grieve while 'cheering' their spouses to survival. They are expected to recognize and identify problems, while reframing their own lives around the illness (Blood et al, 1994).

Mathieson et al (1991) studied 30 laryngectomees and their spouses, comparing their psychological and psychosocial wellbeing. They found that maintenance of a satisfactory sexual relationship was a significant predictor of the spouse's wellbeing. They also found that spouses had higher levels of depression, fatigue and tension than the laryngectomees themselves. They recommend that the spouse's psychological state should be considered separately from that of the patient. After the sexual relationship, the strongest predictors of spousal happiness were changes in friendships and socializing due to the laryngectomy.

Harrison et al (1995) examined the impact of cancer diagnosis on key relatives. The relatives reported high levels of concern. Major concerns included 'patient's illness', 'patient's physical state', 'patient's reaction to illness', 'patient's treatment', 'self feeling upset or distressed', 'effect of illness on others' and 'the future'. These concerns were matched to the patients' own concerns; overall, relatives had higher concern scores than the patients. The greatest discrepancy was about the patient's emotional reaction to the illness; 95% of relatives were concerned, compared to only 18% of the patients themselves. Forty-eight per cent of relatives showed significant psychological morbidity. The highest scores were on the anxiety and insomnia, and somatic symptoms. Female relatives and those with higher concern scores showed higher levels of psychological morbidity. The authors conclude that relatives regard themselves as helpless observers who can do little to influence their loved one's illness and treatment. In contrast, patients can resolve concerns by setting themselves goals, for example, having their operation, or completing their treatment. They recommend that healthcare professionals see relatives separately to patients at least some of the time, as they may have concerns that are significantly different to, and more severe than, those of the patients themselves. They point especially to the need for counselling relatives to raise emotional issues with the patient.

Watt-Watson and Graydon (1995) studied 44 head and neck cancer patients and their caregivers after surgery and found that caregivers identified major caregiving demands related to physical care, treatment regimes and imposed changes from the disease. Concerns included practical issues such as 'need to know about mouth care' and 'need suggestions for food', as well as emotional and social issues such as dealing with anger, tiredness and uncertainty. They felt they had no one to rely on for help and perceived a lack of support from professionals. Their needs for physical and psychological support were very evident from their qualitative responses.

Blood et al (1994) examined 75 spouses of laryngectomees for levels of caregiver stress and burden over time from diagnosis. During the first 6 months after diagnosis, spouses reported significantly high levels of strain and caregiver burden. This was slightly lower during the second 6 months, but still significant. After 12 months, levels of strain and burden lowered and plateaued. The authors recommend that support meetings may be helpful for spouses during the first year after laryngectomy to avoid caregiver burnout.

Educating significant others

Richardson et al (1989) point out that, although social support has been widely shown to have a positive influence on adjustment and rehabilitation, it is not always beneficial. People who are potential sources of support may actually provide negative feedback, accentuating, rather than minimizing, the disability. The support person may become impatient and resentful.

Whilst there is much evidence to show the positive effects of social support, the possible negative effects should not be forgotten. Negative effects can occur when the relationship hampers self-esteem, autonomy and ability to make choices. Negative effects can also be seen when an individual receives more support than they can provide, which leads to feelings of dependency and indebtedness (Bottomley & Jones, 1997). These factors can lead to resentment in the relationship.

Relatives should therefore be assessed, coached and supported carefully. What to expect when they first see the patient postoperatively can be a major anxiety and their initial reactions will be carefully read by the patient. They may be the first 'mirror' the patient uses to 'see' his/her disfigurement.

'The first night when my husband came I watched his face so carefully as he walked toward me to see what his reactions were' (patient's recollection of surgery).

The family should also be educated to give positive reinforcement to encourage the patient's rehabilitation. This includes preparation for both verbal and non-verbal reactions to the patient. Initial reactions to the alaryngeal voice (electronic or tracheoesophageal) can be crucial; a negative reaction, such as 'You sound like a Dalek!' can be devastating to the patient's self-esteem. Adverse facial reactions are particularly difficult to control, and will be noted by the patient first trying out an oesophageal voice, or eating with the family for the first time.

Reminders to encourage independence in the patient are often helpful; for example, relatives may often be tempted to speak for the patient with speech difficulty, so preventing practice with voice rehabilitation, or to allow social avoidance to become ingrained by doing tasks such as shopping which would normally help the patient to regain social confidence. The patient may often feel smothered by well meant attempts to help, and sometimes the nurse needs to act as an advocate and tactfully suggest that the patient is given some personal space and independence.

The family should be educated about emotional problems post-operatively as well as physical care. They will then be better prepared to cope with mood swings and strong emotion after discharge (Herzon & Boshier, 1979). Spouses may often be the target for cancer survivors' anger and negative feelings (Sanchez-Salazar & Stark, 1972).

Ongoing support and follow-up

Research on long-term problems in head and neck cancer patients clearly demonstrates that physical problems and psychosocial distress persist way beyond discharge after surgery and the end of radiotherapy. This has important implications for the organization of follow-up services for head and neck cancer patients. Patients should always be referred to the community nursing team, who are in the best position to provide ongoing support for the family. Patients should also have open access to a specialist head and neck cancer nurse (Edwards, 1997), dietitian and speech and language therapist. Patients who demonstrate specific psychological problems may also require referral to the local mental health team.

Additional evidence for ongoing support and effective organization of outpatient clinics is provided by a study of 40 patients attending a maxillofacial oncology unit for follow-up. Telfer & Shepherd (1993) detected significant levels of psychological distress and physical problems in the sample. Patients found the consultation very stressful; many were preoccupied with physical symptoms, believing them to be evidence of recurrence. The authors concluded that patients needed more personal counselling and support, and recommended that patients have access to a Macmillan nurse at all clinics, as well as psychologists as necessary. They also noted that many patients are made more anxious and miserable by prolonged waits in unpleasant hospital environments; efficient appointment systems with attractive waiting areas are therefore also an important factor.

Table 3.3.5: Support resources for patients and families

Organization	Address
Changing Faces	1 & 2 Junction Mews London W2 1PN Tel 020 7706 4232 Fax 020 7706 4234 E-mail: info@faces.demon.co.uk
CancerBACUP	3 Bath Place, Rivington Street, London EC2A 3JR Cancer information service 0808 800 1234 http://www.cancerbacup.org.uk
Cancerlink	17 Britannia Street, London WC1X 9JN Tel. 020 78332451
Macmillan Cancer Relief	Anchor House, 15/19 Britten Street London SW3 3TZ Helpline 0845 6016161
Let's Face It	Christine Piff, 14 Fallowfield, Yateley, Surrey GU17 7LW
National Association of Laryngectomee Clubs	6 Rickett Street, Fulham, London SW6 1RU Tel. 020 7381 9993 Fax 020 7381 0025
British Red Cross Camouflage Service	National Headquarters, 9 Grosvenor Street, London SW1X 7EJ

Summary

Head and neck cancer has enormous psychosocial consequences for the patient and their significant others. Using evidence in the literature, and assessment tools such as the Hospital Anxiety and Depression Scale (Zigmond & Snaith, 1983), concerns checklists and quality of life measurements (see Chapter 3.1), the nurse can anticipate those most at risk of problems and instigate coping strategies to help patients deal with the effects of their treatment. The management of psychosocial factors is highly skilled, and requires careful planning and evaluation. Some strategies, resources and tools have been suggested in this chapter. The psychosocial aspects of care for these individuals is just as important as their physical care. This care is needed far beyond the end of medical treatment and nurses in both the hospital and community must work together, employing creative interventions to ensure patients enjoy a good quality of life rather than merely endure survival.

Strategy for practice

- Provide evidence-based psychological interventions to promote positive coping strategies.
- Provide regular specialist cancer nursing support during radio-therapy; this is the hardest point of the patient's cancer journey.
- Ensure that all appropriate products and interventions are used to minimize disfigurement and dysfunction.
- Provide group support and training.
- Provide education and support for significant others.
- Provide information of relevant support groups (see Table 3.3.5).
- All your patients should be able to confidently answer the question 'What happened to your face/voice?' (Clarke, 1998).

Section Four
Oncological treatment modalities in head and neck cancer

Chapter 4.1
Surgical treatment of head and neck cancer: general principles and care

GRAHAM BUCKLEY

Introduction

Surgery and radiotherapy are the principal forms of treatment for head and neck cancer. They are usually used with the intention of cure but in some circumstances are also useful for palliation. They may be used alone or in combination. The choice of treatment depends on the type of tumour, the extent of the tumour and on the medical condition and preferences of the patient. Accurate diagnosis and tumour staging are essential components of the decision-making process (see Chapter 1.2). This chapter will give a background to head and neck surgery, with the general principles of resection, reconstruction and neck dissection. Postoperative care is covered in detail.

Resection and reconstruction

Background

The major advances in recent years have not, for the most part, resulted in major improvements in overall survival. They have, on the other hand, significantly reduced the debilitation and improved both the functional and cosmetic outcomes for patients. These changes have come about for two main reasons: firstly a better understanding of the pathology of tumour spread has resulted in modifications of resection techniques, and secondly improvements in tissue transfer have resulted in the ability to reconstruct even major defects. This is well illustrated by the approach to oral and oropha-ryngeal cancer. It was originally thought that these tumours metasta-sized to cervical nodes through lymphatics that passed through the mandible, and that the lymph nodes had to be removed in continuity with the primary tumour. The 'commando' operation evolved to deal with these tumours. The name was a condensation of combined mandibular and oropharyngeal resection but was coined by the resi-dents of the American surgeon John Conley to reflect its heroic nature. Although the operation was effective at tumour control, the cosmetic and functional effects could be devastating. It is now known that tumour spread to the nodes is embolic and that the lymphatics do not pass through the mandible. Consequently very few patients now require mandibular resection. In those cases where mandibular resection is necessary, the use of free tissue transfer has meant that more appropriate and functionally superior reconstruction of the operative defect can be carried out at the time of resection.

The operative procedures for head and neck cancer comprise three related steps: access, resection and reconstruction. Surgical access may be endoscopic or require an external approach. The aims are to maximize exposure of the tumour to allow safe and complete resection and to minimize morbidity from the procedure itself. The technique of resection requires detailed knowledge of the pathology of tumour spread and judgement about how much normal tissue to remove with the tumour to ensure complete exci-sion. This cannot be compromised because morbidity is seldom greater than that from local tumour recurrence. Reconstruction aims to restore the defect created by resection of the tumour to as near normal as possible. Tissue replacement aims to replace, as far as possible, like with like. The first major advance in head and neck reconstruction was the deltopectoral fasciocutaneous flap (Bakamjian, 1965). This meant that it was possible to create a skin-lined tube to replace the pharynx. Its major drawback was that the transfer of the flap had to be delayed to allow it to develop a blood supply from the surrounding tissues. For the patient this meant several weeks in hospital with a salivary fistula. The introduction of the pectoralis major myocutaneous flap by Ariyan in 1979 had a major impact (Ariyan, 1979). This had a vascular pedicle and could be rotated to and used in almost any head and neck site. It meant that single-stage reconstructions could be carried out; it rapidly became the workhorse in head and neck reconstruction. It still has a very important role but its bulk restricts its versatility at some sites. This is not a problem, however, if it is used as a myofascial flap. The development of microvascular techniques means that we now have the ability to reliably transplant free flaps and reconnect their vascular supply. The tissue used for reconstruction can therefore be matched much more closely with the defect, with dramatic functional and cosmetic benefits.

Types of reconstruction

1. *None*. Some defects will heal without any intervention. Defects of the hard palate, nasal mucosa and some tongue and laryngeal resections require no specific reconstruction.
2. *Primary closure*. Small defects may sometimes be closed directly without any functional impairment. This is often the case after partial or total laryngectomy and some partial pharyngectomy defects.
3. *Grafts*. A graft is a tissue transferred to another site without a blood supply. It is revascularized by establishing capillary connections with the surrounding tissue. Skin grafts are the most frequently used. Full thickness skin is used on occasions but most grafts are split thickness because of the reliable revascularization and minimal morbidity at the donor site. Skin grafts are most often used to repair skin defects but may also be used at mucosal sites, for example the posterior pharyngeal wall.
4. *Flaps*. A flap is vascularized tissue that is transferred to another site. Pedicled flaps retain their own blood supply. Free flaps are revascularized by microvascular anastomosis with vessels at the recipient site.

   Pedicled flaps. The defect after resection of a skin tumour is often best repaired by using a local skin flap. Pedicled myocutaneous flaps are used for large pharyngeal defects. The pectoralis major and the latissimus dorsi myocutaneous flaps are the most common.

   Free flaps. The use of microvascular anastomosis allows great versatility in the use of tissues for reconstruction. The fasciocutaneous radial flap is frequently used for oral or pharyngeal defects. Mandibular resection is most reliably reconstructed by using free flaps with a bone component. The most common are fibula, iliac crest, radius and scapula. The free jejunal flap is frequently used for reconstruction after total pharyngectomy.

Management of the cervical lymph nodes: neck dissection

The operation of radical neck dissection was first performed by Crile in 1905. It evolved because it was recognized that simple node excision was often followed by tumour recurrence. The deep cervical lymph nodes are contained within the deep cervical and prevertebral layers of fascia and it was recognized that they could be completely removed within the 'sandwich' formed by the fascial layers (Crile, 1906). The operation had a major impact on survival in head and neck cancer, but there was a price to pay. The operation also removes the sternomastoid muscle, internal jugular vein, cervical plexus and accessory nerve. Consequently, cervical pain and shoulder drop are relatively frequent afterwards. It is now widely accepted that the non-lymphatic structures can often be preserved, unless they are invaded by tumour, without compromising survival. This operation is referred to as the modified radical (functional) neck dissection. It was introduced by Suarez in Argentina (Suarez, 1963) and was popularized in Europe by Bocca (Bocca, 1967).The procedure is more difficult and time-consuming but there is a marked reduction in postoperative morbidity. Pathological studies of radical neck dissection specimens have shown that microscopic tumour deposits occur in a large proportion of patients with tumours at some locations. The site of these metastases follows a predictable pattern that depends on the site of the primary tumour (Lindberg, 1972; Shah, 1990). The Sloan-Kettering Memorial Hospital in New York introduced a system of classification of the cervical lymph nodes into levels which is now widely used (see Figure 4.1.1) (Robbins et al, 1991). These are useful in planning both surgical treatment and radiotherapy. The operation of selective neck dissection is often used now to remove these nodes in high-risk tumours. The particular node groups removed depend on the primary tumour. In laryngeal carcinoma, for example, the upper, middle and lower jugular nodes (levels II, III and IV) would be removed (Candela et al, 1994). All non-lymphatic structures are preserved by these operations and consequently there is a low incidence of postoperative pain or functional impairment.

Classification of neck dissection

A neck dissection may be selective or comprehensive (Robbins et al, 1991). A *selective neck dissection* involves the removal of those lymph

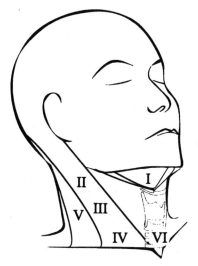

Figure 4.1.1: Cervical lymph node levels.

node groups that are first involved in the spread of a particular tumour. A full description would include the node groups removed. Some of the commoner patterns of selective neck dissection are named, for example the jugular neck dissection (levels II, III and IV) and the supraomohyoid neck dissection (levels I, II and III). A *comprehensive neck dissection* removes node levels I–V. If the sternomastoid muscle, internal jugular vein and accessory nerve are also removed it is termed a *radical neck dissection*. If any or all of these structures are preserved the term *modified radical neck dissection* is used. An *extended neck dissection* also removes node groups other than the cervical nodes, for example the mediastinal nodes.

Pre-operative assessment of the neck

If there is palpable lymph node enlargement then fine-needle aspiration cytology is a rapid, sensitive and specific way of diagnosing squamous carcinoma. Computerized tomography, magnetic resonance imaging and ultrasound combined with fine-needle aspiration have all been utilized to assess nodal disease in the neck with no palpable metastases. They all result in approximately the same accuracy and detect more nodes than palpation alone (Van den Brekel, 1996). Since the decision to treat the N0 neck is largely based on the site and stage of the primary tumour, preoperative imaging does not often alter the treatment of the neck in practice.

Surgical technique

The principle underlying all the forms of neck dissection is the complete removal of nodes within the fascial layers of the neck. The operation is usually carried out through a transverse cervical incision which may be modified to incorporate a vertical limb, depending on the extent of the dissection. Skin flaps are elevated to expose the deep cervical fascia. The platysma muscle is usually preserved with the skin flap. Superficial nerves including the mandibular branch of the facial and the cervical cutaneous nerves are preserved as far as possible. The posterior limit of the dissection is the trapezius muscle for a comprehensive dissection and the cervical plexus for most types of selective dissection. The prevertebral fascia is elevated from the prevertebral muscles as far as the carotid sheath, which it is continuous with. The fascia is dissected from the internal jugular vein, vagus nerve and carotid artery. The fascia extends along the branches of the external carotid artery, which are also preserved. The dissection of the submandibular area usually includes the submandibular salivary gland. The accessory and hypoglossal nerves cross the fascial planes but can be dissected free unless invaded by tumour. The paratracheal and superior mediastinal nodes are removed in tumours involving the subglottic larynx and lower hypopharynx. A full dissection of the superior mediastinum requires a sternotomy. This is sometimes necessary for nodal disease in this area, usually in relation to tumour recurrence around the tracheostome after laryngectomy.

Applications

1. Comprehensive neck dissections are usually used for nodal metastases. Postoperative radiotherapy is often required. If one group of nodes is involved there is a high likelihood of microscopic deposits in the other groups. The neck dissection should therefore remove all potentially involved nodes. A modified radical or radical dissection is used depending on the extent of involvement of non-lymphatic structures.
2. Selective neck dissections are used to remove high-risk node groups in tumours with a known propensity to metastasize. Tumours at some sites, such as the pharynx and supraglottic larynx, may have a 50% or greater likelihood of microscopic metastases even if there is no node enlargement. Previous studies

have identified the nodes that different tumours initially involve. These node groups are removed by selective neck dissection.

3. Extended neck dissections are used to remove nodes beyond the lateral cervical group. Tumours of the subglottic larynx, hypopharynx and thyroid gland, for example, may spread to the paratracheal or superior mediastinal nodes.

Postoperative shoulder disability; neck dissection morbidity

Loss of shoulder function is a distressing consequence of radical neck dissection. It is caused by resection of the accessory nerve, which supplies the trapezius muscle. The trapezius muscle is of major functional importance because it provides the primary supportive and rotatory actions of the shoulder girdle mechanism. Paralysis of the trapezius muscle results in a well-recognized 'shoulder syndrome' involving pain, weakness and deformity of the shoulder girdle. The entire shoulder girdle drops downward and forward (Remmler et al, 1986). The patient experiences difficulty with activities requiring raising of the hands above shoulder level (e.g. brushing hair, hanging up washing, reaching into cupboards). The shoulder becomes painful and stiff (Short et al, 1984). Arthritis and capsulitis of the joint develop. Occasionally, if radical neck dissection has been combined with radiotherapy to the supraclavicular nodes, the clavicle is weakened and fracture occurs due to the unbalanced muscular forces acting on it (Strauss et al, 1982). Patients undergoing modified neck dissections, with preservation of the accessory nerve, will also experience weakness of the trapezius, but this has been shown to resolve between 6 and 12 months post-surgery (Remmler et al, 1986).

The long-term implications of shoulder disability may seem inconsequential compared to survival from cancer, but they should not be underestimated. However, Hillel et al (1989) point out that shoulder disability is often overlooked because it is not part of the routine head and neck examination at follow-up visits, and because 'patients rarely persist in mentioning shoulder problems during follow-up visits'. Clinical experience shows that this may be one of the most distressing disabilities from the patient's point of view, as the following vignettes show.

Joan was 69 when she underwent partial pharyngectomy and a right radical neck dissection. She was a widow and lived alone. She was very independent and enjoyed church activities, looking after her grandchildren and eating out with friends. Her neck dissection caused severe pain and loss of function in her right shoulder. She was no longer able to wash and groom her hair. She could not perform household cleaning such as vacuuming, dusting higher shelves, hanging up washing, reaching into higher cupboards. She did not feel she could safely cope with her grandchildren. Most distressingly, she was unable to drive because she could not turn the steering wheel effectively. This meant it was difficult to go to church and drive her friends on outings to their favourite cafes. Joan was therefore experiencing a complete loss of her former independence and social life. She also experienced pain which woke her up during the night, and could not effectively be controlled by analgesics because she experienced too many side effects from the high doses required. Coping strategies to help Joan included weekly visits to the hairdresser to have her hair washed and styled, a home help to do the heavy housework, and a floor-standing clothes drying rack. She had weekly sessions from a faith healer and homeopathic remedies which helped with the pain. Attendance allowance was successfully applied for and this helped to pay for taxis, as Joan had to sell her car. However, Joan found it very hard to accept her loss of independence and felt she was now 'useless' to her family and to the world in general.

Bill was 49 when he underwent partial laryngectomy and radical left neck dissection. He worked as a fork lift truck driver in a factory. At home, he lived with his wife and enjoyed DIY. He was still paying a mortgage on his house, and was not insured for illness and disability. Bill experienced severe loss of strength and mobility in his shoulder postoperatively, as well as pain. Despite physiotherapy he found that he was no longer able to perform his heavy manual work, and thus lost his job, with a significant drop in income. Sadly, he had to sell his house and move into council accommodation. Due to the loss of his job, his home, his financial independence and his physical strength he became very depressed, despite the success of his cancer treatment.

All patients who have undergone modified or radical neck dissection should be referred for physiotherapy as this is essential for preventing or minimizing long-term disability (Blessing et al, 1986; Fialka & Vinzenz, 1988). Physiotherapy involves instruction in an exercise regime aimed at maintaining the range of motion in the shoulder joint. Initially, passive exercises maintain the joint's mobility. This is followed by a programme of exercises to strengthen the remaining muscles (the scapular retractors and elevators), and range of motion exercises to increase scapulo-humeral joint motion (Saunders & Johnson, 1975). Myocutaneous flaps (pectoralis major, trapezius, rhomboids) also cause physical disability in the shoulder and similarly require physical therapy, to maintain joint motion and strengthen remaining muscles (Har-El et al, 1990).

The often severe pain caused by neck dissection can require referral to a specialist pain management team (see Chapter 2.11 on pain). Lymphoedema is another distressing consequence of neck dissection, especially after bilateral neck dissection; Chapter 2.9 describes the management of lymphoedema.

Technical aspects

Incisions in head and neck surgery

The neck is a solid structure and consequently skin flaps have to be raised as the first part of most operative procedures. Incisions are designed to maximize access and minimize cosmetic or functional deformity. Skin flaps should be carefully planned to avoid compromising their vascular supply. The skin flaps are usually elevated in the relatively avascular plane deep to the subcutaneous platysma muscle. Transverse incisions are preferred, the level depending on the site of the pathology. For example, a low 'collar' incision is used for thyroid tumours and mid-cervical for laryngeal. Access to the posterior triangle for radical or modified radical neck dissection usually requires a vertical extension to the clavicle.

Wound closure, drains and dressings

Several suture materials are available for wound closure, ranging from absorbable sutures to stainless steel clips. There is no clear advantage of one method over another. Additional closure of the subcutaneous tissues is both unnecessary and may increase the rate of wound infection. The strength of the closure comes from the dermis and full strength is not regained for around 6 weeks. There is therefore some logic in using a hydrolysable subcuticular single layer closure.

Suction drains are used to prevent the accumulation of blood or serous fluid under the skin flaps and should be of adequate size ($\frac{1}{4}$ in.). The trocar ends of drains should be left on until the skin incisions have been closed. Otherwise blood drawn in by capillary action may clot and block the drain tubing.

Dressings are not necessary in most circumstances and may obscure the wound, masking early diagnosis of a haematoma.

Preparation and postoperative care in head and neck cancer

Consent and counselling

Time is necessary for truly informed consent. The counselling required is obviously dependent on the nature of the procedure and the personality of the patient. Informed consent is not obtained on a brief discussion the day before surgery, and this is not the appropriate time to discuss surgical complications. This information should have been given well before admission with time for information to be absorbed and the consequences of surgery to be appreciated by the patient. Chapter 1.2 describes these issues in detail.

Preparation for surgery

A dental assessment is necessary in patients undergoing radiotherapy to the mouth or salivary glands (see Chapter 2.2). This is usually carried out prior to surgery. Some patients are in a poor nutritional state and benefit from nasogastric feeding before surgery (see Chapter 2.4). Many patients require postoperative nasogastric feeding. A fine-bore nasogastric feeding tube is more comfortable and is easier to insert prior to the operation. Communication difficulties should be anticipated and discussed with the patient before surgery so that an appropriate postoperative method can be established (see Chapter 2.5). The patient should have received appropriate interventions for tobacco and alcohol problems (see Chapter 1.3).

Preoperative investigations such as chest X-ray and scans will have been obtained before admission (see Chapter 1.2). Most patients will require a biochemical profile, full blood count and ECG. The nurse should check that all the relevant X-rays, scans and test results are on the ward and accompany the patient to theatre. Blood is cross matched according to the nature of the operation.

Postoperative care

Most patients will require high-dependency nursing for the first 24–48 hours. The nurse should be conversant with postoperative fluid and circulation monitoring, care of the wound drains, tracheostomy care and the complications that may arise after head and neck surgery. Particular attention should be given to communication in this group of patients. Antibiotic prophylaxis on induction and for the immediate postoperative period will be used for most patients.

Monitoring and lines

The following are standard for major head and neck procedures:

1. two peripheral intravenous lines
2. a central venous line
3. an arterial line
4. rectal and skin temperature probes
5. urinary catheter.

Routine monitoring includes:

1. ventilation details
2. heart rate (ECG), blood pressure, central venous pressure
3. fluid balance
4. central and peripheral temperature.

Within 45 minutes of arrival on the intensive care/high-dependency ward, the following are checked:

1. haemoglobin (Hb), packed cell volume (PCV) and clotting
2. arterial gases
3. urea and electrolytes
4. blood sugar in diabetics
5. urine, blood, protein and sugar; urea and electrolytes and osmolarity.

PCV, gases and potassium are checked every 2 hours for the first 4 hours or until stable. In diabetics, blood sugar is checked hourly for the first 4 hours, and then 2-hourly if stable.

Airway

Patients usually have a tracheostomy or reinforced endotracheal tube in situ. The head should be kept in a neutral position and the tube position should be verified by chest X-ray within the first few hours after surgery. A tracheostomy tube will usually be sutured into position to avoid displacement and pressure of tapes on the neck skin or flaps. Tracheostomy suction will be necessary because of the increased tracheobronchial mucus secretion. This is carried out as required — usually half-hourly initially. Humidification of inspired air or oxygen will be required. A cuffed tracheostomy tube will normally be used.

Cuff pressure should be checked and adjusted hourly to 20–30 cm water. In most cases the cuff can be deflated after 12 hours.

Displacement or obstruction of the tube may be indicated by a persistent air leak (unresolved by inflation of the cuff with small volumes of air (< 10 ml) to a pressure of 20–30 cm water), failure to ventilate or a sudden change in airway pressure or hypoxaemia. If displacement is suspected, the patient should be gently manually ventilated with 100% oxygen. A suction catheter should be passed down the tube to detect any obstruction. A smaller tracheostomy tube, a 7.0 mm tracheal tube and tracheal dilators should be available. In an urgent situation, if the tracheostomy tube is displaced or blocked, a smaller tracheostomy tube should be inserted. However, if the situation is stable the surgical team should be informed first.

Airway management is discussed in more detail in Chapter 2.1.

Ventilation

Patients may require overnight ventilation after surgery. Hypocapnia should be avoided, and blood gases should be kept at a PaO_2 of 10.0–18.0 kPa and $PaCO_2$ of 4.5–6.5 kPa. Assuming that the blood gases are acceptable, and the chest X-ray does not show any major abnormality, patients are usually weaned off ventilation during the first postoperative day. If blood gases deteriorate, ventilatory support should be resumed early.

Fluid management

A clear record of intraoperative fluids and blood loss should be transcribed into the ward records. Intravenous fluids are used until the patient is able to swallow or commence nasogastric feeding. This is usually on the day after surgery or 48 hours at the latest. For those patients who will require postoperative feeding, a fine-bore nasogastric tube is preferable.

Fluid replacement preference varies from centre to centre and the recommendations cannot be taken as inviolable. Fluid balance and circulatory state are monitored using heart rate and blood pressure, central and peripheral temperature and urine output. Central venous pressure can be helpful in some circumstances but can be misleading; pulmonary wedge pressure is preferred in complex situations (Sibbald & Keenan, 1997). Normally blood loss is replaced in theatre and so replacement of water loss is the principal postoperative requirement. Fluid overload is a very real possibility in many postoperative head and neck cancer patients, and so caution should be observed with both sodium containing crystalloid and colloid infusion (Schierhout & Roberts, 1998). Twenty-four-hour replacement for adults and children can be calculated as follows:

0–10 kg = 100 ml/kg
10–20 kg = 1,000 ml + 50 ml/kg for every kg above 10
> 20 kg = 1,500 ml + 20 ml/kg for every kg above 20
i.e. for a 70 kg adult approximately 2,500 ml.

Sodium replacement is not necessary for the first 24 hours and water is provided by giving 5% dextrose. Thereafter requirements are 1–2 mEq/kg/day. This will replace obligatory sodium losses and suppress aldosterone secretion enough to prevent potassium wasting. Potassium losses are approximately 40 to 60 mEq/day in an adult, therefore, replacement with 0.5 to 1 mEq/kg/day is usually enough to maintain potassium balance in a patient with normal kidneys. Other electrolytes are supplemented as indicated by clinical assessment and laboratory testing. Tissue perfusion is monitored by measuring core and peripheral temperature. The core-peripheral temperature difference should be zero by 6 hours after the operation. A converging temperature difference should indicate a satisfactory circulatory state. Urine output will normally be 0.5–1.5 ml/kg/hour. Rates lower than this suggest renal failure, low flow states, or hypovolaemia. Rates higher than this suggest overhydration, diabetes insipidus, osmotic diuresis, or post-obstructive diuresis.

Temperature

Body temperature is measured centrally using a rectal probe and peripherally using a big toe probe (unless the patient has peripheral vascular disease). The probe foot should neither be specifically exposed or insulated. Initial control of heat loss is important to prevent flap cooling and a compromise in oxygenation. Patients will have cooled below the temperature achieved in theatre during transfer to the high-dependency/intensive care ward. Heat loss can be controlled by a warming blanket, space blanket, warmed intravenous fluids and humidified gases, avoiding draughts and increasing the environmental temperature. The peripheral temperature will normally warm to approach the central temperature within 6 hours. If this does not occur and the trend is not improving it is most often due to hypovolaemia. It may be associated with tachycardia, hypotension, and poor urine output (< 0.5 ml/kg/hour). A less frequent cause is reduced cardiac output with peripheral vasoconstriction. This may be associated with fluid overload. The central venous pressure may be high, but can be unreliable. A vasodilator and/or diuretic may be useful in this situation. Peripheral vasoconstriction may also be related to poor analgesia with restlessness.

A central pyrexia may result from hypovolaemia, inadequate sedation, blood transfusion or early sepsis. If the central temperature remains above 38°C in the presence of a full circulating volume and adequate analgesia and sedation, paracetamol or chlorpromazine (in 2.5 mg increments up to a dose of 25–50 mg) can be given. If there is no response a Glyceryl Trinitrate (GTN) patch or infusion may be needed. Patients should not be exposed, fanned or tepid-sponged to reduce a high central temperature.

Alimentary feeding

Patients are seen prior to surgery by a dietitian who will have prescribed an enteral feeding regime. The nasogastric tube is aspirated to check for position and gastric status prior to feeding. Enteral feeding can usually be commenced within 24 hours of the operation if there are no contraindications, such as:

1. vomiting: if patients are nauseated or vomiting, anti-emetics are given according to the cause. Prochlorperazine is given for opioid-induced emesis, metoclopramide for gastric stasis (in the absence of pyloric obstruction). If emesis persists, ondansetron may be indicated in some cases
2. excessive gastric aspirate
3. abdominal distension
4. absent bowel sounds.

A full-strength proprietary feed providing approximately 2,400 kCal per day can normally be used by 48 hours.

See Chapter 2.4 for more information on nutrition.

Analgesia and sedation

Analgesia is provided by opioid infusion (usually morphine or alfentanil). Sedation is provided by propofol infusion supplemented by Diazemus or midazolam intermittently. Opioid and propofol infusions should be prepared prior to transfer from theatre. Although muscle relaxants may occasionally be required, it is obvious that patients should never be awake and paralysed. The free flap is very sensitive to endogenous and exogenous catecholamines. Patients must not be allowed to become too lightly sedated as this results in release of catecholamines and vasoconstriction, with reduction in flap blood flow. Inadequate sedation may also be associated with hypertension and coughing, which should be treated urgently as it may cause bleeding and haematoma formation.

Wound drains

Suction drainage is usually used after head and neck operations. The purpose of the drains is normally to prevent the accumulation of blood. The drain is removed when wound drainage is less than 30 ml per day. When there is a persistent but stable serous drainage it is preferable to remove the tube.

Flap monitoring

Postoperative flap monitoring is by direct observation. This applies particularly to free flaps. A visible flap should be examined at least every 15 minutes for the first 12 hours following surgery. A small proportion of flaps undergo vascular failure, which will lead to flap death if left uncorrected. A flap is unlikely to be salvaged after 3–5 hours of ischaemia. Rapid action is therefore essential if there is any doubt about viability.

A free flap should be regularly examined for:

1. Colour: flaps should be an appropriate pink or red colour depending on the donor site.
2. Blanching and capillary return: skin flaps will blanch when pressed with an instrument. The white patch produced will disappear as the capillaries refill; this normally happens within 1–7 seconds of blanching.

3. Temperature: where appropriate a temperature probe should be placed on the flap. An acute cooling of the flap of 2°C or more, over an hour or less, in the presence of a stable skin/core temperature difference may indicate a change in flap blood flow.
4. Swelling: all free flaps swell in response to ischaemia during their transfer. However, flaps that suddenly become grossly swollen, particularly with a blue or mottled appearance, have suffered a thrombosis of their venous drainage. The flap will fail to blanch and cooling will occur.
5. Muscle twitch: it is difficult to use the above techniques to monitor free muscle flaps which are commonly used to reconstruct lower limb defects; these flaps may be totally or subtotally covered by a skin graft. Free muscle flaps will respond to direct stimulation from a peripheral nerve stimulator; this response is rapidly attenuated if the flap vasculature is interrupted. See Chapter 2.7 for more information on flap and wound care.

Complications of head and neck surgery

Specific complications are discussed in the appropriate sections in Chapter 4.2. There are some complications that are common to most head and neck operations. General complications may occur after any operative or anaesthetic intervention. The most frequent cardiovascular complication is heart failure, but this should be avoidable in most cases by careful postoperative fluid management. Myocardial infarction, deep vein thrombosis and pulmonary embolism are relatively infrequent. Chest infection may result from postoperative aspiration and is managed by tracheobronchial suction and/or chest physiotherapy. Intestinal ileus or obstruction are very infrequent even after free jejunal transfer. Urinary retention is common in older male patients and managed in the first instance by catheterization.

Local complications that are specific to the surgery are usually classified according to the time of occurrence.

Within the first 24 hours

Haemorrhage

This may be apparent from increased wound drainage, swelling or visible bleeding from the mouth or tracheostome. Blood loss can be considerable before there is an alteration in blood pressure. Haemorrhage is treated by blood replacement and a rapid return to the operating theatre to stop the bleeding. Bleeding may also be due to hypertension or coagulation problems which must be rapidly diagnosed and treated. Carotid haemorrhage is discussed in Chapter 2.8.

Airway obstruction

A preliminary tracheostomy will have been carried out before most operations on the mouth, larynx and pharynx. If there is increasing obstruction then the airway should be secured as soon as possible. Endotracheal intubation or tracheostomy are used according to circumstances.

Flap failure

If the arterial anastomosis fails a flap will become pale and will not refill after blanching on pressure. Hypovolaemia, hypotension or peripheral vasoconstriction will also cause pallor and should be corrected in minutes rather than hours. In the absence of these general problems, extreme pallor indicates arterial failure of the flap, which will require immediate surgical exploration. A venous failure is more common and manifests with flap congestion and bluish discoloration. This situation necessitates an immediate return to theatre. Haematoma formation may lead to obstruction of the flap vasculature, and therefore require evacuation in theatre.

Pneumothorax

This may result from damage to the cervical or mediastinal pleura during surgery or, more likely, during central line insertion! Respiratory difficulty with no evidence of airway obstruction should raise the possibility. Clinical diagnosis is usually straightforward and can be radiologically confirmed by chest X-ray unless there is rapid deterioration. Treatment is by insertion of a chest drain connected to an underwater seal.

Raised intracranial pressure

This may be associated with bilateral radical neck dissection, but this is rarely carried out nowadays. If it occurs following skull base procedures then it is likely to be due to intracranial bleeding. The warning signs are headache and restlessness with a slowing pulse and rising blood pressure often with arrhythmias. If bleeding is suspected the patient should be returned to theatre.

Cerebrovascular accident

The combination of carotid manipulation in a high-risk group of patients runs a risk of embolism with cerebral arterial occlusion.

From 1 to 14 days

Wound infection/dehiscence

Although cervical skin flaps usually need to be raised for surgical exposure, skin necrosis is infrequent because of its blood supply. The principal local risk factors are poorly planned incisions, previous surgery or radiotherapy and pressure from haematoma or external dressings. A poor nutritional state, blood loss, diabetes, cardiorespiratory disease, liver disease and renal failure are general risk factors. Treatment of skin flap necrosis is by meticulous local cleaning and debridement as necessary. Antibiotics are used if cellulitis supervenes. Skin grafting or flap replacement may be required later.

Oral or pharyngeal fistula

The predisposing factors are similar to those for skin necrosis. Saliva may leak into the wound drains through the incisions or form a local abscess. A small localized fistula will usually close spontaneously. The patient is maintained on nasogastric feeding until closure occurs. A large dehiscence is better treated by early repair. This type of fistula is likely to be associated with relative ischaemia of the surrounding tissue and will require a vascularized flap for closure. The pectoralis major myocutaneous flap is used most frequently.

Secondary haemorrhage

This is associated with infection from a skin breakdown or fistula. It may occur from the internal jugular vein or from the carotid artery. The bleeding is severe but is almost always heralded by minor bleeding in the preceding 48 hours. The best policy is aggressive treatment of the underlying cause. If rupture of the carotid artery or jugular vein does occur then immediate control is obtained by pressure and the patient immediately returned to theatre. Ligation of the vessel is the only safe option in this situation. If the carotid artery is ligated there is a high incidence of hemiplegia in patients who survive. Carotid haemorrhage is discussed in Chapter 2.8.

Chyle leak

This complication arises from damage to the thoracic duct low on the left side of the neck. It is best avoided by recognizing injury and ligating the duct. It may not manifest itself postoperatively until feeding begins when wound drainage increases dramatically and turns milky. Ligation of the duct is feasible if the problem is recognized in the first 24 hours. After this time it is best managed conservatively by intravenous feeding.

Late complications

Lymphoedema

A degree of lymphoedema is frequent after combined surgical and radiotherapy treatment but it is not usually severe or troublesome. Management is conservative by cutaneous massage. This can be taught to the patient and carers. See Chapter 2.9 on the management of lymphoedema.

Persistent or recurrent disease

Although this is theoretically avoidable by following oncological principles, it will on occasions occur in practice. It is not often salvageable.

Subcutaneous fibrosis

Subcutaneous or sternomastoid fibrosis is more frequent with combined surgery and radiotherapy. The tight sensation can occasionally be troublesome. There is, unfortunately, no effective treatment.

Summary

Head and neck surgery can be extremely debilitating and disfiguring, leaving the patient with both functional and psychosocial problems. However, major improvements in conservation surgery and reconstructive techniques mean that patients can now enjoy much improved quality of life and surgical outcomes. The importance of being treated by an experienced head and neck surgical team cannot be understated. Skilled critical care nursing is essential for the patient's survival in the postoperative period. This chapter has given an overview of the general principles of head and neck surgery and critical care; specific tumour site surgery is described in the next chapter.

Chapter 4.2
Surgical management at specific sites

GRAHAM BUCKLEY

Introduction

This chapter describes the surgical procedures used at each specific head and neck site: resection, reconstruction, neck management, postoperative care and complications. This information can be used to help the nurse understand the side effects that the patient will experience and the nursing interventions required. It can also be used when coaching patients preoperatively and postoperatively, as well as for preparing written patient information.

Oral cavity and oropharynx

Early tumours are successfully treated by either surgical excision or brachytherapy (see Chapter 4.3). The choice depends on the site of the tumour and the anticipated functional result. Small tumours of the palate, buccal mucosa or anterior tongue may be approached through the mouth. Laser resection is useful to minimize bleeding in this situation (Panje et al, 1989). Larger tumours require more extensive access, which is usually obtained by dividing the mandible. This may be achieved by midline division of the lower lip and osteotomy of the mandible in a paramedian position, medial to the mandibular foramen (shown in Figure 4.2.1) (McGregor & MacDonald, 1983). Although other approaches may be used, this has the advantages of wide access, preservation of the innervation of the lower lip and better preservation of the periosteal blood supply to the mandible (with better healing).

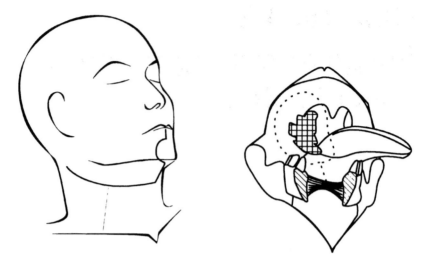

Figure 4.2.1: Paramedian mandibulotomy for excision of oral and oropharyngeal tumours.

Tumour resection

This aspect requires careful judgement. The tumour must be removed with a margin of normal tissue to prevent local recurrence. The size of the margin depends on the tumour size and site. Spread into the tongue muscle, for example, may be extensive and necessitate a margin of 2 or 3 cm. Spread to the mandible is relatively uncommon. It may be obvious on plain X-rays or computerized tomograph, but can sometimes be difficult to assess preoperatively. The most common site of invasion is on the alveolar ridge with early invasion of the inferior alveolar nerve (McGregor & MacDonald, 1988). The tumour may spread along the nerve beyond the confines of the mandible. If this type of invasion is present, the lateral segment of the mandible is removed along with the whole length of the inferior alveolar nerve. Tumours of the oropharyngeal wall are removed by full thickness excision with adjacent parapharyngeal or retropharyngeal lymph nodes. Tumours of the tongue base may spread extensively within the tongue muscle and are usually advanced at the time of presentation. The proximity of the lingual vessels means that total glossectomy may be required for complete removal. This results in severe aspiration and consequently a total laryngectomy is usually also necessary. An option is to carry out a supraglottic laryngeal resection and close the larynx as a vocal shunt to preserve voice but prevent aspiration.

Reconstruction

Small lesions of the tongue may not require any form of reconstruction after excision. If any of the floor of the mouth has been resected, however, attempts at primary closure are likely to result in reduced tongue mobility. This can have devastating effects on speech and swallowing. Reconstruction is primarily aimed at maintaining tongue mobility. The most frequently used method is a radial forearm fasciocutaneous flap (Soutar et al, 1983). This versatile flap is often also useful for oropharyngeal defects (see Figure 4.2.2). The

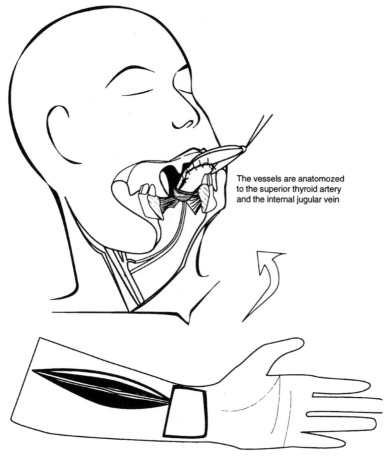

The vessels are anatomozed to the superior thyroid artery and the internal jugular vein

The flap is raised on the radial artery and accompanying deep veins

Figure 4.2.2: Reconstruction of a defect in the floor of the mouth and tongue using a free radial forearm fasciocutaneous flap.

pectoralis major myofascial flap is also used, and has the advantage of rapidly being covered by mucosa with a potential for return of sensation. Several techniques have been described to reconstruct the mandible. The most reliable method is a free flap with a vascularized bone component. Fibula, iliac crest, scapula and radial bone are the most frequently used. The pectoralis major and latissimus dorsi myocutaneous flaps are used for high-volume defects, particularly large pharyngeal resections (see Figure 4.2.3). They are also optimal for reconstruction of the defect following a total glossectomy. Mandibular closure is usually achieved using titanium miniplates.

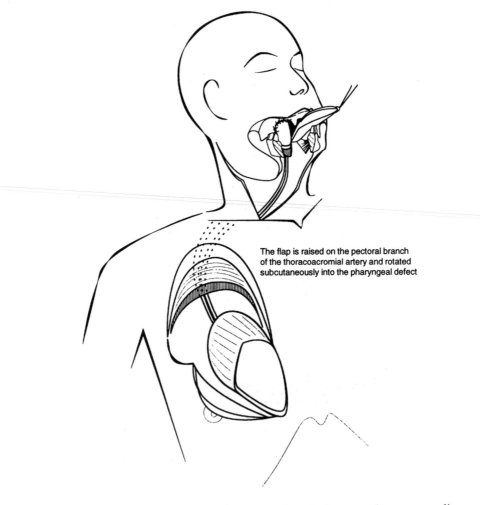

The flap is raised on the pectoral branch of the thoracoacromial artery and rotated subcutaneously into the pharyngeal defect

Figure 4.2.3: Reconstruction of a defect in the oropharynx using a pectoralis major myocutaneous flap.

Cervical nodes

The likelihood of cervical lymph node metastases is related primarily to the site and size of the tumour. Tumours of the tongue and floor of the mouth have a much higher likelihood than tumours of the upper alveolus and hard palate (Shah et al, 1990). Tumours of the posterior oral cavity and oropharynx have a particular propensity to metastasize. The more advanced T-stage tumours are more likely to metastasize. The most significant factor here is the depth of tumour invasion, approaching 50% for tumours invading more than 2 mm (Spiro et al, 1986). Confirmed metastases are usually treated by radical or modified radical dissection. Selective neck dissection is used in those tumours with a high chance of microscopic metastases.

Postoperative care

Most patients will have a temporary tracheostomy and nasogastric tube. Tube feeding will normally be possible the day after the operation. If reconstruction with a flap has been carried out then regular observation should be carried out (see Chapter 2.7). Meticulous oral hygiene is essential in preventing wound infections (see Chapter 2.2). Oral intake commences on the fourth postoperative day with liquids followed by a soft diet. The tracheostomy is removed when the airway is clear — usually 2 to 3 days after the operation (see Chapter 2.1).

Rehabilitation of swallowing can be a problem after resection of oropharyngeal tumours. This depends on the size and site of the defect. Palatal resection is difficult to reconstruct in a satisfactory way because its dynamic function cannot be replaced. Initial nasal regurgitation of fluid is frequent but does improve with time. Resections extending down to the vallecula or hypopharynx can result in postoperative aspiration because of the absence of sensation in flaps used for reconstruction. This is not usually severe and improves during the first few weeks after surgery. See Chapter 2.3 on eating and swallowing problems.

Complications

Salivary fistula from the mouth or pharynx may occur but is infrequent unless there is necrosis of the flap. Non-union or osteonecrosis of the mandible may occur at the site of the mandibular osteotomy. The risk is increased if there has been prior radiotherapy or if the overlying soft tissue has broken down. It is treated with antibiotics, removal of dead tissue and re-fixation of the mandible. If there is insufficient vascularized soft tissue to cover the area then a flap should be used.

Larynx and hypopharynx

Laryngeal tumours are subclassified by site into supraglottic, glottic and subglottic. The most common histological type by far is squamous carcinoma, but adenocarcinoma and sarcomas do occur rarely. Supraglottic tumours present with pain on swallowing and do not affect the voice until the vocal cords are invaded. They are frequently large by the time of presentation and metastases to the cervical nodes, either obvious or occult, occur in 30–70% depending on stage. Glottic tumours cause hoarseness at an early stage. This will often result in quicker referral and diagnosis and therefore prognosis tends to be better. Nodal metastases usually only occur in T3 and T4 tumours. Subglottic tumours are very rare and, according to some investigators, may represent inferior spread from the undersurface of the vocal cord. They have a worse prognosis than other sites, which may in part be explained by their proclivity to metastasize to the paratracheal lymph nodes. Hypopharyngeal carcinomas develop from the pyriform fossa, postcricoid region or posterior pharyngeal wall. They produce little in the way of symptoms initially and late stage presentation is common. Their behaviour is similar to that of supraglottic laryngeal tumours with aggressive local spread and frequent cervical lymph node metastases.

Early laryngeal tumours may be treated with surgery or radiotherapy. The choice of treatment is influenced by the site and size of the tumour, by local expertise and by the medical condition and preferences of the patient. Supraglottic tumours are better controlled surgically in all but the earliest stages (DeSanto, 1985; Robbins et al, 1988; Lee et al, 1990; Mendenhall et al, 1996). Treatment by partial laryngectomy may however cause a degree of aspiration, at least initially, and so it is important to take into account the patient's respiratory status and their motivation. Endoscopic resection offers the lowest morbidity treatment and is being utilized with increasing frequency for early glottic cancer. Partial laryngectomy may offer better local control of those glottic tumours that invade the vocal cord musculature (Glanz et al, 1989). Advanced disease presenting with stridor or with invasion of the laryngeal framework will usually necessitate total laryngectomy and will often require postoperative radiotherapy. Hypopharyngeal cancer is notoriously aggressive and most would accept that combined surgery and radiotherapy offers the best chance of local control of disease. This will require a partial pharyngolaryngectomy for early tumours and total pharyngolaryngectomy for advanced disease.

Endoscopic resection

This is one of the earliest described treatments for laryngeal carcinoma. It is the treatment offering the lowest morbidity, in many cases being carried out as a day case procedure. It is most applicable to early-stage tumours confined to the vocal cord. Recently its indications have been extended to the treatment of more advanced glottic and even some supraglottic and hypopharyngeal tumours (Steiner, 1993; Zeitels et al, 1994), although its role in this situation is still controversial. Excision is carried out under general anaesthesia using a rigid laryngoscope and operating microscope. Laser excision is particularly useful for the excision of more advanced tumours as well as debulking larger tumours that present with stridor. This latter indication may avoid the need for tracheostomy in this situation.

Partial laryngectomy

This term covers a spectrum of procedures ranging from simple resection of a vocal cord to extensive subtotal laryngectomies. A temporary tracheostomy is usually required and carried out at the start of the procedure, followed by the neck dissection if necessary.

Supraglottic tumours: supraglottic laryngectomy (see Figure 4.2.4a)

Removal of part or the whole of the supraglottic larynx is carried out through a suprahyoid or infrahyoid pharyngotomy. This separates the base of the tongue from the larynx with entry into the pharynx through the vallecular mucosa. The approach may be extended along the pharyngeal wall for tumours of the pyriform fossa or aryepiglottic fold. The mucosal tumour is removed with the underlying pre-epiglottic or paraglottic space. Direct closure of the defect is usually possible.

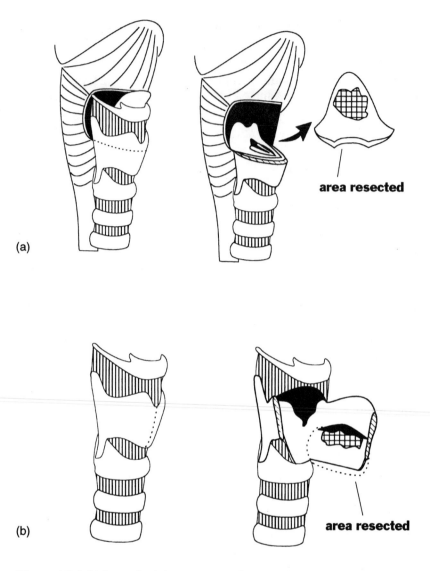

(a)

(b)

area resected

Figure 4.2.4: (a) Supraglottic laryngectomy; (b) vertical partial laryngectomy.

Glottic tumours: vertical partial laryngectomy (see Figure 4.2.4b)

The approach used depends on the site of the tumour. Small glottic tumours are usually approached by division of the thyroid cartilage. Larger tumours may require division of the cricothyroid ligament and thyrohyoid membrane. This can be used bilaterally for tumours extending across the anterior commissure. The extent of resection is dictated by the extent of the tumour. This may range from simple excision of the vocal cord to resection of the entire glottic larynx with the underlying paraglottic spaces (Mohr et al, 1983). Reconstruction is unnecessary after cordectomy. A resection of the cord and para-glottic space can be reconstructed using a sternohyoid muscle flap. The epiglottis can be used to reconstruct the entire glottis in exten-sive bilateral resections. In this case the cricoid is approximated to the hyoid bone, a reconstruction known as a cricohyoidoepiglot-topexy (Laccourreye et al, 1989).

Multiregional tumours: subtotal and near-total laryngectomy (see Figure 4.2.5)

This group includes tumours that have spread to involve the supra-glottic and the glottic larynx. The usual approach is the same as that for supraglottic tumours. The extent of resection is deter-mined by the tumour. This type of procedure is often termed a subtotal laryngectomy. If an extensive supraglottic/glottic resec-tion has been carried out, reconstruction is usually by approximat-ing the hyoid bone to the cricoid cartilage as a cricohyoidopexy (Laccourreye et al, 1990) (see Figure 4.2.5). An alternative is to close the laryngeal remnant on itself, leaving a narrow channel between the trachea and the pharynx. This procedure is known as a near-total laryngectomy (Pearson et al, 1980). This vocal shunt allows speech and, because it is innervated, will prevent aspiration. The major disadvantage is that a tracheostomy is required for breathing.

Total laryngectomy (see Figure 4.2.6)

This is used for large tumours invading the laryngeal framework or subglottic region. The larynx is detached from the base of the tongue and the hypopharynx, and the trachea is divided. The pharynx is then closed primarily. A transverse closure is now generally preferred because it is thought to result in better post-laryngectomy speech acquisition. The tracheal stump is sutured to the skin as an end tracheostome.

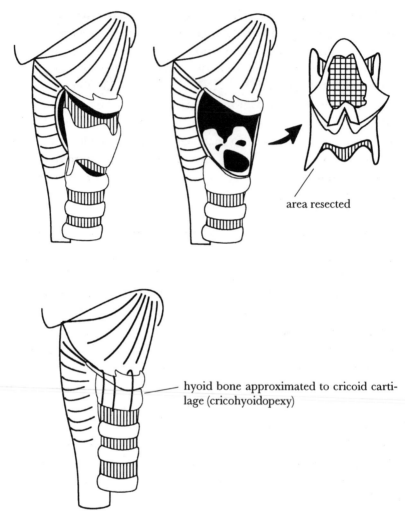

area resected

hyoid bone approximated to cricoid cartilage (cricohyoidopexy)

Figure 4.2.5: Subtotal laryngectomy with cricohyoidopexy.

Partial pharyngectomy

A suprahyoid pharyngotomy is used to expose the tumour and is extended as the tumour is visualized. The tumour is resected with the full thickness of the pharyngeal wall. If the tumour arises on the medial wall of the pyriform fossa, then a partial supraglottic laryngectomy will also be necessary. Small defects may be closed primarily but most require reconstruction with a flap. A radial forearm free flap or pectoralis major myocutaneous or myofascial flap are used according to the size and site of the defect.

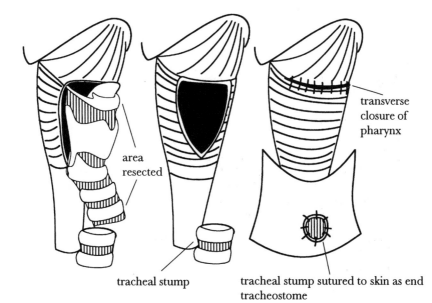

Figure 4.2.6: Total laryngectomy.

Total pharyngectomy

Extensive tumours may necessitate removal of the whole of the hypopharynx. Reconstruction in most centres is carried out with a free jejunal flap (see Figure 4.2.7). Some surgeons recommend a tubed free radial forearm fasciocutaneous flap for shorter defects. Replacement by gastric transposition is now less common but is necessary if the oesophagus is also resected.

Voice restoration after laryngectomy

An ingenious device was used to attempt voice restoration after the very first laryngectomy in 1874. However, the initial mortality of the operation was so high that surgeons and their patients were content with survival alone. Oesophageal speech has been the mainstay of rehabilitation for most of this century but it is only satisfactory in a minority of patients. The concept of creating a fistula between the trachea and oesophagus was introduced in 1927 by a laryngectomee Hamburg butcher who carried out his own operation using a heated icepick! After the Second World War several surgeons attempted to create similar fistulas, but all met with the problems of either rapid spontaneous closure, or worse, a persistent saliva leak into the

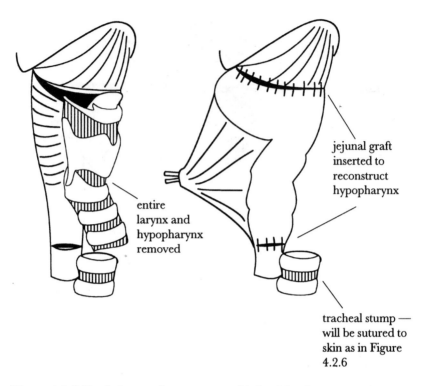

jejunal graft
inserted to
reconstruct
hypopharynx

entire
larynx and
hypopharynx
removed

tracheal stump —
will be sutured to
skin as in Figure
4.2.6

Figure 4.2.7: Total pharyngolaryngectomy with free jejunal reconstruction.

trachea. In the early 1970s this was overcome by introducing a valved prosthesis, but the design was complex and bulky. Singer and Blom introduced a simple silicone valve in 1978 (Singer & Blom, 1980) and several variations on the original design are currently used.

The tracheoesophageal fistula is created either at the time of laryngectomy or as a secondary endoscopic procedure. A replaceable silicone prosthesis is placed in the fistula. This acts as a one-way valve: occlusion of the tracheostome directs expired air into the oesophagus but does not allow oesphageal contents to leak the other way. The vibration induced in the oesophagus produces the noise necessary for speech. Speech quality varies according to the closure technique and pharyngeal muscle tone. Tracheoesophageal voice restoration can also be used after pharyngolaryngectomy with good results.

See Chapter 2.5 for more detailed information on tracheoesophageal speech.

Cervical nodes

Cervical lymph node metastases are present in one-half to two-thirds of patients presenting with supraglottic or hypopharyngeal tumours (McGavran et al, 1961; Cummings, 1974; Kirchner, 1975; Andre et al, 1977). These are treated by modified radical neck dissection. Selective neck dissection is used in those patients with no evident metastases, since approximately half will have microscopic disease. Midline disease may spread to both sides of the neck, requiring bilateral neck dissection. The likelihood of nodal spread is low in T1 and T2 glottic cancer, and neck dissection is only used for evident metastases. More advanced tumours are treated in the same way as supraglottic and hypopharyngeal tumours. Those tumours with extension to the subglottis or postcricoid region have a higher chance of metastases in the paratracheal and superior mediastinal nodes. Removal may necessitate total thyroidectomy.

Postoperative care

Partial laryngectomies and pharyngectomies present no unique immediate problems. A temporary tracheostomy will usually be necessary and is removed as soon as the airway is adequate (see Chapter 2.1). Swallowing can be commenced immediately after a vertical partial laryngectomy. After a partial pharyngectomy or partial pharyngolaryngectomy aspiration may occur initially. This tends to be worse with liquids and may be overcome by using thickeners. Swallowing after total laryngectomy can commence after 3 or 4 days, initially with clear liquids progressing to solids. See Chapter 2.3 for more information.

Following total pharyngolaryngectomy, patients are ventilated overnight. Careful monitoring of fluid balance is necessary for optimum perfusion of the free jejunal flap. Nasogastric feeding can normally be started after 24 or 48 hours and a barium swallow is carried out on the fourth postoperative day to check the integrity of the anastomoses. Swallowing can start if this is satisfactory.

Complications

Pharyngocutaneous fistula is the most significant specific complication. It may manifest by saliva in the wound drains, local abscess formation or leakage from the skin incision or around the tracheostome. A small fistula will usually heal spontaneously, but a dehiscence of the pharyngeal suture line will require a vascularized flap. Stenosis of the tracheostome after laryngectomy or pharyngolaryngectomy results from chondritis of the tracheal cartilage. This is usually the result of a fistula. (See Chapter 2.1 for management of the laryngostome.) A number of techniques have been described to correct the problem and all seem to work in the hands of their originators! Generally speaking the problem can only be effectively solved by excision of the stenosed trachea and refashioning of the stoma.

Salivary glands

Salivary tumours occur in the parotid, submandibular or sublingual major salivary glands or in minor salivary glands throughout the upper aerodigestive tract. Figure 4.2.8 shows the major salivary glands.

For practical purposes sublingual tumours are indistinguishable from minor salivary tumours and the management is the same. Most salivary tumours arise from the gland epithelium and may be benign or malignant. In the parotid gland approximately 90% are benign, falling to 50% in the submandibular gland and 20% in the minor glands (Eveson & Cawson, 1985). Tumours present as a swelling in the

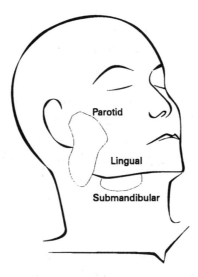

Figure 4.2.8: Position of the major salivary glands.

affected gland. Pain or rapid enlargement suggest malignancy; skin invasion or involvement of related nerves (facial paralysis for example) are specific diagnostic signs. Preoperative diagnosis may not be possible but fine-needle aspiration cytology is sometimes helpful. Imaging by computerized tomography (CT) or magnetic resonance imaging (MRI) is useful for disease localization and identification of the site of parapharyngeal swelling if a deep lobe parotid gland tumour is suspected (Kraus et al, 1992; Leverstein et al, 1995). The treatment of benign tumours is by excision. The treatment of salivary carcinoma depends on the histological type. Broadly speaking tumours can be subdivided into low-grade and high-grade types (Seifert & Sobin, 1992). Low-grade tumours are treated by surgical excision. High-grade tumours are treated by surgical excision followed by postoperative radiotherapy. The natural history of salivary carcinoma differs from squamous carcinoma. It has a high rate of both local recurrence and distant metastases (Spiro, 1986). These can present years after the original tumour and disease can sometimes be present in a quiescent state for a long period. The steady decline in survival even after 15 or 20 years means that it is difficult to ever be certain of curing the disease.

Parotid tumours

The facial nerve is divided into a superficial and a deep part. This nerve emerges from the skull base at the stylomastoid and enters the medial surface of the gland. It divides into its separate branches to the facial muscles within the substance of the gland. Most tumours arise superficial to the nerve. Both benign and malignant tumours should be removed with a cuff of normal gland. 'Shelling out' of tumours results in a high recurrence rate and should be avoided (Woods et al, 1975; Maran et al, 1984). The facial nerve is identified at an early stage in the operation of parotidectomy and is dissected through the gland. Once this is accomplished the tumour can be safely removed. A nerve stimulator is useful to check the functional integrity of the nerve or one of its branches.

A total parotidectomy is needed for tumours arising in the deep lobe. After the facial nerve has been identified and the superficial part of the gland removed, the deep lobe is removed by dividing the supplying branches of the external carotid artery. Although this approach is suitable for small tumours, larger tumours may require division of the mandible for surgical access to the parapharyngeal space.

Extensive malignant tumours with facial nerve invasion are treated by total parotidectomy (Theriault & Fitzpatrick, 1986). The facial nerve is resected and reconstructed if possible by immediate nerve grafting. If this is not possible further facial reanimation procedures may be utilized at a later date (Harrison, 1985). Some of these tumours invade the adjacent skull base and a partial or total petrosectomy may be indicated.

Submandibular gland tumours

Tumours are removed by complete excision of the gland (Byers et al, 1973). This is carried out through a cervical incision. This is approximately 4 cm below the mandible to avoid damage to the mandibular division of the facial nerve which crosses the upper part of the gland. Damage to the nerve causes paralysis of the depressor muscles of the lower lip. The gland is removed by division of the facial vessels and separation of its attachment to the lingual nerve in the floor of the mouth.

Minor salivary gland tumours

Preoperative diagnosis can usually be made by biopsy, since the overlying epithelium is removed during subsequent excision. Benign tumours are treated by simple excision. Malignant tumours are treated in a similar way to a squamous carcinoma at the same site (Jones et al, 1998). Salivary carcinoma excites little tissue reaction and consequently it can be difficult to establish tumour limits. A wider margin of normal tissue may therefore be required for these tumours.

Cervical nodes

Cervical node metastases from a salivary carcinoma are treated by a comprehensive neck dissection. Most salivary carcinomas have a low metastatic rate to the cervical nodes and so selective neck dissection is not usually necessary (Kelley & Spiro, 1996).

Postoperative care and complications

Most patients are able to leave hospital one or two nights after submandibular or parotid gland excision. Postoperative bleeding after submandibular gland excision may result in oedema of the floor of the mouth and tongue and threaten the airway. This is managed by immediately securing the airway by intubation or tracheostomy and stopping the bleeding.

Damage to the adjacent mandibular branch of the facial nerve (causing paralysis of the depressors of the lower lip), the lingual nerve (anaesthesia of the tongue) or hypoglossal nerve (paralysis of the same side of the tongue) are uncommon complications of submandibular gland excision. The facial nerve is at greatest risk during the excision of deep lobe parotid tumours, particularly since the nerve may be stretched over large tumours. A degree of temporary facial paralysis is frequent in this situation but recovers provided the nerve is undamaged. Frey's syndrome or parotid sweating may occur after parotidectomy because of regrowth of parotid secretomotor nerve fibres into skin sweat glands. This results in sweating of the facial skin during salivation. This probably occurs frequently but is rarely noticeable or significant. If symptomatic, then local application of antiperspirants is effective. Failing this some patients benefit from intratympanic division of parasympathetic glossopharyngeal nerve fibres.

Nasal cavity, sinuses and nasopharynx

Nasal and paranasal sinus tumours are diverse in histology. Benign tumours typically present with nasal obstruction and are treated by excision. Inverting papilloma is an important and relatively common benign tumour that arises from the lateral nasal wall. Although benign, it recurs locally if incompletely excised and may be associated with the subsequent occurrence of squamous carcinoma (Harrison & Lund, 1993). The most frequent malignant tumours are squamous carcinoma and adenocarcinomas. Other less frequent tumours include melanoma, bone, cartilage and soft tissue sarcomas, olfactory neuroblastoma and lymphoma. Tumours arising in the sinuses usually present only after invasion of neighbouring structures. They are therefore almost always advanced by the time of presentation. Extension occurs into the nose with obstruction and bleeding, the orbit with diplopia and proptosis, the cheek with swelling, the oral cavity with loosening of the teeth or the cranial cavity with headache or invasion of cranial nerves III–VI. The extent of these tumours is usually best defined by a combination of CT and MRI (Lloyd et al, 1987). Treatment is by excision and postoperative radiotherapy. The extent of resection depends on the stage and site of the tumour.

Nasopharyngeal carcinoma is uncommon in the UK. It differs in aetiology and behaviour from squamous carcinoma at other sites. Although it can occur at any age, its peak incidences are in adolescence and in the fourth and fifth decades. It is not smoking-related, but genetic predisposition and the Epstein–Barr virus have been implicated in its aetiology (Andersson-Anvert et al, 1977). It presents in a similar way to sinus tumours. It also often presents with hearing loss due to Eustachian tube invasion or with cervical node metastases. It is highly radiosensitive and the role of surgery is predominantly in treating cervical node metastases. Recurrent primary disease is also sometimes amenable to surgical treatment.

Approaches

Transfacial

Small tumours of the nasal septum may be resectable transnasally. This exposure may be extended by utilizing an incision at the alar base. Similar small benign tumours arising on the lateral nasal wall can be approached transnasally. The improved visualization with rigid nasal endoscopes has facilitated this approach. More extensive exposure is required for most malignant tumours of the maxillary sinus or lateral nasal wall. A lateral rhinotomy incision will expose the medial wall of the maxilla and can be extended through the midline of the upper lip or along the inside of the lower eyelid to expose the whole maxilla. This latter approach, the Weber-Fergusson incision, is often used for maxillectomy (Figure 4.2.9). More recently the midfacial degloving approach has been described (Maniglia, 1986). A combination of an intraoral incision and nasal incisions allows the elevation of the midfacial skin from the maxilla and will often obviate the need for facial incisions or at least allow smaller, cosmetically better incisions.

Craniofacial

Approaching the ethmoid sinus from above, as well as from below, allows resection of ethmoid tumours in one piece and with surrounding bone (Ketcham et al, 1963). This has had a major impact on the local control of these tumours (Cheeseman & Lund,

1986). A midline forehead or bicoronal scalp incision can be used (see Figure 4.2.9). The latter gives a better exposure and is cosmetically superior. A flap of frontal bone is removed and the frontal lobes of the brain elevated extradurally from the floor of the anterior cranial fossa. This exposes the cribriform plate, roof of the ethmoid and roof of the orbit. Dural elevation can extend to the optic chiasm if necessary. This approach is usually used in combination with a transfacial approach for craniofacial resection of ethmoid tumours.

Lateral

Tumour extension from the maxillary sinus or the nasopharynx into the infratemporal fossa may require a lateral approach for en-bloc resection (Figure 4.2.9). This entails removal of the glenoid fossa and dislocation or resection of the head of the mandible. Removal of the zygomatic arch exposes the infratemporal fossa. The approach may be extended by using a mastoidectomy for resection of the Eustachian tube (Fisch, 1983) or by using a middle fossa craniotomy (Sekhar et al, 1987) for larger tumours invading the floor of the middle cranial fossa.

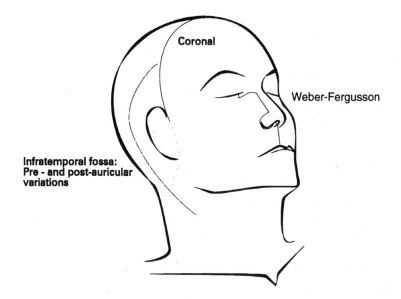

Figure 4.2.9: Incisions used to access paranasal sinuses.

Resection and reconstruction

Maxillary sinus tumours: maxillectomy

The maxilla is removed either through a Weber–Fergusson incision or a midfacial degloving approach. The latter may require additional smaller facial incisions to facilitate exposure. Facial flaps are elevated and osteotomies of the palate, orbit, zygoma and pterygoid plates are fashioned. The maxilla is then removed after transection of the pterygoid muscle attachments. When oncologically possible preservation of part of the hard palate or the orbital rim is functionally and cosmetically better. Large defects can be dealt with using a free rectus abdominis muscle flap. The best functional result with palatal defects is often to simply use a palatal obturation on a denture plate.

Ethmoid and frontal sinus tumours: craniofacial ethmoidectomy

Craniofacial and transfacial approaches are combined so that osteotomies of the ethmoid complex can be carried out from above and below. The ethmoid/frontal sinus block is then delivered inferiorly and removed. The principal reconstructive problem is separation of the cranial and nasal cavities. A vascularized pericranial or galeopericranial flap can be raised during the approach and is ideal for this purpose.

Nasopharyngeal tumours

Benign tumours, for example nasopharyngeal angiofibroma, are usually approached anteriorly. Small tumours may be resectable using an endoscopic transnasal or a transpalatal approach. A midfacial degloving approach is preferable for larger tumours, provided they do not extend far into the infratemporal fossa. Access to the nasopharynx is achieved by resection of the medial maxilla or maxillary osteotomies. A more extensive exposure is necessary for larger benign or malignant tumours. This entails a combination of a lateral and an anterior approach in most cases. No reconstruction is usually necessary unless the cranial cavity has been opened, in which case temporalis, free rectus abdominis or other muscle flaps are usually used.

Extended resections

Tumours arising in the maxillary or ethmoid sinuses may invade the orbit. Resection of the orbital contents is necessary when tumour has extended through the orbital periosteum. Larger tumours invading the skull base may present difficult problems and require a combination of superior, lateral and anterior approaches. The temporary removal of large areas of the craniofacial skeleton employed in the facial translocation approach give excellent access to large complex tumours (Janecka et al, 1990).

Postoperative care

Observation of the airway and for signs of bleeding are important for the first 12 hours. Intracranial bleeding is very infrequent after craniofacial resection. It is signified by an alteration in conscious level, hypertension, cardiac arrhythmias and bradycardia and necessitates return to the operating theatre.

Complications

The most significant initial complication is bleeding, either into the pharynx or intracranial. A cerebrospinal fluid (CSF) leak or intracranial air may occur if there is a defect in the dura. Provided there is a vascularized reconstruction healing is rapid. Late scarring and contracture can occur after maxillectomy. The severity of this is reduced by the avoidance of facial skin incisions, when possible, and by appropriate reconstruction. Removal of the medial wall of the orbit may result in displacement of the eye with diplopia. Late correction of this is very difficult and avoidance by suitable reconstruction is the best solution when this is possible.

See Chapter 2.10 on the management of altered sensory function after craniofacial surgery.

Ear and temporal bone

Malignant tumours of the ear and temporal bone are rare and often present at a late stage. The temporal bone is anatomically complex and the mode of presentation of tumours depends on the particular structures that are invaded. Early symptoms of tumours arising in the ear canal are hearing loss and pain. Invasion of the mastoid bone and middle ear may affect the facial nerve, causing facial weakness or paralysis. A complete sensorineural hearing loss and loss of balance will result from invasion of the inner ear and unilateral headache from dural invasion. CT and MRI scanning are complementary in the investigation of temporal bone tumours (Horowitz et al, 1994). The most frequent malignant tumour is squamous carcinoma. Adenocarcinomas and sarcomas are less common primary tumours. The temporal bone may also be invaded by tumours arising from adjacent sites such as the parotid gland and the overlying skin. Relatively low-grade tumours such as basal cell carcinoma may become highly invasive and difficult to treat once there is invasion of the temporal bone. The glomus jugulare tumour deserves special mention. Although this tumour is usually benign it displays invasive behaviour and malignant change can be difficult to predict. It arises from chemoreceptor cells in the jugular bulb and invades the floor of the middle ear, initially causing hearing loss and pulsatile tinnitus (Fisch, 1982). It may invade the temporal bone or extend into the cranial cavity. The most effective treatment is surgical removal, but radiotherapy may be used in older patients to prevent further growth.

Malignant tumours of the temporal bone have a poor prognosis but one that has improved from approximately 5% 5-year survival to around 40–50% (Liu et al, 1993) in recent years. This has resulted from the combined use of complete excision and postoperative radiotherapy. Although the morbidity of treatment can be considerable, palliation of persistent or uncontrolled disease in the temporal bone is extremely difficult.

Partial temporal bone resection

Tumours that are confined to the ear canal can be completely removed by a lateral temporal bone resection. A transmastoid approach is used. A post-auricular skin flap is raised and the ear canal transected close to the pinna. If the tumour also involves the pinna then the whole or part of the pinna is resected in continuity. The middle fossa dura and the facial nerve are exposed by removal of the overlying bone and the portion of temporal bone lateral to the facial nerve removed. The defect is then either closed directly or by a muscle flap, often the free rectus abdominis (Tiwari, 1985).

Involvement of the jugular bulb, most commonly by a glomus jugulare tumour, is removed by a temporocervical approach (Fisch, 1978). The sigmoid sinus and facial nerve are exposed from the mastoid bone and the internal carotid artery and internal jugular vein from a neck dissection. The facial nerve lies superficial to the jugular bulb crossing the surgical access. This problem has been solved by the temporary or permanent transposition of the intact facial nerve using the infratemporal fossa approach. Division of the internal jugular vein and the sigmoid sinus then allows the jugular bulb to be removed.

Subtotal temporal bone resection

Invasion by malignant tumours beyond the confines of the ear canal necessitates a removal of the petrous temporal bone (Sataloff et al, 1987). The facial nerve is usually involved by these tumours and will require resection followed by nerve grafting. The approach is by a wide post-auricular flap. The temporal bone is exposed on its superior surface by a middle fossa craniotomy. The usual anterior limit is the internal carotid artery which is exposed after resection or displacement of the head of the mandible. The carotid artery and jugular vein are exposed by an upper neck dissection. The posterior limit is usually the sigmoid sinus, but if this is involved, then the transverse sinus is exposed and divided in the posterior fossa. The temporal bone is removed by division of the bone at the petrous apex. Involved dura is resected and repaired using a fascial graft. Reconstruction requires a vascularized flap to seal the cranial cavity and prevent meningitis. The rectus abdominis free flap is ideal for this purpose.

Postoperative care

Close observation for signs of intracranial haemorrhage is important in the immediate postoperative period. CSF leak may occur but will rapidly settle if a vascularized flap has been used for reconstruction. If the Eustachian tube is not adequately sealed this complication may be evident as CSF rhinorrhoea or a salty taste.

Complications

Intracranial bleeding is signified by an alteration in level of consciousness, hypertension, cardiac arrhythmias and bradycardia, and necessitates a return to the operating theatre. A CSF leak or intracranial air may occur if there is a defect in the dura. Provided there is a vascularized reconstruction, healing is rapid. Both these complications are only likely if there has been a resection of the dura.

More extensive resections in which the posterior and middle cranial fossae have been opened are correspondingly more likely to develop significant complications. Retraction of the dominant temporal lobe may result in temporary dysphasia.

See Chapter 2.10 on the management of altered sensory function after craniofacial surgery.

Summary

Each head and neck cancer operation causes specific problems for the patient and family. Individualized preparation for each operation is thus essential, and there is scope for the development of patient information booklets for each site. Acute complications require careful monitoring by the nurse, appropriate interventions and comprehensive teamwork from the various professionals involved to ensure optimum recovery and maximum quality of life.

Chapter 4.3
Radiotherapy for head and neck cancer

STEVEN EDWARDS

Introduction

Radiotherapy is the therapeutic use of *ionizing* radiation in the treatment of disease; most notably the treatment of cancer. Radiotherapy is used frequently in head and neck cancer, both as first-line treatment and as part of a combined modality treatment approach consisting of surgery and postoperative radiotherapy. It is therefore important that nurses working in head and neck oncology have a good understanding of this treatment modality.

Radiotherapy is a local treatment, only affecting the tissues or organs targeted by the radiation. It can be given with radical intent (to cure) or palliatively (for symptom control). In head and neck cancer, radical radiotherapy is used as a first-line treatment for early tumours, inoperable tumours, for patients who are unfit for surgery, and frequently as postoperative treatment for those with advanced (stage 3 and 4) tumours, metastatic lymphatic disease, or for tumours where excision margins are not clear. Some tumour sites in the head and neck are known to present a high risk of lymphatic spread, and the neck is therefore electively irradiated even though the patient may not have any clinical evidence of disease.

Increasingly, within the context of head and neck cancer there is a new subset of treatment intent: radical palliation. Here the intent of the treatment is to palliate symptoms but the planning and treatment is, to all intents and purposes, the same as that used for radical radiotherapy. The rationale for this is that local control is tremendously important for people with head and neck cancer, as uncontrolled local tumours cause such unpleasant and difficult problems. Thus most patients with head and neck cancer will receive radical radiotherapy, whereas only one-third of general oncology patients do so.

There are three main types of radiotherapy — external beam radiotherapy, brachytherapy and radioactive isotopes.

Radiobiology

Cell damage

The energy particles within the radiation beam (electrons or photons), interact directly and indirectly with the target cells to produce highly charged electrons, known as free radicals. Hence the term ionizing radiation. These free radicals damage nuclear DNA. If this damage is not repaired, the target cell will no longer be able to produce daughter cells, and the tumour stops growing.

Tolerance of normal tissue

High-energy radiotherapy damages all living cells that it interacts with; however cancer cells have a more impaired repair mechanism than normal cells. Although normal cells *are* damaged by radiotherapy, they are more able to recover from this damage than cancer cells. It is this difference in ability to repair radiotherapy damage that is the basis of radiotherapy. There is a point/dose level at which radiotherapy damage to normal/healthy tissue cannot be reversed or repaired (the tolerance dose). The radiation dose that can safely be delivered to tumours is generally determined by the radiation tolerance of the surrounding normal tissues.

Tolerance dose varies from tissue to tissue (and tumour to tumour). It is dependent on factors such as the volume (amount) of organ or tissues to be irradiated, the dose per treatment and the treatment schedule to be employed. Techniques such as conformal radiotherapy and intensity beam modulated radiotherapy can be used to spare normal tissues as much as possible thus allowing a lethal tumour dose to be delivered with minimum side effects.

Doses and fractionation

The unit for measuring dose in radiotherapy is the Gray (Gy). It is the measure of Radiation Absorbed Dose. The typical total dose needed to treat squamous cell carcinoma of the head and neck is in the region of 55–70 Gy. The total dose of radiotherapy is given by means of individual doses — this is known as fractionation. Splitting the total dose into individual equal treatments (fractions) provides a means of safely getting the dose into the target area. Fractionation also allows hypoxic cells within the tumour to become re-oxygenated as the tumour shrinks. Cellular damage by radiotherapy is greatest in the presence of oxygen, therefore where there are hypoxic cells, radiotherapy is less effective. Most solid tumours have a hypoxic portion, often at the centre of the tumour mass. Imagine that the tumour mass is a doughnut, with the hole representing the hypoxic centre. With each dose of radiotherapy a part of the outer solid portion of the doughnut is removed, while at the same time the hole (representing the hypoxic portion of the tumour) is shrinking. Fractionation also allows normal tissues to recover/repair radiotherapy damage (see Table 4.3.1).

Table 4.3.1: The four Rs of radiobiology

Repair	Cells can repair themselves after radiation damage. Their ability to repair depends on the dose given. Normal cells have a better ability to repair than tumour cells
Reoxygenation	Hypoxic cells are radioresistant. Tumours often contain hypoxic cells at their centre. As the tumour shrinks, the cells in the centre are reoxygenated and killed by further doses of radiation
Repopulation	Cells which survive a dose of radiation repopulate the area. Repopulation of normal tissues is essential. Repopulation of tumour cells is undesirable. Rapidly dividing tumour cells, such as squamous cell cancers of the head and neck, should be given the least opportunities possible to repopulate (i.e. unplanned gaps in treatment should be avoided)
Redistribution	Cells have varying sensitivity to radiation, depending on which stage of the cell cycle they are in. Cells are more sensitive in the mitotic phase. Cells which are in resistant phases of the cycle when a dose of radiation is given will be killed by later doses, as they move into mitosis

In the UK it is standard practice to deliver the total dose of radio-therapy by means of equal daily doses, treating on Monday to Friday, with a break for the weekend. In the UK, the dose per fraction is usually 2.75–3 Gy for head and neck cancer. A radical course of treatment can last from 4–6 weeks. Work has shown that doses of greater than 2 Gy per fraction give improved responses in laryngeal cancer because it reduces repopulation by tumour cells (Yu et al, 1997). Work in Denmark has shown that 6 fractions per week, plus the use of a hypoxic cell sensitizer (Nimorazole) resulted in a signifi-cant increase in head and neck tumour control. This is now a stan-dard treatment in Denmark (Overgaard et al, 1997). Fractionation and overall treatment time is often influenced not only by factors such as providing the optimum chance of cure, but also by economic factors such as the adequate provision of treatment facilities in a particular region.

Cell kinetic studies (Tucker & Chan, 1990) have led to a debate about the value of standard fractionation schedules (e.g. 2.75 Gy per fraction, five times a week) in the treatment of squamous cell carci-nomas, when radiotherapy is the first-line treatment. If treatment is given using more than one treatment (fraction) a day, this is known as hyperfractionation. The fractions must be more than 6 hours apart to ensure repair of normal tissues, especially the spinal cord and the dose per fraction tends to be smaller than the standard dose. A number of clinical trials have looked at altered fractionation sched-ules, as a means of improving local control and/or survival. The most notable example is the Medical Research Council Continuous Hyperfractionated Accelerated Radiotherapy (CHART) Trial (Saunders et al, 1989). The CHART trial compared a conventional fractionation regime of 66 Gy in 33 daily fractions (control group) with the CHART regime of 54 Gy in 36 fractions, treating three times a day. The trial did not demonstrate a benefit for early tumours, but suggested a difference in favour of CHART for later stage (T3) disease.

Where treatment is given using less than 5 fractions a week, this is known as hypofractionation. As a rule when hypofractionation is used the dose per fraction is larger than the standard dose. Hypofractionation is rarely used in the radical management of head and neck cancer in the UK (Wiernik et al, 1990).

External beam radiotherapy

What is external beam radiotherapy?

External beam radiotherapy is the type of radiotherapy most used in the management of head and neck cancer. External beam radiotherapy uses machines (linear accelerators) to direct a beam of radiation to the part of the body that is to be treated. A variety of beams can be used including photons, electrons, neutrons, or gamma rays. Photons and electrons are delivered by megavoltage linear accelerators and are generally used in the treatment of head and neck cancer. Gamma rays and neutrons are rarely used in head and neck cancer treatment.

The energies of the machines typically used in external beam radiotherapy range from 4 million volts to 20 million volts (1 million volts is typically written as MV for megavolts), hence the term megavoltage. For comparison, the energy of the standard diagnostic X-ray machine used to take chest X-rays is about 75,000 volts. External beam radiotherapy does not make the patient radioactive, and it is perfectly safe for them to be with other people, including children, throughout their treatment.

The planning process

To ensure that treatment is given as accurately and safely as possible, the patient attending for external beam radiotherapy will pass through a series of steps. These include:

- the mouldroom
- the simulator
- treatment planning
- treatment
- treatment verification.

The first step in the planning process for the head and neck patient having external beam radiotherapy, is a visit to the mouldroom to have a beam direction shell (BDS) made. The BDS, also known as a 'jig' or 'mask', ensures that the patient's head is in a fixed position (immobilized) throughout the planning and treatment process. Good immobilization means that at each treatment the radiotherapy beam is accurately and reproducibly directed at the target area throughout the course of treatment. In the head and neck region small changes in the position of the neck or chin can greatly affect the accuracy of beam placement. This has been shown to affect tumour control rates. Research suggests that immobilization of the patient with a BDS during treatment increases the local control rate, especially where the area being treated is small (Robertson et al, 1993). The beam direction shell also ensures that the marks outlining the target area (the field) are placed on the mask as opposed to the patient's face or neck. Some patients find the BDS very claustrophobic and experience panic attacks. The management of this 'mask phobia' is outlined in Chapter 3.3.

The next stage in the planning process involves the patient having a series of X-rays taken on the simulator wearing the BDS. The simulator is an X-ray machine with the same shape and movements of a treatment machine. Using a combination of patient history, clinical examination and radiological imaging (e.g. magnetic resonance imaging or computerized tomography), the clinical oncologist will mark an outline of the target area (the field) on to the X-rays taken by the simulator. This field indicates the area to be treated, including prophylactic nodal irradiation, and encompasses the known extent of the tumour plus a clinical margin for microscopic disease as well as a small margin for reproducibility of the daily treatment set-up on the machine. Prophylactic lymph node irradiation of the neck and supraclavicular nodes is often given; this needs to be explained to the patient, as they often worry that the cancer has spread, or is more extensive than they thought, when they see that their neck and clavicles are being irradiated.

Treatment planning involves designing the optimal arrangement of radiotherapy beams to cover the target with a uniform tumouricidal dose whilst avoiding or minimizing the dose to surrounding normal tissues. One of the primary aims of the radiotherapy planning process is to ensure maximum damage to the tumour, with minimal serious injury to normal tissues. At the most basic level this is achieved by limiting the amount of normal tissue that is to be treated to a high dose level. An arrangement of two, three or four beams approaching from different directions but converging on the tumour may be required. Hence the need for good immobilization. Treatment plans of multiple beams are drawn up using computerized data describing the characteristics of the beam and enabling rapid addition of their effects at a point. With the advent of 3-D imaging processes and planning systems the extent of the tumour can now be accurately defined (tumour localization) and treatment planned in three dimensions. State of the art information technology will soon provide software programs that will be able to design biological models of treatment based on normal tissue complication probability and tumour control probability data.

Once the planning is complete, the patient returns to the simulator for a series of films, again wearing the BDS, to check or verify that the instructions to deliver the treatment are correct and that the proposed volume of treatment is correct. During treatment delivery on the linear accelerators electronic imaging of the irradiation fields, or films, can be taken whilst the patient is being treated to verify accuracy. During treatment the patient will be monitored continually and assessed.

Side effects of external beam radiotherapy

Radiotherapy is associated with a broad spectrum of side effects. These side effects can be either acute (short term) or late (long term). Acute reactions occur during the course of treatment. They can be severe, but are often temporary in nature, resolving a few weeks after completion of treatment. Late effects occur months or even years after treatment and are permanent. The damage sustained will vary in relation to (amongst other things) total dose, fractionation, volume of irradiated tissue, presence of hotspots or areas of slight overdosage and intrinsic *radiosensitivity* of the specific tissue.

Radiosensitivity refers to the relative vulnerability of cells to damage by ionizing radiation. Different tissues, cancerous and normal, have different sensitivities. Some tissues can be damaged by relatively low radiation doses and are said to be radiosensitive. Other tissues can withstand high doses of radiation with minimal effect and are said to be radioresistant. The Bergonie and Tribondeau (1906) principle provides an insight into the basis of radiosensitivity. In general it states that ionizing radiation is more effective against cells that are actively dividing and undifferentiated. Ancel and Vitemberger (1925) modified this hypothesis by proposing that the inherent vulnerability of any cell to damage by ionizing radiation is the same, but that the time of the appearance of radiation-induced damage differs among different types of cells. In short, cells that divide quickly would express the damage sooner and appear 'sensitive', compared with those that divide slowly and express their damage later and thus appear 'resistant'. In clinical terms, stem cells, such as those found in the oral mucosa and skin, quickly express radiation damage during a course of radiotherapy, and as such are radiosensitive. At the opposite end of the radiosensitivity scale, nerve cells and muscle cells, which do not divide and are highly differentiated, are affected later in the course of treatment (as the total radiotherapy dose rises) and as such are radioresistant.

The key to recognizing, and effectively treating, radiation damage in the head and neck patient lies in understanding the effect of radiotherapy on normal tissues. In describing the effects of radiotherapy it must be emphasized that only the tissues lying within the target area will be affected. For example, a patient with a T1 tumour of the larynx will only have a field that measures 5 cm by 5 cm to cover the larynx. A patient with a nasopharyngeal tumour, with a high risk of lymphatic metastases, will have a field measuring 16 cm by 12 cm, covering an area from the base of the skull to the clavicles. Thus, this patient will experience a much higher morbidity than the patient with the small field.

Skin reactions

First and second weeks of radiotherapy

No obvious radiation effects occur during the first or second weeks, except for the occasional appearance of a faint erythema after the first few radiation doses, and progressive dryness of the skin. Transient erythema may be seen in some patients during the first week, which is probably caused by capillary dilatation and increased vascular permeability. After about 2 weeks epilation (hair loss) may start; complete hair loss is related to the radiation dose to the skin.

Third week

The skin turns red and becomes warm and oedematous. This is called erythema. There is dilatation of the vessels in the upper dermis, obstruction of arterioles by fibrin thrombi and associated inflammatory infiltration initially consisting of leucocytes later replaced by macrophages, eosinophils, plasma cells and lymphocytes. The patient may report a sensation of burning and tenderness. Erythema is clearly limited to the radiation field.

Fourth and fifth weeks

Depending on the treatment schedule, the skin reaction may progress from dry desquamation to the exudative phase — moist desquamation. The dermis is denuded and responds with marked inflammation and the oozing of serum. Patients may suffer from considerable discomfort during this period.

Sixth week

About 1 week after the termination of radiotherapy, recovery and re-epithelialization begins. Healing is through re-epithelialization which occurs from islands of less affected basal layer, starting from the margins or from regenerative foci in the centre of the radiation field.

Seventh and eighth weeks

Three to 4 weeks after the end of radiotherapy recovery is usually complete. The increased pigmentation usually apparent at the end of a course of radiotherapy will gradually disappear during the following months.

Three months to a year

The typical late stage of skin reaction after radiotherapy is mild skin atrophy with a somewhat glossy appearance. The sebaceous skin glands do not usually recover after a course of fractionated radiotherapy. This lack of the oily secretions from the sebaceous glands causes a drying of the skin.

One year onwards

After about a year, tiny varicose veins (telangiectasia) occasionally become visible. Telangiectasia is dilatation of small blood vessels, especially in the skin, producing a purplish, blotchy spidery appearance. The incidence and severity of skin telangiectasia depends on the radiation dose and the radiotherapy technique used, it increases in frequency as time goes on.

See Chapter 2.6 for management of the skin during radiotherapy.

Lymphatic damage

The exchange between the blood and the medium in direct contact with the tissues is controlled by a selectively permeable barrier. The anatomical substrate of this barrier is the lymphatic capillary wall and primarily the endothelium. Increases in lymphatic vascular permeability have been observed after irradiation with 60 Gy (Mann et al, 1981). Increases in permeability are demonstrated, at the cellular level, by the presence in the extravascular space of an increasing amount of intravascular material; clinically, this would manifest as localized lymphoedema. Abnormal accumulations in the extravascular space, due to cellular damage in the endothelial barrier and/or impaired removal by the lymphatic drainage, may be responsible for lymphoedema. Alteration in the transverse contour of the normal neck means that a high radiation dose is given in this area, therefore the lymphatics are most damaged in this area, resulting in the development of submental oedema, or 'dewlap'. Patients who have neck dissection plus nodal irradiation are particularly at risk of lymphoedema; severe facial lymphoedema occurs in patients who have bilateral neck dissections plus irradiation.

See Chapter 2.9 for management of lymphoedema.

Mucous membranes

Mucous membranes are rapidly proliferating tissues and hence manifest radiation injury early. Acute radiation-induced side effects on mucous membranes result from reproductive killing of stem cells in the basal layer of the epithelium. Death of these cells cause, after a lag period, mucosal denudation. This denudation triggers the stem cells that survive the radiation damage into accelerated proliferation in an attempt to offset this induced cell depletion and to repopulate the tissue. Capillaries may be dilated and the endothelium swollen. These effects cause an observable erythema. Atypical fibroblasts may appear in the submucosa during the acute phase but are more commonly seen later. The magnitude and length of denudation depends on numerous dose and fractionation factors.

Two weeks onwards

Approximately 2 weeks into a course of fractionated radiotherapy, erosion and desquamation of mucosal epithelium occur (mucositis). The denuded surface becomes covered with a pseudomembrane of fibrin, cell debris and leucocytes. Mucositis within the oropharyn-geal region leads to dysphagia.

Six to eight weeks

Regeneration and repopulation of the epithelium are usually completed within a month of the end of a 4-week course of radio-therapy, although the epithelium remains thin and sometimes more pale than before irradiation. Microscopically, there is atrophy of the basal layers of the stratified squamous epithelium. There is fibrosis of the lamina propria and submucosa.

Months to a year

As part of the repair process following ulceration, tissues may be replaced by granulation tissue. Some capillaries are telangiectasic and arterioles can have thick hyalin walls. Partly on account of the progressive scarring and vascular compromise, the oral mucosa remains susceptible to even minor trauma. Potentially serious chronic ulceration may develop even months after radiotherapy. Some of the persistent oral mucosal changes are related to other complications of radiotherapy of the area, namely xerostomia, dental caries and osteoradionecrosis (Baker, 1982; Fajardo, 1982; Berthong, 1986).

See Chapter 2.2 on mouth care and the section on pain manage-ment during radiotherapy in Chapter 2.11.

Xerostomia

One or more of the major salivary glands are frequently in close proximity to primary tumours of the head and neck region and to the pathways for the lymphatic spread of these tumours. Therefore, it is frequently impossible to avoid including all or part of these tissues in radiation fields.

First day of treatment onwards

Irradiation of the major salivary glands can produce an acute clini-cal syndrome of swelling, tenderness and pain in one or more of the glands. These symptoms are more frequently associated with the submandibular gland than the parotid, although it may be similarly affected. Dryness of the mouth (xerostomia) and difficulty in swallowing (dysphagia) may develop. These early reactions can occur within 12 hours of the first radiotherapy dose, but are more commonly encountered during the first or second week of standard fractionated radiotherapy. Initial symptoms may develop after a dose of 10–20 Gy of fractionated radiotherapy. The acute syndrome usually subsides spontaneously within days of development, despite permanent alteration in the volume and physical properties of the saliva, which becomes viscous and sticky. Accompanying the acute physical changes are the subjective complaints of loss of taste or decreased taste sensitivity, unusual taste sensations and diminished appetite. Although some patients experience subjective improvement of xerostomia several years after treatment, objective recovery of salivary flow is not usually demonstrated (Parsons, 1984). A total dose of 40–60 Gy will induce complete xerostomia in about 80% of patients (Marks et al, 1981).

Side effects secondary to xerostomia

Dental caries
The rate of tooth decay and periodontal disease increases dramatically after radiotherapy to the oral cavity. Dental caries is a chronic infectious disease caused by agents of the indigenous oral flora (Shaw, 1987). Although early investigators attributed dental decay to direct radiation injury of teeth, it is now accepted that the deterioration of the teeth following irradiation is secondary to xerostomia (Parsons, 1984). The reduced amount of saliva and its increased viscosity is less effective in removing particulate matter from the mouth. Diminished secretory antibodies and the lowered pH favour the growth of cariogenic bacteria and yeast (Marks et al, 1981; Kuten et al, 1986). Dental caries result from the dissolution of enamel and dentine by acids produced by metabolism of food residues by these organisms, which colonize the surfaces in the altered oral environment (Shaw, 1987).

See Chapter 2.2 on mouth care.

Taste dysfunction

Alteration of taste usually appears 2–3 weeks after the start of radiotherapy (Mossman et al, 1982). Taste dysfunction can affect digestion due to impaired stimulation of digestive enzyme secretion and decreased gastric contractions (Schiffman, 1983a). These factors may compromise the overall health of the patient and impair the recovery of radiation injury (Mossman et al, 1982; Chencharick & Mossman 1983). It is difficult to determine the relative contributions of direct radiation damage to taste buds and secondary damage to taste buds caused by xerostomia, since salivary glands and taste buds are frequently irradiated simultaneously.

See Chapter 2.10 on altered sensory function.

Spinal cord

For the clinician, the potential of radiation damage to the spinal cord (radiation myelopathy) is an important dose-limiting factor when planning head and neck radiotherapy. Although there is no definitive tolerance dose for the spinal cord, it is generally accepted that radiation damage to the spinal cord can occur when the spinal cord is included in the treatment area and receives a dose greater than 45 Gy in 22–25 daily fractions (Schultheiss & Stephens, 1992).

Loss of myelin (demyelination) from individual nerve fibres and necrosis (malacia) of groups of nerve fibres are the consistent features of clinically induced radiation myelopathy. Grossly, the radiation damaged spinal cord may be swollen or atrophic and may contain areas that are discoloured by necrosis and haemorrhage (Schultheiss & Stephens, 1992).

Within 4–6 weeks of radiotherapy, patients can present with tingling shock-like sensations affecting the shoulder, trunk and extremities, known as Lhermitte's syndrome (1929). The symptoms usually regress after 1–5 months. Lhermitte's syndrome is also known as transient radiation myelopathy (Jones, 1964).

Long-term damage to the spinal cord can present 8–48 months after radiotherapy. Initially, the signs may include sensory deficit and diminished temperature sensation, clumsiness and lower extremity weakness. These can progress to changes in gait and difficulty in walking, and if severe can culminate in complete paraplegia or quadriplegia. The prognosis of a radiation myelopathy patient depends on the height of the lesion up the spinal cord and the age of the patient. Patients with cervical myelopathy have the poorest prognosis, with 55% of them dying at 18 months, compared to 25% of patients with thoracic lesions. Young patients have a better prognosis than older patients (Schultheiss et al, 1986).

Any risk of spinal cord dose causing myelopathy is unacceptable and radiation may be given in several phases with reduction in field size to reduce normal tissue damage in subsequent phases. If treatment is required to the neck, after reaching spinal cord tolerance dose, electrons can be used instead of photons as they deposit energy in a more superficial manner, avoiding more damage to the spinal cord.

Trismus

Trismus may occur if the muscles of mastication, notably the masseter, medial pterygoid and temporalis, are included in the radiotherapy beams and receive a dose of 60 Gy or more. When muscle is affected/damaged by radiotherapy it is repaired by dense, disorganized collagen. The result is progressive fibrosis and limitation of mandibular opening.

See section on trismus management in Chapter 2.2.

Osteoradionecrosis

Osteoradionecrosis (bone death) is one of the most devastating complications of radiotherapy in the head and neck. Bone death is thought to occur secondary to vascular insufficiency caused by radiation damage to local blood vessels and affects the mandible most frequently (Million & Cassisi, 1994, pp. 251–253). The differential diagnosis in any form of necrosis is recurrence, and it is important that trauma through biopsy does not precipitate worsening necrosis. Conservative management includes antibiotic therapy and hyperbaric oxygen treatment, but may ultimately necessitate hemimandibulectomy (Koka et al, 1990). The incidence of osteoradionecrosis of the mandible in curative radiotherapy has been quoted as being as high as 30% (Ang et al, 1991). A recent article reporting on the results of an 8-year review quotes an incidence rate of 4.7% (Toljanic et al, 1998). Significant causative factors include radiotherapy dose, proximity of tumour to bone and dental status of the patient. Osteoradionecrosis is rarely seen under 60 Gy. The incidence is 1–2% up to 70 Gy and 9% above 70 Gy. Carious teeth should be extracted prior to radiotherapy, as the incidence of osteoradionecrosis is known to be greater when extractions are carried out post-radiotherapy (Beumer et al, 1983b). A gap of at least 10 days is required for adequate healing before the start of radiotherapy.

See Chapter 2.2 on mouth care.

Cartilage chondritis

Inflammation of the laryngeal cartilage(s), particularly the arytenoid cartilage, occurs in the first 3 months following radiotherapy in most patients with laryngeal cancer and resolves within a year. Post-irradiation laryngeal oedema is important because it is often difficult to distinguish between patients with persistent or progressive arytenoid oedema and patients with tumour recurrence. The incidence of post-irradiation laryngeal oedema is noted to be highest in patients with supraglottic disease as opposed to glottic disease (Ichimura et al, 1997). Chronic cartilage chondritis lasting more than a year after radiotherapy tends to occur when larger treatment fields are used (Inoue et al, 1992) and at doses of more than 70 Gy (Ichimura et al, 1997). Necrosis of laryngeal cartilage is a serious late side effect of radiotherapy; however, it is rarely seen where megavoltage radiotherapy has been used. The incidence of laryngeal necrosis is in the region of 1 to 2%. Deep biopsy post-radiotherapy to eliminate the diagnosis of recurrence can precipitate necrosis.

Eye

Conjunctivitis may be a problem in patients having radiotherapy near to the eye, where the eye is to receive a total dose of 50 Gy or more. The probability of developing a radiation-induced cataract depends on the total dose and the amount of the lens irradiated. A cataract is defined as the loss of normal transparency of the lens of the eye. Cataracts usually develop about 2 to 3 years after the lens has been irradiated to a dose of 5 Gy or more. Because cataracts can now be easily treated, they are of less concern than they used to be.

The acute effects of radiotherapy on the cornea are normally temporary. Punctate keratitis may occur with doses of 30–50 Gy in 4–5 weeks (Merriman et al, 1972). Punctate keratitis is characterized by multiple small defects on the corneal epithelium. Symptoms include irritation of the eye with tearing. The use of megavoltage equipment, because of its ability to spare superficial tissues, is less damaging. Late effects include atrophy of the lacrimal gland and impaired tear production, if the cornea has received doses of 50–60 Gy. The result is a dry eye.

Ears

If the ears are included in the treatment area the canals, eardrums and Eustachian tubes can become inflamed and erythematous. At doses of about 40 Gy serous otitis media may result from obstruction of the Eustachian tubes. This causes significant hearing impairment and occurs frequently in patients having radiotherapy for nasopharyngeal and parotid cancers.

See Chapter 2.10 on the management of hearing impairment.

Hypothyroidism

Damage to the thyroid gland (leading to hypothyroidism) is common after radiotherapy to the head and neck. This injury may be a result of radiotherapy (Liening et al, 1990) or surgery and radiotherapy given in combination (Vrabec & Heffron, 1981; Donnelly et al, 1995). The incidence of hypothyroidism is highest when the whole thyroid gland is in the target volume, for example when the larynx or hypopharynx is being treated. Tami et al (1991), reporting on 100 consecutive patients receiving treatment for head and neck cancer, found that in the 10 patients treated with surgery alone, none were hypothyroid. Of those treated with radiotherapy alone, 28% developed hypothyroidism. Those treated with both surgery and radiotherapy became hypothyroid in 40% of cases. These results were borne out by a study by Donnelly et al (1995), who assessed the thyroid function of 27 laryngeal cancer patients, who had undergone total laryngectomy with ipsilateral hemithyroidectomy. All the patients treated with surgery alone had normal thyroid function. Abnormal results were found in 45% of patients who had received combined treatment (surgery and radiotherapy). Tell et al (1997) found a high incidence of hypothyroidism occurring up to 3 years after radiotherapy. The incidence increased in patients who had undergone laryngectomy. There is clinical (Alexander et al, 1982) and experimental (Cannon, 1994) data to show that hypothyroidism in combination with surgery and radiotherapy adversely affects wound healing.

It is important to monitor thyroid function at follow-up even many years after radiotherapy. Side effects include tiredness and lethargy and are entirely treatable (see Chapter 5.1 for thyroid function and hormone replacement therapy).

Pituitary and hypothalamus function

The pituitary gland and hypothalamus are irradiated during treatment of nasopharyngeal and paranasal sinus cancers. This may cause damage to these organs which leads to deficiency of:

- growth hormone; this does not affect adults, but must be treated in children
- adrenocorticotrophin; causing symptoms of weakness and fatigue, and in severe deficiency, epigastric pain, diarrhoea and hypotension
- gonadotrophins; causing amenorrhea, impotence, absence of body hair, testicular atrophy and decreased libido
- thyrotropin; causing hyopthyroidism
- prolactin; causing amenorrhea and galactorrhoea
  (Parsons, 1994).

Biochemical checks for evidence of hypopituitarism and hypothalamism should be carried out at follow-up, with referral on to an endocrinologist as required.

Temporal lobe necrosis

There is a small risk of temporal lobe necrosis occurring as a late effect of nasopharyngeal irradiation (around 10 years post-treatment). The risk is related to the dose of radiation given per fraction; the risk at 2.5 Gy per fraction is 4.6% (Lee et al, 1998).

Pregnancy

Radiation is very harmful to the developing foetus and therefore female patients in their reproductive years should be advised to use a reliable form of contraception whilst undergoing radiotherapy. Pregnancy would contraindicate radiotherapy and a termination of pregnancy may be advised for a patient requiring radiotherapy.

Summary

To summarize this section, radiotherapy is a highly technical treatment that entails very unpleasant side effects for the patient. Patients undergoing radiotherapy experience a high level of emotional and psychosocial problems and therefore require a correspondingly high

level of support from specialist cancer nurses throughout their radiotherapy experience and beyond. Chapter 3.3 outlines in detail
psychosocial support during radiotherapy.

Brachytherapy

What is brachytherapy?

Brachytherapy is the use of radioactive substances to deliver high
doses of radiation to a tumour with minimal doses to the surrounding tissue. This allows for enhanced tumour control with minimal
toxicity to the surrounding area. Brachytherapy is performed by
using a radioactive isotope as a 'source' of radiation. The source is
placed by an experienced oncologist very near to the tumour, either
into the tissues surrounding it (interstitial) or in the cavity next to the
tumour (intracavity). The amount and spacing of the implants
containing the source are carefully calculated by a medical physicist,
who also calculates the length of time they need to be left in place.

Sources used in brachytherapy

The most commonly used source in head and neck cancer brachytherapy is iridium (^{192}Ir), which has a half life of 74.5 days. Iridium is
supplied in the form of wires, which can be used in interstitial implants,
or incorporated into applicators. For example, the tissue surrounding a
small tumour of the tongue can be implanted with iridium wires in the
form of needles, hairpins, sutures or loops (interstitial brachytherapy)
or a tumour in the nasopharynx can be treated by inserting an applicator which carries a radioactive source (intracavity brachytherapy). The
time taken for an iridium implant or application to deliver the optimum dose of 65 Gy to a tumour is usually about 5 to 6 days.

Another isotope that may be used in brachytherapy is Iodine-
125. This is supplied in the form of 'seeds' which can be implanted
permanently. Gold-198 is also supplied in the form of 'seeds' for
permanent implantation.

Low dose rate brachytherapy

Implantation of the above isotopes into the tissues delivers a dose of
radiation over a period of days and is therefore known as low dose
rate brachytherapy. There are several techniques for delivering interstitial low dose rate brachytherapy:

- Plastic tube technique: needles are placed within the tissue around the tumour to act as guides for plastic tubes and for placement verification by X-ray. When placed to the satisfaction of the oncologist, the needles are replaced by the plastic tubes and iridium wires are inserted into these at a later time (manual afterloading). Tubes are sometimes used to loop over the surface of a lesion to deliver radiation to the surface. The tubes are held in position by plastic tube spacers and the system is secured by metal buttons. This system is often used in the tongue and floor of the mouth.
- Guide gutter technique: the guide gutters are inserted into the tissue, their correct placement is checked by X-ray, the iridium wires (as hairpins or single pins) are then inserted into the guides, and the guides are removed leaving the pins in situ. The pins are secured by sutures. This system is often used in the tongue.
- Hypodermic needle technique: the needles are inserted, placement checked and tailor-made plastic templates or tubing are attached to hold them in position. The iridium wires are then loaded into the needles and secured by lead caps crimped over the needle tips. This system is used for external lesions such as carcinoma of the lip or nose.
- Silk suture technique: a braided silk thread with a cylindrical cavity containing an iridium wire is inserted into the tissues using a needle. The suture ends are tied and taped to the skin. This technique is used for lesions of the lower eyelid, ear or nasal bridge and other areas where anatomical curvatures must be met (the iridium wire is very pliable and so will bend to the curve).
- Tailored moulds: areas with superficial lesions which are difficult to implant can have an acrylic resin mould of the area made. The mould incorporates plastic tubes which are loaded with iridium wires before being applied to the lesion. Areas such as the pinna, or a maxillectomy cavity can be treated in this way. The mould must be held carefully in position with packing or tape. (Gerbaulet et al, 1993.)

High dose rate brachytherapy

In circumstances when the implant or applicator is amenable to connection to a remote afterloading system, high dose rate brachytherapy can be given. This can cut treatment time down to a few minutes per day, although interstitial afterloading catheters must be kept in place. The benefits of this technique are in the reduction of radiation exposure of staff. The patient does not have to be isolated with restricted visiting and if the treatment is via a removable applicator, outpatient attendance is possible.

The radioactivity administered by this type of brachytherapy is not absorbed by the body, so body fluids and waste are not radioactive.

The role of brachytherapy in head and neck cancer

Primary treatment

Brachytherapy often allows for tumour control without the need for surgery. Resection of organs such as the lip, oral tongue, base of tongue, floor of mouth and other sites can cause considerable functional and cosmetic morbidity. For small (T1 and T2 N0) tumours, brachytherapy offers the opportunity to give a lethal tumour dose without the more widespread toxicity of external beam radiotherapy. It therefore is the treatment of choice in these situations (Harrison, 1997). For low dose rate, typically doses of 65 Gy are delivered over 6 days. The tumour must be small, well defined, accessible and in a site that allows geometric stability. The geometric arrangement of the sources is dictated by a set of rules known as the Paris System. This delivers a maximum dose to the tumour volume. Local control rates of 90% or more are obtained with this treatment.

Combination with external beam radiotherapy and surgery

For larger T2 and T3 tumours in the base of the tongue, a combination of external beam radiotherapy and brachytherapy is often utilized. The external beam treatment provides irradiation to the primary site with a generous margin, and includes irradiation of the neck. A dose of around 50 Gy can be given via external beam and this is followed by an implant to give an extra 20 to 30 Gy to the tumour site only (Harrison, 1997). Iridium wires are used with the plastic loop technique (Harrison et al, 1992; Pernot et al, 1996; Horwitz et al, 1996). Patients who have positive neck nodes may have a neck dissection as part of their treatment.

High dose rate intracavity brachytherapy has been used in nasopharyngeal carcinoma, using a specially designed flexible nasal applicator and on an outpatient basis (Levendag et al, 1998). This treatment is very superficial and used as a boost after external beam irradiation or to retreat an area of recurrence.

The use of Iodine-125 seeds in the base of the tongue, oropharynx and nasopharynx has been described by some authors (Horwitz et al, 1996; Horwitz et al, 1997; Harrison, 1997) (via a transnasal, transoral or transpalatal approach).

Occasionally, an implant is used after excisional biopsy of T1 lesions in the floor of the mouth or tongue (Ange et al, 1975; Mendenhall et al, 1989).

Recurrent disease

In certain situations of local or nodal recurrent disease, especially when prior radiation has been given, brachytherapy can be used to re-irradiate a small area. Brachytherapy may be used in combination with salvage surgery for recurrence; for example, nodal recurrence may be treated by excision and reconstruction of the neck with brachytherapy implant loops inserted into the tumour bed during surgery. These are loaded with iridium at a later date to treat any incompletely excised disease. After treatment, they are easily removed by being pulled out.

Recurrent disease in the nasopharynx can be successfully retreated with intracavity brachytherapy (Hwang et al, 1998) and occasionally, Iodine-125 seeds (Park et al, 1991). Schafer et al (1996) describe the palliative treatment of a tracheostomal recurrence using brachytherapy; a tracheostomy tube was used as an applicator for the iridium wires. Local recurrences after maxillectomy can be treated using a specially made obturator as applicator for sources.

Complications of brachytherapy

The side effects and complications associated with brachytherapy depend on the site being treated.

Acute complications

- infection
- haemorrhage
- the main complications for brachytherapy in combination with salvage surgery for the neck are skin ulceration and wound breakdown (Harrison, 1997). Carotid rupture occurs occasionally, with fatal consequences
- pain
- mucositis (limited to the immediate area)
- Chang et al (1996) report foul odour due to nasopharyngeal crusting after nasopharyngeal brachytherapy.

Late complications

Major complications after oral brachytherapy are *soft tissue necrosis* (Pernot et al, 1997) and *osteoradionecrosis of the mandible* (Lozza et al, 1997). Steps are taken to avoid this occurring by careful placement of the implants and calculation of the dose. Biopsy of an area to diagnose recurrence should also be avoided prior to brachytherapy. Authors also propose that risk of necrosis can be reduced by the use of a 'spacer' (a dental guard or shield) to reduce the dose to the mandible, made from acrylic resin by the prosthetics team. Miura et al (1998) report a significant reduction in the dose to the mandible and the incidence of osteoradionecrosis when a spacer was used. However, in practice these are very difficult to use as their placement causes difficulty in imaging during the insertion procedure and changes in the dosimetry due to altering the position of the tongue. In addition, they are very uncomfortable to wear, and the patient must frequently remove the device for comfort, to eat and to perform oral hygiene.

Major complications of nasopharyngeal brachytherapy include *palate* or *sphenoid sinus floor perforation* and *nasopharynx necrosis* (Chang et al, 1996). However, these complications are extremely rare, except in cases of retreatment of previously irradiated patients.

Nursing care of the individual undergoing brachytherapy

There are three primary factors in radiation protection when caring for an individual with a radioactive source: time, distance and shielding. It is beyond the scope of this chapter to discuss these in more detail, and the reader is referred to generic texts on cancer nursing and their local radiation protection guidelines for more information.

It is vital that the nurse checks that the patient is suitable for brachytherapy treatment at the initial nursing assessment. He/she must be relatively capable of self-care and thus able to comply with radiation protection requirements. For example, elderly patients who require a high level of physical care, or confused patients who cannot be relied upon to stay in isolation or perform self-care, are not suitable. Careful alcohol dependency assessment must be carried out and appropriate action taken to prevent acute alcohol withdrawal occurring post-implantation, as delirium would inevitably mean the unacceptable exposure of staff to radiation (see Chapter 1.3). As with external beam irradiation, a dental assessment and treatment must be carried out prior to implantation (see Chapter 2.2).

Because the nurse can spend only very limited time with an individual once they have an active source in situ, thorough education and preparation prior to the procedure are absolutely essential. This includes preparation for the psychological and emotional effects of being isolated for several days. Evidence shows that isolation can have negative psychological effects on patients, but that a structured preparatory information programme reduces anxiety and depression (Gammon, 1998).

Specific nursing management for head and neck brachytherapy patients includes the following:

- Pain. The implant procedure will cause acute pain, which is managed as acute surgical pain by intravenous opiate therapy using a patient-controlled analgesia system. As pain reduces, analgesics will be titrated downwards accordingly (see Chapter 2.11 for information on pain management). Oral medication is usually sufficient by the second postoperative day.
- Oral hygiene. An intraoral implant is a surgical wound and thus puts the area at risk of infection. Additionally mucositis will develop after 10 to 14 days. Oral hygiene must therefore be scrupulous, using an oral care protocol (see Chapter 2.2).
- Displacement of sources. The implant should be inspected four times per day to check that the sources are all present and remain correctly positioned. Often, the presence of intraoral implants can only be discerned by the sutures holding them in place. The nurse handing over the patient at the shift change should show the next nurse the position and number of sutures holding in the implant so that their appearance and situation are known. A diagram in the nursing notes may also be helpful. Additionally, the patient should be asked to use a bowl, rather than the sink, when performing oral care in case a source is dislodged and lost down the plughole. If a source is dislodged, it should be placed in a lead box using long-handled forceps and the oncologist advised immediately.
- Wound care. If the implant is through the skin, the entry sites should be kept clean and dry, and observed for signs of infection. This is particularly important if the brachytherapy is being given as a boost after external beam radiotherapy, as moist desquama-

tion is often present, increasing the risk of infection. Frequent cleansing of the site with normal saline may be required.

- Postoperative oedema. The tongue may become very swollen after an implant. Severe oedema may be treated with corticosteroids. Base of tongue implants may cause oedema which compromises the airway, and occasionally patients may undergo a temporary tracheostomy prior to the procedure in order to protect the airway (Harrison, 1997). It is important that the patient is completely recovered from the insertion procedure, and that there are no signs of airway problems, before manual afterloading of the iridium wires is performed; this is therefore often done after 24 hours rest. See Chapter 2.1 for management of airway problems.
- Appearance. Patients who have facial implants, and their significant others, should be prepared for the appearance of their face once the implant is in situ.
- Nutrition. Chewing may be a problem if an oral implant is in situ, therefore the patient will require a soft/liquidized diet and supplements. In some circumstances, for example if severe oedema occurs, nasogastric feeding may be required. See Chapter 2.4 on nutritional management.

Removal of the implant is carried out on the ward by a senior member of the medical team and the nurse caring for the patient. Premedication with an analgesic is necessary as removal can be temporarily painful. If the skin's integrity has been damaged, a dressing will be required until the wound has healed.

Aftercare

Side effects of brachytherapy are exactly the same as for external beam radiotherapy, occurring after 10 to 14 days, and should not be underestimated. The area irradiated is small but the dose is much higher and is defined inhomogeneously, so some areas close to the source will receive double the prescribed dose — in the region of 130 Gy.

By the time acute tissue reaction occurs, the patient will have had the implant removed and been discharged home, and therefore will require coaching from the nurse prior to discharge on the expected side effects depending on the tumour site (acute mucositis, erythema, pain, crusting of the nose/lip). Thus for individuals who have had oral implants, oral hygiene must continue for several weeks post-implant, until the reaction has settled. Painkillers will be required to manage this painful mucositis and should be provided on discharge with coaching on how to achieve pain control. The patient will require close observation and support, so community and outpatient nursing support are essential. The tongue is a particularly sensitive structure, and individuals who have had tongue implants will experience pain and discomfort at the tumour site for several months. Clinical experience has shown that these patients experience high levels of anxiety post-discharge, as the side effects often lead to fear that the tumour is progressing and has not responded to treatment.

At the time of writing, there does not appear to be any research on the individual's experience of brachytherapy, nor the nursing management of this group of patients.

Radio-iodine treatment

Radioactive isotopes may be administered systemically. Radioactive iodine (^{131}I) is an isotope used in the treatment of papillary and follicular thyroid tumours, as these cells selectively take up iodine to manufacture thyroid hormones. See Chapter 5.1 for detailed information.

Summary

In the management of head and neck cancers, radiotherapy can be used as the first and only line of treatment or in combination with surgery, and/or chemotherapy. Combined modality treatments have improved the cure rates for even advanced disease. However, the acute effects of such treatment can be very debilitating and late effects are usually quite marked. An understanding of the impact of the disease, and its therapy, is vital if healthcare professionals are to provide consistent and accurate information about the likely consequences of treatment, and to guide practice in the effective management of these side effects.

Chapter 4.4
Chemotherapy for head and neck cancer

Introduction

Cytotoxic drugs act against tumour cells by interfering with cell division, thereby slowing down or reversing the growth of the cancer. They do this at various phases in the cell cycle; different drugs have effects at different phases. Thus a combination of different drugs with effects on different phases is usually given to have maximum effect.

Cytotoxic drugs cannot differentiate between normal cells and cancer cells, so when introduced into the body, they will inhibit the division of normal cells, for example the bone marrow, the gastrointestinal epithelium, the skin and hair follicles, as part of the normal processes of growth and repair. The extent to which this occurs is known as the dose-limiting toxicity of the drug. In addition to this toxicity, individual drugs have specific toxicities against body organs; for example cardiac damage, neurotoxicity, liver and renal impairment.

It is beyond the scope of this chapter to give an in-depth coverage of cancer chemotherapy. The reader is referred to specific texts on cancer chemotherapy for this information. The following section will give an overview of the use of chemotherapy in squamous cell cancer of the head and neck.

The role of chemotherapy in head and neck cancer

In head and neck cancer, chemotherapy may be used in several different circumstances.

Recurrent and metastatic disease

Chemotherapy is a standard treatment for recurrent and metastatic head and neck cancer. The goal of this treatment is palliation. Several randomized trials have demonstrated that a combination of cisplatin and 5-fluorouracil (5-FU) is more effective than any other agents currently being used in head and neck cancer. Response rates of 30 to 60% are reported with expected survival of 4 to 10 months (Amrein, 1990; Guthrie et al, 1990; Forastiere, 1994). Thus it can be given to patients with recurrent or metastatic disease with a reasonable expectation of good palliation.

Carboplatin/5-FU has slightly lower response rates but has the advantage of less neurological and renal toxicity, and easy outpatient administration (Forastiere, 1994). However, carboplatin is much more expensive.

Low-dose methotrexate is occasionally used for palliation in head and neck cancer.

Induction (neoadjuvant) chemotherapy

Induction chemotherapy is given in advanced squamous cell head and neck cancer prior to definitive surgery or radiotherapy, with the aims of improving local control and surgical resectability, eliminating micrometastasis and evaluating the chemosensitivity of the tumour for subsequent treatment. Cisplatin and 5-FU combination therapy has shown a superior response in clinical trials (Hughes & Frenkel, 1997). However, Munro (1995) and Harari (1997) caution that reports of high response rates do not translate into improved survival rates, and the literature should be interpreted carefully. Neoadjuvant chemotherapy does not improve survival. Munro (1995) goes on to propose that induction chemotherapy may even stimulate resistance to radiotherapy by accelerating repopulation of certain tumour cells.

Trials have shown that patients who have a complete response to induction chemotherapy and go on to have radiotherapy alone, instead of surgery and radiotherapy, have a comparable survival. This exciting finding gives scope for organ preservation in selected patients, and is also an option for patients who refuse surgery (Jacob et al, 1987; Department of Veterans Affairs, 1991; Lefebvre & Sahmoud, 1994). The Department of Veterans Affairs Laryngeal Cancer Study Group trial (1991) and the EORTC trial (Lefebvre & Sahmoud, 1994) demonstrated no significant differences in survival in patients who received induction cisplatin/5-FU and radiotherapy or total laryngectomy and radiotherapy. Munro (1995) argues that these trials did not provide any evidence that chemotherapy plus radiotherapy was any better than radiotherapy alone.

Adjuvant chemotherapy

Trials of maintenance chemotherapy with platinum/5-FU combination after standard treatment for head and neck cancer have not produced any consistent evidence of a beneficial effect.

Concurrent chemoradiotherapy

Concurrent chemoradiotherapy is one of the most recent developments in oncology. Chemotherapy given in combination with radiotherapy has been trialled with improvements in disease-free and overall survival in some head and neck patients. Possible mechanisms for enhancement of radiation effects include inhibition of sublethal damage, selective radiosensitization of hypoxic cells, reduction of tumour bulk giving improved tumour blood supply and reoxygenation and recruitment of cells into a more radiosensitive proliferative phase (Fu & Phillips, 1991).

Platinum and platinum/5-FU combinations again are reported as particularly successful (Forastiere, 1994). Concurrent chemotherapy has better success rates for advanced head and neck cancer than induction/neoadjuvant therapy (Merlano et al, 1992; Weissler et al, 1992; Vokes et al, 1992; Munro, 1995). Chemoradiotherapy for nasopharyngeal cancer has been reported as increasing 3-year survival rate by 30% in a recent trial (El-Sarraf et al, 1998), and for a group of patients with advanced oral, oropharyngeal, hyopharyngeal and laryngeal cancers, increasing the 3-year survival rate by 19% (Wendt et al, 1998). However, not all trials have produced such high success rates. Acute toxicity in these trials was extremely high and all the authors conclude that much more supportive care is needed for patients undergoing concurrent chemoradiotherapy. Munro (1995) points out that if concurrent chemotherapy increases morbidity to the extent that overall treatment time is prolonged, or radiotherapy has to be curtailed, there may be little overall gain.

Single-agent platinum and radiotherapy is less toxic as platinum does not have mucosal toxicity, whilst 5-FU greatly enhances mucosal toxicity. As yet, optimum drug combinations, drug doses, radiation doses and schedules remain unknown.

Other agents

Other agents that are occasionally used in head and neck cancer include:

Methotrexate, bleomycin, carboplatin, ifosfamide, paclitaxel (Taxol), mitomycin C, gemcitabine, docetaxel (Haas et al, 1976; Cervellino et al, 1991; Forastiere, 1993; Hughes & Frenkel, 1997; Fountzilas et al, 1997; Colevas et al, 1997). These have been used alone and in various combinations with varying response rates; some act as radiosensitizers, and others are hypoxic cell sensitizers. Trials with these drugs are ongoing.

Nursing the head and neck cancer patient undergoing chemotherapy

The drugs commonly used in head and neck cancer and their side effects are shown in Table 4.4.1. Nursing management of the main problems associated with these drugs is discussed below.

Education

A major nursing responsibility is to teach the patient and significant others about the expected side effects of the cytotoxic drugs they are to receive, in order to ensure that informed consent has been obtained, to prepare the patient for any unpleasant effects and to coach them on prevention of problems, early detection and coping strategies.

Bone marrow suppression

The consequences of bone marrow suppression are infection, bleeding and anaemia.

• Infection is a very serious complication and the cause of many cancer deaths (Wilkes, 1996). Thus nursing care and patient education is directed towards the prevention of infection, or early detection and treatment. The single most important risk factor for infection is a decreased neutrophil count.

Table 4.4.1: Commonly used cytotoxic drugs in head and neck cancer

Drug	Method of administration	Side effects	Other information
Carboplatin	IV infusion over 30–60 minutes	Acute effects: nausea, vomiting Later effects: bone marrow depression, nephrotoxicity (infrequent), mild stomatitis, mild diarrhoea, mild hepatotoxicity, neurological/otological toxicity (rare), mutagenicity	70% of drug excreted in urine within 24 hours Patient must use contraception if sexually active
Cisplatin	IV infusion over 1–6 hours	Acute effects: metallic taste, nausea and vomiting, diarrhoea Later effects: nephrotoxicity, bone marrow depression, otological toxicity (tinnitus, high frequency hearing loss), peripheral neuropathy (rare), hyperuricaemia, cardiac toxicity (rare), mutagenicity	Interacts with aluminium Sensitive to strong sunlight Mainly excreted via kidneys Urine output should be at least 100–150 ml per hour; pre- and post-hydration are given, forced diuresis may be needed Renal function is closely monitored Patient must use contraception if sexually active
5-Fluorouracil (5-FU)	IV infusion	Acute effects: diarrhoea, occasional nausea, coronary spasm, cerebellar ataxia Later effects: chemical phlebitis and brown discoloration of veins, bone marrow depression, stomatitis, palmar/plantar erythema, hyperpigmentation, brittle nails and nail loss	Excreted as respiratory CO_2 Very short life (30 mins)

Methotrexate	IV bolus or IV infusion	Acute effects: gingivitis, stomatitis, dizziness, blurred vision, malaise, mild nausea (rare) Later effects: bone marrow depression, erythematous rashes, pruritus, photosensitivity, hepatotoxicity, cystitis, pulmonary changes, renal failure (high dose)	Doses > 70 mg/m^2 require folinic acid rescue High-dose methotrexate regimes require forced alkaline diuresis to prevent renal toxicity. Excreted in urine

Information from Lilly Oncology (1993) and Barton Burke et al (1996).

- Low platelet counts (thrombocytopaenia) predispose the patient to bleeding. Drugs that contain aspirin, and therefore interfere with platelet function, should be avoided. The patient should be alert to the signs of bleeding and avoid injuries, injections etc. whilst the platelet count is low.
- Anaemia will cause fatigue, dizziness, breathlessness and activity intolerance. The patient will need help to identify coping strategies until this has been corrected by red cell transfusions.

Mucositis

Mucositis is specified by its anatomic location. In the oral cavity it is stomatitis, in the oesophagus it is oesophagitis and in the intestines it is proctitis and usually results in diarrhoea.

- The management of stomatitis is discussed in Chapter 2.2.
- Oesophagitis is managed by maintaining patient comfort via use of analgesics, preventing secondary infection (e.g. *Candida*) and maintaining optimum nutrition (see Chapter 2.4).
- Diarrhoea is managed by maintenance of fluid and electrolyte balance, maintenance of nutrition and promotion of patient comfort by perianal skin care and administration of anti-diarrhoea medications.

Nausea and vomiting

Cisplatin and carboplatin have high emetic potential. 5-FU and low-dose methotrexate have low emetic potential. There are several mechanisms by which cytotoxic drugs cause nausea and vomiting. Briefly these are as follows:

- The cytotoxics cause mucosal injury in the intestines which then release serotonin ($5\text{-}HT_3$). $5\text{-}HT_3$ then stimulates $5\text{-}HT_3$ receptors on the gastrointestinal vagal afferent fibres, which in turn stimulate the vomiting centre. $5\text{-}HT_3$ antagonists (e.g. ondansetron, granisetron) have been very effective in the prevention of this process, thus reducing chemotherapy-induced nausea and vomiting significantly.
- The cytotoxics stimulate the chemoreceptor trigger zone (CTZ). This then stimulates the vomiting centre.

- Anxiety can also stimulate the vomiting centre via a cortical pathway through the hypothalamus. This pathway is probably responsible for anticipatory nausea and vomiting.

Anti-emetic therapy should be given prior to chemotherapy so that the receptors in the CTZ can be effectively blocked before the cytotoxic drugs enter the bloodstream (Wilkes, 1996). They should continue to be administered until the drug's duration of action has ended. There are many anti-emetic drugs, but it is beyond the scope of this chapter to describe them.

Alopecia

Most people associate chemotherapy with hair loss, and this can be one of the most emotionally distressing side effects of some chemotherapy regimes. However, none of the drugs listed above cause alopecia, so the head and neck cancer patient is thankfully spared yet another onslaught on their appearance and body image.

Specific organ toxicity

The main organ toxicity in platinum-based therapy is renal impairment. Renal function will be measured prior to commencement of therapy and will be monitored carefully throughout treatment regimes. Intensive pre-hydration and post-hydration is given with cisplatin. Diuretics may also be given. Signs of toxicity will indicate a dose reduction or cessation of treatment.

The other main toxicity is to hearing, and management of impaired hearing is discussed in Chapter 2.10.

All patients undergoing platinum chemotherapy will be at risk of mutagenicity and therefore should receive counselling about the effects of treatment on their sexual function and advised to use contraception as appropriate.

Summary

Individuals undergoing chemotherapy for head and neck cancer present a great challenge to the nurse. They may have to cope with chemotherapy in addition to the news that their cancer has recurred and is now incurable. They may be having chemotherapy prior to radical radiotherapy or surgery, or chemotherapy and radiotherapy together. All these treatment modalities have significant morbidity in the head and neck; when used together, they will cause the patient several distressing physical problems in addition to the psychological and emotional problems which will invariably be present. Nurses will need an array of knowledge and skills to deal with all these problems and to coach the patient and family through them. For those interested in reading further in this subject Barton Burke et al (1996) is recommended.

Section Five
Thyroid cancer

Chapter 5.1
Cancer of the thyroid gland

TRICIA FEBER
GRAHAM BUCKLEY

Introduction

Thyroid cancer is a very rare malignancy occurring in the younger age groups, particularly in females (Dow et al, 1997a). Differentiated thyroid cancer is a slow-growing disease with excellent 10- and 20-year survival rates. However, despite the good prognosis, survivors must undergo long-term surveillance to monitor for recurrence. This surveillance necessitates regular periods of induced hypothyroidism. The thyroid gland has effects on almost every cell in the body, and absence of it has a profound impact on the body and the person. Thus thyroid cancer survivors experience a significant negative impact on their quality of life and wellbeing, which is often over-looked by clinicians. The potential role of nurses in improving quality of life by support, education and facilitation of coping strategies for this group of individuals is tremendous. However in many centres, nursing input for this group is very minimal. This chapter aims to give an understanding of the anatomy and physiology of the thyroid gland, an understanding of thyroid cancer and its treatment, and to explore the nursing interventions required to support the patient. Parathyroid cancer, an extremely rare malignancy, is also covered briefly in this chapter.

489

Anatomy and physiology of thyroid and parathyroid glands

Martini 1992d

The thyroid gland curves across the anterior surface of the trachea just below the thyroid cartilage. It consists of two lobes that are joined together by the isthmus. The thyroid gland is very well vascularized to supply the glandular cells which it is made up of. The thyroid gland contains large numbers of thyroid follicles which are surrounded by a network of capillaries supplying nutrients and regulatory hormones, as well as taking away thyroid hormones and metabolic wastes released by the follicles.

There are two pairs of parathyroid glands embedded in the posterior surfaces of the thyroid lobes. They contain chief cells which produce parathormone.

Thyroid hormones are all structural derivatives of the amino acid tyrosine to which three or four iodine atoms have been attached. Tetraiodothyronine (thyroxine or T4) contains four atoms of iodine and makes up approximately 90% of all thyroid secretions. Triiodothyronine (liothyronine or T3) is secreted in small amounts and contains three iodine atoms. These two hormones affect almost every cell in the body, influencing cellular metabolism and oxygen consumption. T3 produces a strong and immediate increase in cellular metabolism, but is very short lasting. T4 gradually diffuses into the tissues, producing a gradual long-term effect. Once in the cytoplasm T4 molecules are converted to T3 and have exactly the same effect.

The effects of thyroid hormones are:

- elevation of oxygen and energy consumption, generating heat for adaptation to cold temperatures
- increase of heart rate and force of contraction, causing a rise in blood pressure
- increase in sensitivity to sympathetic stimulation
- maintenance of normal sensitivity of respiratory centres to changes in oxygen and carbon dioxide concentrations
- stimulation of formation of red blood cells
- stimulation of other endocrine tissues
- acceleration of mineral turnover in bones.

The demand for thyroid hormones changes constantly. The follicular cells synthesize thyroglobulin, which contains tyrosine, and store it in the follicle lumen. Iodine from the surrounding interstitial fluids is transported across the cell into the follicle where it binds with the tyrosine molecules to produce T3 and T4, contained within the thyroglobulin molecules. Secretion of T3 and T4 from the follicle occurs when endocytosis brings a small packet of thyroglobulin molecules into the cytoplasm of a follicular cell. Lysosomal enzymes then break this down, releasing the T3 and T4. Approximately three-quarters of these hormone molecules become attached to thyroid-binding globulins as they enter the circulation. The remaining unbound hormones diffuse into the peripheral tissues producing an immediate effect. The bound molecules are gradually released over a week or more, prolonging the effects of thyroid stimulation.

T3 and T4 are released at a low background level until their release is stimulated. Release is mainly controlled by the levels of thyroid stimulating hormone (TSH) in the blood. TSH is released by the anterior pituitary gland, which is stimulated by thyroid releasing hormone (TRH) from the hypothalamus. TRH release is stimulated by decreased blood concentrations of T3 and T4, or a low body temperature.

The thyroid gland also contains C (parafollicular) cells which produce the hormone calcitonin. Calcitonin works alongside parathormone from the parathyroids to regulate calcium ion concentrations in body fluids. Calcitonin inhibits osteoclast activity, decreases the rate of intestinal calcium absorption, and increases the rate of calcium ion excretion. Parathormone has exactly the opposite effect; increasing osteoclast activity, increasing the rate of intestinal absorption, and decreasing the rate of calcium ion excretion.

Calcium ion concentrations must be closely controlled, as even small variations affect cellular operations. Large changes cause acute clinical changes. Nerve and muscle cells are particularly sensitive to changes. If calcium levels rise, they become relatively unresponsive. If levels decrease they become very excitable so that convulsions may occur. Tetany occurs with hypocalcaemia; numbness, tingling and cramps in extremities; stiffness, twitching or spasms in hands and feet; Trousseau's sign, carpopedal spasm induced by inflation of BP cuff to 200 mmHg for 1 minute. A 50% fall in calcium levels usually causes death.

Types of thyroid cancer

There are four types of thyroid neoplasms: papillary, follicular, medullary and anaplastic. Papillary and follicular tumours arise from the follicle, medullary tumours arise from the parafollicular cells and anaplastic tumours arise from differentiated papillary and follicular cells (Wickham & Roham, 1997).

Papillary tumours

Papillary tumours comprise 60 to 70% of thyroid cancers. These tumours are more common in females. Papillary tumours are usually well differentiated and slow growing, with a good prognosis. They are more aggressive in males and older patients. The incidence of distant metastasis in this group of patients is low; Shaha et al (1997) report an incidence of 2.3%. Even with metastatic disease, patients may survive for decades (Wickham & Roham, 1997). Overall, papillary thyroid cancers have an 80 to 90% 10-year survival (O'Doherty & Coakley, 1998).

Follicular tumours

Follicular tumours comprise 20% of thyroid cancers. These tumours are more aggressive and commonly occur in the 50 plus age group. Tumours may be large and invade blood vessels and they are more likely to metastasize (Shaha et al, 1997). Hurthle cell carcinoma is a subtype occurring in older individuals (Wickham & Roham, 1997). Overall, follicular tumours have a 65 to 75% 10-year survival (O'Doherty & Coakley, 1998).

Medullary tumours

Medullary tumours comprise 5 to 10% of thyroid cancers. Medullary cancer of the thyroid is a tumour of the C cells which occurs in sporadic and hereditary clinical settings (Chi & Moley, 1998). For those falling into the hereditary group, some may be associated with multiple endocrine neoplasia (MEN) syndromes, MEN 1 and MEN 2, caused by a genetic abnormality. Genetic testing is used to confirm this in individuals diagnosed with medullary thyroid carcinoma; DNA analysis can then be used to test relatives for risk. Affected relatives are offered annual screening and preventative thyroidectomy (Lips et al, 1994; Wells et al, 1994). Plasma calcitonin levels are a sensitive tumour marker, and are therefore monitored regularly. Patients and their relatives should also be screened for other endocrine tumours. These tumours occur equally in men and women over the age of 50. The tumour's secretion of calcitonin may cause hypocalcaemia and diarrhoea. Fifty per cent of patients have cervical lymph node metastasis at diagnosis, and surgery is the treatment of choice (Chi & Moley, 1998). Prognosis for those with negative cervical nodes is 90%, whilst it is only 42% for those with positive nodes (Wickham & Roham, 1997). Medullary tumours metastasize to lung, liver and bone. Overall 10-year survival is in the range of 60 to 70% (O'Doherty & Coakley, 1998).

Anaplastic tumours

Anaplastic tumours comprise 5 to 10% of thyroid cancers. These tumours occur in the 60 plus age group and grow rapidly, invading neck structures to cause dysphagia and dysphonia. Metastasis to lymph nodes, bone and lung occurs early in the course of the disease and the prognosis is poor, with average survival being 4 to 12 months after diagnosis (Wickham & Roham, 1997).

Aetiology of thyroid cancer

Ionizing radiation is the only clearly identified cause of thyroid cancer (Hall & Holm, 1998). Children who receive external beam head and neck irradiation are at increased risk. The rate of thyroid cancer after the Chernobyl nuclear plant disaster increased from one case per million before the accident, to 100 cases per million 9 years afterwards (Hall & Holm, 1998). Diagnostic X-rays have been implicated in female papillary thyroid cancer; an increased risk was found for female dentists and dental assistants with occupational exposure to X-rays, and also diagnostic X-ray exposure was associated with increased risk (Wingren et al, 1997).

Greater incidence of thyroid cancer in women than men, particularly during the reproductive years, has led to the suggestion that female hormones may increase the risk of thyroid cancer. However, Rossing et al (1998) found no evidence to support this hypothesis when they reviewed 468 cases of female thyroid cancer. Other factors which may be implicated include benign thyroid disease and iodine deficiency (Goldman et al, 1980; Hallquist et al, 1994). High rates of follicular and papillary tumours are noted in areas of endemic goitre (Galanti et al, 1995; Francheschi et al, 1998). Recent evidence shows that prolonged, chronic stimulation of the thyroid by TSH can result in tumours (Hard, 1998).

Akslen & Sothern (1998) report a seasonal variation in the presentation and growth of thyroid cancer; significantly more cases present in late autumn and winter, with tumour diameter and proliferation indicators being highest at this time of year.

Diagnosis and staging

A thyroid tumour typically presents as a painless swelling. Malignant tumours may present with signs of invasion of surrounding structures: invasion of the trachea results in stridor, oesphagus in dysphagia and recurrent laryngeal nerve in hoarseness. Fine-needle aspiration biopsy is the procedure of choice to confirm thyroid malignancy (Rosen et al, 1993; Gharib et al, 1993; Greenspan, 1997). Tumour localization by ultrasound may help increase the accuracy. Sectional imaging (computerized tomography, magnetic resonance imaging) is used to identify the extent of malignant tumours and identification of cervical node metastases. Tables 5.1.1 to 5.1.4 outline staging classification.

Table 5.1.1: Staging classification for thyroid cancer (UICC, 1997)

TX	Primary tumour cannot be assessed
T0	No evidence of primary tumour
T1	Tumour 1 cm or less in greatest dimension, limited to the thyroid
T2	Tumour more than 1 cm but not more than 4 cm in greatest dimension, limited to the thyroid
T3	Tumour more than 4 cm in greatest dimension, limited to the thyroid
T4	Tumour of any size extending beyond the thyroid capsule

Table 5.1.2: Regional lymph node staging (UICC, 1997)

NX	Regional lymph nodes cannot be assessed
N0	No regional lymph node metastasis
N1	Regional lymph node metastasis
N1a	Metastasis in ipsilateral cervical lymph node(s)
N1b	Metastasis in bilateral, midline or contralateral cervical or mediastinal lymph node(s)

Table 5.1.3: Distant metastases (UICC, 1997)

MX	Presence of distant metastasis cannot be assessed
M0	No distant metastasis
M1	Distant metastasis

Table 5.1.4: Stage grouping of thyroid cancer (UICC, 1997)

Papillary or follicular	Under 45 years	45 years and over
Stage I	Any T any N M0	T1 N0 M0
Stage II	Any T any N M1	T2 N0 M0
		T3 N0 M0
Stage III		T4 N0 M0
		Any T N1 M0
Stage IV		Any T any N M1
Medullary (all ages)		
Stage I	T1 N0 M0	
Stage II	T2 N0 M0	
	T3 N0 M0	
	T4 N0 M0	
Stage III	Any T N1 M0	
Stage IV	Any T any N M1	
Undifferentiated (all ages)		
Stage IV	Any T any N any M	

Treatment

The treatment of thyroid carcinoma is primarily surgical, either by lobectomy or by total thyroidectomy depending on the histology and tumour stage (Shah et al, 1992). Some small differentiated tumours are treated by thyroid lobectomy. Thyroxine is normally given postoperatively to suppress tumour development in the remaining thyroid lobe. Larger differentiated tumours are treated by total thyroidectomy. Treatment with radioactive iodine (^{131}I) is given postoperatively to ablate thyroid micrometastases (see below) (Ahscraft & Van Herle, 1981). Medullary carcinoma is treated by total thyroidectomy (Brunt & Wells, 1987). External beam radiotherapy is occasionally used to attempt to control anaplastic, recurrent or metastatic disease. It is useful in the palliation of painful bone metastases.

Surgery

Thyroidectomy

The thyroid is approached through a low transverse cervical incision. The recurrent laryngeal nerve is identified and the branches of the inferior thyroid artery and veins are divided; preserving, if possible, the supply to the parathyroid glands (Karlan et al, 1984). The procedure is carried out on one side as a lobectomy or on both sides as a total thyroidectomy.

Extended resection

Thyroid tumours may invade the neighbouring larynx, trachea or oesophagus. The trachea is the most frequent site and is managed by sleeve resection and primary anastomosis (Grillo & Zannini, 1986). Partial laryngectomy may be required for laryngeal invasion. Oesophageal invasion is unusual and is treated by excision and reconstruction of the resultant defect.

Cervical nodes

The lymph nodes at greatest risk are those in the paratracheal groove. These are removed with the thyroid gland in malignant disease. Palpable lymphadenopathy is treated by selective or comprehensive neck dissection depending on the site and size of the nodes (Shah, 1986).

Postoperative care and complications

Postoperative nursing care includes the monitoring for and management of the following potential complications:

- Airway obstruction may occur due to haematoma or vocal cord paralysis; observe for stridor and cyanosis and keep emergency tracheostomy set at bedside for the first 12 hours. Compression of the subglottic veins by haematoma may result in subglottic oedema with airway obstruction. This will not be immediately relieved by removal of the haematoma, and intubation is required. The haematoma is evacuated and bleeding controlled.
- The most significant initial complication is bleeding; monitor wound for haematoma (dressings should not be used), output

from drains and vital signs for hypovolaemic shock for the first 12 hours. The drain can usually be removed the day after surgery.

- Thyrotoxic crisis after partial thyroidectomy (thyroid storm); observe for pyrexia, tachycardia, restlessness, delirium.
- Hypoparathyroidism may occur during the first 48 hours, causing hypocalcaemia; observe for muscle hyperreactivity and tetany and monitor serum calcium levels daily. This is corrected by calcium replacement and 1-alpha calcidol (1–2 per day). The parathyroids will be preserved if possible during thyroidectomy; if any of the glands or their blood supply are damaged, they can be autotransplanted to the sternomastoid muscle. However, permanent hypoparathyroidism is occasionally a distressing long-term complication of thyroidectomy. The incidence of hypoparathyroidism is directly proportional to the extent of the thyroidectomy and inversely proportional to the skill of the surgeon (Shaha & Jaffe, 1998).
- Hypothyroidism; this is a long-term effect of thyroidectomy and requires administration of thyroxine at a dose of 100–200 µg per day. Most patients will receive radio-iodine treatment after total thyroidectomy and so thyroxine will not be commenced immediately. T3 replacement (20 µg per day) may be given as an interim measure and must be stopped 2 weeks before ^{131}I treatment. The patient should be told to avoid iodine-containing medicines, fish or added salt prior to treatment. Screen TSH levels periodically.
- Vocal cord paralysis results from damage to the recurrent laryngeal nerve. This causes hoarseness which may not be immediately apparent. If it does not recover, the voice may be improved by medialization of the paralysed cord. This can be carried out temporarily by collagen injection. Endoscopic injection of Teflon or a thyroplasty procedure offer a more permanent solution. Thyroplasty requires an external skin incision but the results are more predictable and voice quality is better than with Teflon injection (Crumley, 1990). Bilateral vocal cord paralysis is fortunately rare. It usually results in stridor which may not be evident at rest. If the paralysis is permanent then tracheostomy with a speaking valve is the standard treatment. Endoscopic arytenoidectomy is an option, but the airway is not as good and the voice may be reduced to a breathy whisper.

Thyroid hormone replacement therapy

Thyroidectomy causes hypothyroidism, and the patient will require lifelong thyroid replacement therapy postoperatively. T3 and T4 can be administered orally, with good absorption from the gut. Absorption is best if the tablets are taken well apart from food. The best indicator of adequate treatment is the plasma TSH (normal range 0.2–6) (Laurence et al, 1997). Periodic screening will always be required.

T4 reaches its maximum effect in about 10 days from the first dose, as it binds to plasma proteins. Its effect lasts for 2 to 3 weeks from the last dose. The dose required to achieve normal plasma levels will vary between individuals, and is somewhere in the range of 100 μg to 200 μg per day. Doses should be increased gradually (to minimize cardiovascular risk due to a sudden increase in metabolic demand) by 25 μg every fortnight to achieve optimum levels (Laurence et al, 1997).

T3 is about five times more potent than T4 and reaches its maximum effect within 24 hours. Its effect lasts for about 24 to 48 hours after the last dose. It is not used in the routine treatment of hypothyroidism because its rapid onset can cause heart failure. It is mainly used in acute situations such as hypothyroid coma and also prior to radio-iodine treatment and uptake scans, so that the patient can be more quickly rendered hypothyroid prior to the procedure (Laurence et al, 1997).

Thyroid replacement therapy is lifelong and the patient must be educated on the importance of taking the replacement therapy and also be aware of the need to remind their doctor to do periodic blood tests.

Parathormone replacement therapy

The parathyroid glands are not only removed for the rare case of parathyroid malignancy, they are often removed alongside total thyroidectomy and therefore replacement of the function of parathormone will be required. Alongside parathormone, Vitamin D promotes the active absorption of calcium from the gut to control the mineralization of bone and to promote renal tubular reabsorption of calcium and phosphate. Administration of natural vitamin D is difficult, however; alfacalcidol (One-Alpha) is a substance which is converted to vitamin D (calcitrol) in the liver. Alfacalcidol can therefore be used to maintain plasma calcium levels after parathyroidectomy. The daily dose is 1–2 µg (Laurence et al, 1997). Periodic screening of calcium levels will always be required (normal range of standard calcium is 2.1–2.9). The patient must be educated on the importance of taking the replacement therapy and also be aware of the need to remind their doctor to do periodic blood tests.

Radio-iodine treatment

What is radio-iodine treatment?

Radioactive isotopes may be administered systemically. Radioactive iodine (^{131}I) is an isotope used in the treatment of papillary and follicular thyroid tumours, as these cells selectively take up iodine to manufacture thyroid hormones. ^{131}I is an effective treatment even for patients with advanced differentiated thyroid cancer at all sites and can cure, on average, 50% of all patients in this group (Pelikan et al, 1997). Medullary and anaplastic cells do not concentrate and retain iodine. Radio-iodine emits mainly beta radiation (90%) which penetrates only 0.5 mm of tissue and thus affects thyroid tissue only, without damaging surrounding structures. However, it also emits some gamma rays which are more penetrating and can be detected with a Geiger counter.

Four to 6 weeks after thyroidectomy, a diagnostic scan with ^{131}I is performed to detect any remaining functioning thyroid tissue and to assess the dose of ^{131}I needed to ablate this tissue. High thyroid stimulating hormone levels (TSH) are required to enhance ^{131}I take-up by tumour cells in residual primary or metastatic tumour. Thus the patient is rendered hypothyroid prior to the procedure. The patient is usually prescribed T3 postoperatively and this is stopped 10 days prior to the procedure. During this time, the patient will experience the signs and symptoms of hypothyroidism, and will therefore have difficulty working and should be advised not to drive or operate machinery (see hypothyroidism and quality of life below).

If the diagnostic scan is positive, an ablative dose of ^{131}I is administered to the individual. The half life of ^{131}I is 8 days, so although the patient is initially highly radioactive, levels quickly fall. ^{131}I is administered orally as a capsule or a drink and is absorbed, metabolized and excreted by the body. The patient and his/her body fluids and waste are therefore radioactive for several days.

Side effects of radio-iodine

- Acute oedema of the throat and neck (thyroiditis) on day 2 or 3 (occasionally)
- salivary gland side effects (Rodrigues et al, 1997); the epithelial cells of the intralobular ducts in salivary glands also concentrate iodine, therefore about 2% of the administered ^{131}I dose is absorbed by the salivary glands. Acute inflammation of the salivary glands may occur. Sialadenitis manifests within a week of treatment and lasts between 3 weeks and 2.5 years, affecting 11.5% of patients. Salivary gland impairment (xerostomia) is a chronic side effect caused by irreversible damage to the acinar cells
- nausea and vomiting
- headache
- fatigue
- sore mouth
- bone marrow suppression
- metallic taste
- fertility; the sperm count may be temporarily reduced (McDougall, 1997), but there do not appear to be any long-term effects on fertility, or any mutagenicity (O'Doherty & Coakley, 1998).

Nursing care of the patient undergoing ^{131}I treatment

It is vital that the nurse checks that the patient is suitable for ^{131}I treatment. He/she must be relatively self-caring and thus able to comply with radiation protection requirements. For example, elderly patients who require a high level of physical care, or confused patients who cannot be relied upon to stay in isolation or perform self-care, are not suitable. Careful alcohol dependency assessment must be carried out and appropriate action taken to prevent acute alcohol withdrawal occurring post-administration, as delirium would inevitably mean the unacceptable exposure of staff to radiation (see Chapter 1.3). Thorough preparation of the patient prior to the administration of ^{131}I is vital, as contact post-administration is very minimal. This preparation should include psychological and emotional preparation for isolation, as well as coaching the patient on self-care management and the expected side effects. Evidence shows that isolation can have negative psychological effects on patients, but that a structured preparatory information programme reduces anxiety and depression (Gammon, 1998).

Radiation protection

The nurse will work closely with the isotope department to manage the patient undergoing ^{131}I treatment. After administration of the ^{131}I by the isotope staff, the patient is highly radioactive. He or she will be nursed in a separate room, with its own toilet and washing facilities. Dose rate measurements are taken daily using a Geiger counter, to determine how much radio-iodine is in the body, and are used to calculate how long visitors can stay, and when the patient is safe to leave their room.

Radio-iodine is excreted from the body in urine, sweat, saliva, faeces, etc. Any objects the patient touches are therefore contaminated and must be kept inside the room until dose rate measurements show they are safe to remove. Thus patients are instructed to wash their own crockery inside the room, and cannot give any items (money, books, etc.) to visitors or staff. Money to pay for daily papers and other essential items should therefore be given to a member of staff prior to treatment and kept in the ward safe. Clothing will be contaminated and must be stored until safe. This can take several days, and patients should be instructed to bring old clothing which they do not mind leaving in storage. Linen will also be stored until safe. The radioisotope department will place a line on the floor over which staff and visitors must not go. If a patient is ill and nursing staff need to enter the room, protective clothing, including long-sleeved gowns, gloves and shoe covers, must be worn and left behind in the room.

The patient should be instructed to shower regularly to remove radioactive sweat from the skin. Disposable mats are placed around the shower, sink and toilet to avoid contamination of the floor. The patient is asked to avoid splashing (men should be requested to sit on the toilet when passing urine). The toilet should be flushed two or three times after use, with specific guidelines varying between centres. Diagnostic tests such as blood, urine and sputum samples are avoided unless absolutely necessary, and in this case must be handled according to local radiation protection guidelines.

Monitoring and controlling side effects

Control of nausea and vomiting is particularly important as vomiting presents a major contamination hazard. Good oral hygiene instructions and the use of artificial saliva can minimize oral problems. Analgesics should be given to control pain. The patient is encouraged to have a high fluid intake (2 litres per day) to flush the ^{131}I out of the body.

The patient will usually need to stay in hospital for between 5 and 8 days, until they no longer present a radiation hazard. On discharge there may still be restrictions on being near to other people, particularly children, for a few days. Because thyroid cancer affects predominantly females in their reproductive years, this restriction can be particularly difficult. Dow et al (1997b) quote a patient saying: 'The most difficult part of treatment was being told to stay away from my young children after radioactive iodine treatment. I dreaded the thought of coming home from the hospital and telling them to keep away from Mommy'.

T3 will be restarted after all radio-iodine has been excreted (approximately 10 days after administration).

Follow-up for thyroid cancer

Thyroid cancer presents the patient with profound effects on lifestyle, not only because of treatment, but also because of the follow up required after treatment. Whole-body radio-iodine scanning and serum thyroglobulin measurements are the primary methods of follow-up surveillance. Serum thyroglobulin is a sensitive tumour marker, but false negative results can be obtained unless thyroid hormone therapy has been withdrawn (Colacchio et al, 1982). Thus both these modalities require the stimulation of residual thyroid tissue by elevated levels of TSH. To achieve elevated TSH levels, the patient must be rendered hypothyroid. Unfortunately the resulting symptoms have a major impact on the patient's family, work and social life (Dow et al, 1997b). The most debilitating period in thyroid cancer surveillance is during the withdrawal of hormone medication. Ninety-four per cent of patients experience fatigue, and 89% report decreased vigour and activity (Meier et al, 1994).

Surveillance procedures

Approximately 3 months after ^{131}I ablation, an isotope scan is done to check for any remaining tumour or thyroid tissue (this shows as areas of increased uptake on the scan). If this scan is negative, it is repeated in another 3 months. With a negative response on this occasion, the patient can go on to T4 therapy and will not be rescanned for 1 year. Thyroglobulin levels will be monitored periodically.

In patients with positive scans, and therefore persistent disease, the ^{131}I treatment is repeated at a higher dose. Another follow-up scan is done at 3 months; if this is positive, external beam radiotherapy is given. External beam radiotherapy is also useful for the treatment of residual, recurrent and nodal disease in differentiated thyroid cancer (Lin et al, 1997). Thyroid cancer recurrence is associated with significant emotional morbidity, because of the continued need for induced hypothyroidism in addition to ongoing concerns about cancer recurrence (Kaplan, 1990).

Hypothyroidism and quality of life

The physical signs of hypothyroidism include hair loss, facial puffiness, fluid retention, constipation, cold intolerance, headaches, fatigue, malaise, sluggishness, fibromyalgia, weight gain and confusion. Hypothyroidism also causes a cluster of neuropsychiatric symptoms including irritability, depression, clouded thinking, dysphoria, a sense of powerlessness, inability to concentrate, and difficulty with social role management (Dzurec, 1997). Furthermore, thyroid-related symptoms such as these may often be experienced before thyroid function tests become abnormal.

Dow et al (1997a and b) are the only authors who have investigated the impact of thyroid cancer survivorship in detail. Quality of life in this group of patients is important as survivorship is high. However, there may be little in the form of support for these patients. Dow et al (1997a) report the following patient experience as an example of this:

> One thing that always stands out in my mind about my cancer experience is that having thyroid cancer made me feel as if I didn't really fit in as a cancer patient. No support groups seemed to apply to me (because) ... I wasn't going through chemotherapy or radiation treatments. But I did have cancer and that is very scary. Doctors and others seem to treat thyroid cancer very lightly (in the emotional sense) (because) ... it is usually quite curable. I had cancer but I felt that people thought, 'oh well it's just thyroid cancer'. That's not how it felt to me.

Dow et al (1997b) studied quality of life in 34 thyroid cancer survivors to evaluate the impact of thyroid hormone withdrawal. The greatest differences in quality of life were experienced between peak withdrawal on the day of scanning, and the time when thyroid hormone replacement kicked back in. There was significant impact on physical wellbeing, with patients experiencing symptoms including fatigue, appetite loss, pain, disturbed sleep, constipation, decreased motor skills, fluid retention and increased sensitivity to cold. Qualitative data from the same patients (Dow et al, 1997a) revealed the devastating effects of hormone withdrawal:

> Coping with the physical effect consumes all trains of thought to function and accomplish even the simplest task ... Body scans for thyroid cancer are extremely difficult, not as a procedure, but being deprived of thyroid hormone is difficult physically and emotionally. It becomes difficult to cope with life — taking care of the kids, housework, etc. — on a daily basis because of being extremely tired, lacking energy and desire to do anything. When off synthyroid, I stop caring about things and my quality of life becomes much worse.

Negative psychological impact was felt in areas including coping, happiness, sense of control, satisfaction, concentration, usefulness, appearance, anxiety and depression. In addition, patients identified fear of the results of the scanning procedure. One patient in Dow et al's study (1997a) is cited:

> My cancer was diagnosed a year and a half ago. My check-up with two whole body scans was an experience I shall never forget. I keep thinking there's got to be a better way to prepare a patient for a test, a more humane way that doesn't incapacitate a human being. I've been in a deep depression for 3 weeks now. To be without needed therapy for 6 weeks is very poor medicine indeed.

Another patient commented: 'I live a normal life except when my medication is taken away. Then I feel like hell'.

Social impact was also measured, with significant negative impacts on family relationships, socializing and sexuality. Subjects had difficulty performing usual household tasks and meal preparation. At work, patients identified major changes in motivation, productivity, and quality of work. Participants described going to work and then literally having to be carried home. These changes are particularly significant as thyroid cancer is a cancer affecting working adults with families and presents major disruptions in daily life for both patient and family. From the qualitative study (Dow et al, 1997a), comes the following comment:

> Quality of life is my ability to do the things which make me and the people around me happy. This has been terrible. Because of losing my voice (after thyroidectomy), I can't even talk to my friends. I can't even go to a movie because my driving isn't good enough. I can't concentrate well enough to drive.

Even after resumption of thyroid medication, participants commented that balancing their medication and getting back to normal function was a process that took several weeks:

> Cancer has changed my quality of life by taking control over how I feel physically at times. I feel like I lose large chunks of time going through the process of becoming hypothyroid and then coming back to normal. Last year I did not feel completely normal for months.

The significant negative impact of thyroid surveillance procedures implies that individuals need anticipatory education about the effects of hormone withdrawal and facilitation of coping strategies, so that they can adjust their social, work and home activities accordingly during this critical time. Thyroid cancer survivors need access to educational materials on management of symptoms relating to fatigue, decreased concentration, sleep disturbances and other physical effects (Dow et al, 1997a). Patients also need reassurance that the emotional and psychological changes they experience are organic and reversible. The authors suggest that the use of their Quality of Life Thyroid tool may help to evaluate the otherwise non-complaining or quiet patients so that appropriate support, education and counselling can be offered.

Cancer of the parathyroid gland

Cancer of the parathyroid gland is extremely rare. It is commonly linked to familial MEN 1. The patient presents with hypercalcaemia. Immunoassay will reveal raised parathormone levels. Radiotherapy and chemotherapy are ineffective, therefore surgery is the treatment of choice. Resection includes the adjacent thyroid lobe and isthmus. Neck dissection is also performed. Postoperative care focuses on maintaining and monitoring calcium levels and teaching the patient and family self-care management. In uncontrolled and recurrent disease, hypercalcaemia is a major problem and is controlled by administration of calcitonin and biphosphonates. These may only be effective for a limited time and uncontrolled hypercalcaemia is usually the cause of death (Hakaim & Esselsytn, 1993; Shane, 1994).

Summary

The thyroid and parathyroid glands are very important endocrine glands which affect almost every cell in the body. Malignancies of these glands are rare. Surgery and radio-iodine therapy are the treatments of choice, although there is a wide variation in treatment between different centres. Lifelong hormone replacement therapy is essential post surgery and the patient will require education on self-care management. Lifetime management of thyroid function after treatment imposes great demands and challenges on the individual and family (Baker & Feldman, 1993), perhaps even greater than during treatment. However, because survivors are viewed as 'cured' they may not have the same access to support groups as other cancer patients, and their hypothyroid symptoms of fatigue, difficulty concentrating and low mood may be easily dismissed as non-life-threatening. This is an aspect of care that may frequently be over-looked because the patient has minimal contact with nursing staff during hospitalization, and no major physical reasons for contact with nurses after treatment. However, this is a client group that would benefit from emotional, psychological and educational support from the nurse. There is minimal attention to these problems in the nursing literature, and this is identified as an area in which research and development is needed.

Strategy for practice

- Provide people with thyroid cancer with verbal and written information about all side effects including hypothyroidism, and suggest coping strategies.
- Identify sources of support for patients with young families and discuss childcare needs prior to radio-iodine treatment.
- Monitor thyroid function regularly.
- Provide information about support groups.
- Consider carrying out research and development in this area.

Patient information resources

The British Thyroid Foundation
PO Box HP22
Leeds LS6 3RT

CancerBACUP
3 Bath Place
Rivington Street
London EC2A 3JR

References

Aaronsson NK, Bullinger N, Ahmedzai S (1988) A modular approach to quality of life assessment in cancer clinical trials. Recent Results in Cancer Research 111: 231–49.

Abram SE (Ed) (1989) Cancer Pain. Boston: Kluwer.

Abrams RA, Hansen RM (1989) Radiotherapy, chemotherapy, and hormonal therapy in the management of cancer pain: putting patient, prognosis and oncologic options in perspective. In Abram SE (ed) Cancer Pain. Boston: Kluwer.

Ackerman M (1985) The use of bolus normal saline instillations in artificial airways: is it useful or necessary? Heart and Lung 14 (5): 505–6.

Ackerman M (1993) The effect of saline lavage prior to suctioning. American Journal of Critical Care 2 (4): 326–30.

Ackerstaff AH, Hilgers FJM, Aaaronson NK, Balm AJM (1994) Communication, functional disorders and lifestyle changes after total laryngectomy. Clinical Otolaryngology 19: 295–300.

Adamietz IA, Mose S, Harberl A et al (1995) Effect of self-adhesive, silicone coated polyamide net dressing on irradiated human skin. Radiation Oncology Investigations 2: 277–82.

Adams JF, Lassan LF (1995) Leech therapy for venous congestion following myocutaneous pectoralis major flap reconstruction. ORL–Head and Neck Nursing 13(1): 12–14.

Aday LA (1993) At Risk In America: The Health and Health Care Needs of Vulnerable Populations in the United States. San Francisco: Jossey-Bass.

Addy M, Slayne M, Wade W (1992) The formation and action of plaque: an overview. Journal of Applied Bacteriology 73: 269–78.

Agur A (1991) The cranial nerves. Chapter 9 in Grant's Atlas of Anatomy. Baltimore: Williams & Wilkins.

Ahmedzai S, Brooks D (1997) Transdermal fentanyl versus sustained release morphine in cancer pain: preference, efficacy and quality of life. Journal of Pain and Symptom Management 13 (5): 254–61.

Alexander I (1985) Alcohol-antabuse syndrome in patients receiving metronidazole during gynaecological treatments. British Journal of Clinical Practice 39 (7): 292–3.

Alexander MV, Zajtchuk JT, Henderson RL, (1982) Hypothyroidism and wound healing. Archives of Otolaryngology 108: 289–91.

Al-Khafaji BM, Nestok BR, Katz RL (1998) Fine-needle aspiration of 154 parotid mass-
    es with histologic correlation: ten-year experience at the University of Texas MD
    Anderson Cancer Center. Cancer 84(3): 153–9.

Allison R, Vongtama V, Vaughan J, Kyu HS (1995) Symptomatic acute mucositis can
    be minimized or prophylaxed by the combination of sucrulfate and fluconazole.
    Cancer Investigation 13 (1): 16–22.

Amagasa T, Yokoo E, Sato K et al (1985) A study of the clinical characteristics and treat-
    ment of oral carcinoma in situ. Oral Surgery Oral Medicine Oral Pathology 60:
    50–55.

American Dietetic Association Report (1987) Position of the American Dietetic
    Association: issues in feeding the terminally ill patient. Journal of the American
    Dietetic Association 87: 78–85.

Amrein PC (1990) Cisplatin and 5-FU vs. the same plus bleomycin and methotrexate in
    recurrent squamous cell carcinoma of the head and neck. Proceedings of the
    American Society of Clinical Oncology 9: 175.

Ancel P, Vitemberger P (1925) Sur la radiosensibilité cellulaire. C R Soc Biol 92: 517.

Andersen PE, Kraus DH, Arbit E, Shah JP (1996) Management of the orbit during ante-
    rior fossa craniofacial resection. Archives of Otolaryngology Head and Neck
    Surgery 122 (12): 1305–7

Andersson-Anvert M, Forsby N, Klein G, Henle W (1977) Relationship between the
    Epstein–Barr virus and undifferentiated carcinoma: correlated nucleic acid hybridisa-
    tion and histopathological examination. International Journal of Cancer 20: 486–94.

Anderton A, Aidoo IF (1990) Decanting — a source of contamination of enteral feeds?
    Clinical Nutrition 9: 157–62.

Anderton A, Nwoguh CE (1991) Problems with the reuse of enteral feeding systems — a
    study of the effectiveness of a range of cleaning and disinfection procedures. Journal
    of Human Nutrition and Dietetics 4: 25–32.

Andre P, Pinel H, Laccourreye H (1977) Fréquence et prognosis des adenopathies du
    cancer du sinus piriforme. Journal Français Otorhinolaryngologie 26: 419–31

Ang KK, Stephens LC, Schultheiss TE (1991) Oral cavity and salivary glands. In
    Scherer E, Streffer C, Trott K (eds) Radiopathology of Organs and Tissues. Berlin:
    Springer-Verlag, pp 283–311.

Ange DW, Lindberg RD, Guillamondegui OM (1975) Management of squamous cell
    carcinoma of the oral tongue and floor of mouth after excisional biopsy. Radiology
    116: 143–6.

Anon (1994) Practice Guidelines. Hearing loss. ORL — Head and Neck Nursing 12 (3):
    24–5.

Appleton J, Machin J (1995a) Treatment and management of swallowing disorders. In
    Working with Oral Cancer 1st edn. Bicester: Winslow Press.

Appleton J, Machin J (1995b) Anatomy, physiology and medical aspects. In Working
    with Oral Cancer 1st edn. Bicester: Winslow Press

Argyle M (1972) The psychology of interpersonal behaviour. New York: Penguin.

Ariyan S (1979) The pectoralis major myocutaneous flap: a versatile flap for reconstruc-
    tion in the head and neck. Plastic Reconstructive Surgery 63: 73–81.

Aronson EA (1990a) Anatomy and physiology of phonation. In Clinical Voice Disorders
    3rd edn. New York: Thieme Stratton Inc.

Aronson EA (1990b) Organic voice disorders: neurologic disease. In Clinical Voice
    Disorders 3rd edn. New York: Thieme Stratton Inc.

Aronson EA (1990c) Psychogenic voice disorders. In Clinical Voice Disorders 3rd edn. New York: Thieme Stratton Inc.

Ashcraft MW, VanHerle AJ (1981) Management of thyroid nodules II, scanning techniques, thyroid suppressive therapy and fine needle aspiration. Head Neck Surgery 3: 297–322.

Asklen LA, Sothern RB (1998) Seasonal variations in the presentation and growth of thyroid cancer. British Journal of Cancer 77 (7): 1174–9.

Audit Commission (1993) What Seems To Be The Matter: Communication Between Hospital and Patients. NHS Report No. 12. London: HMSO.

BACUP (1995) The Right To Know : A Guide to Information and Support for People Living with Cancer. London: BACUP.

Baile WF, Gibertini M, Scott L, Endicott J (1992) Depression and tumour stage in cancer of the head and neck. Psycho-Oncology 1: 15–24.

Baile WF, Gibertini M, Scott L, Endicott J (1993) Prebiopsy assessment of patients with suspected head and neck cancer. The Journal of Psychosocial Oncology 10 (4): 79–91.

Bakamjian VY (1965) A two-stage method of pharyngoesophageal reconstruction with primary pectoral skin flap. Plastic Reconstructive Surgery 36: 173.

Baker BM, Fraser AM, Baker CD (1991) Long term postoperative dysphagia in oral/ pharyngeal surgery patients; subjects' perceptions vs videofluoroscopic observations. Dysphagia 6: 11–16.

Baker C (1995) A functional status scale for measuring quality of life outcomes in head and neck cancer patients. Cancer Nursing 18 (6): 452–7.

Baker CA (1992) Factors associated with rehabilitation in head and neck cancer. Cancer Nursing 15 (6): 395–400.

Baker DG (1982) The radiobiological basis for tissue reactions in the oral cavity following therapeutic X-radiation. Archives of Otolaryngology 108: 21–24.

Baker K, Feldman J (1993) Thyroid cancer: a review. Oncology Nursing Forum 20: 95–104.

Bale S (1997) Wound dressings. Chapter 6 in Morison M, Moffat C, Bridel-Norton J, Bale S (eds) Nursing Management of Chronic Wounds 2nd edn. London: Mosby.

Balfe DM, Koehler RE, Setzen M et al (1982) Barium examination of the oesophagus after total laryngectomy. Radiology 143: 501–8.

Bandura A (1977a) Social Learning Theory. New York : Prentice Hall.

Bandura A (1977b) Self-efficacy: towards a unifying theory of behaviour change. Psychological Review 84: 191–215.

Banks V, Jones V (1993) Palliative care of a patient with terminal nasal carcinoma. Journal of Wound Care 2 (1): 14–15.

BAPEN (1996) Standards and Guidelines for Nutritional Support of Patients in Hospitals — a report by a working party of the British Association for Parenteral and Enteral Nutrition. Maidenhead: British Association of Parenteral and Enteral Nutrition.

Barendregt JJ et al (1997) The healthcare costs of smoking. New England Journal of Medicine 337 (15): 1052–7.

Barkvoll P, Attramadal A (1989) Effect of nystatin and chlorhexidine digluconate on Candida albicans. Oral Surgery Oral Medicine Oral Pathology 67: 279–81.

Barton Burke M, Wilkes GM, Ingwersen KC (1996) Cancer Chemotherapy. A Nursing Process Approach. Boston: Jones & Bartlett.

Bastow MD (1996) Complication of enteral nutrition. Gut 27(Supplement 1): 51–5.

Beck S (1979) Impact of a systematic oral care protocol on stomatitis after chemotherapy. Cancer Nursing (June): 185–99.

Beddar SM, Aikin JL (1994) Continuity of care: a challenge for ambulatory oncology nursing. Seminars in Oncology Nursing 10 (4): 254–63.

Bedi R (1996) Betel quid and tobacco chewing among the United Kingdom's Bangladeshi Community. British Journal of Cancer 74 (Supplement XX1X): S73–S77.

Benko I et al (1997) A case of fibrin sealant application for closing benign tracheaesophageal fistula. Acta Chir Hung 36 (1–4): 5–26.

Benner P (1984) From Novice To Expert Excellence and Power in Clinical Nursing Practice. California: Addison-Wesley.

Benner P, Wrubel J (1989) The Primacy of Caring: Stress and Coping in Health and Illness. California: Addison-Wesley.

Benninger MS (1992) Medical liaisons for continuity of head and neck cancer care. Head and Neck 14: 28–32.

Benowitz NL (1997) Treating tobacco addiction — nicotine or no nicotine? The New England Journal of Medicine 337 (17): 1230–31.

Berger A, Henderson M, Nadoolam W et al (1995) Oral capsaicin provides temporary relief for oral mucositis pain secondary to chemotherapy/radiation therapy. Journal of Pain and Symptom Management 10 (3): 243–8.

Bergner M, Bobbitt RA (1981) The sickness impact profile: development and final revision of a health status measure. Medical Care 19: 787–805.

Bergonie J, Tribondeau L (1906) De quelques resultats de la radiothérapie et essai de fixation d'une technique rationelle. C R Acad Sci (Paris) 143: 983 cited in Mettler Jr FA, Upton AC (eds) Medical Effects of Ionising Radiation. London: WB Saunders.

Bernstein E F, Sullivan F J, Mitchell J B et al (1993) Biology of chronic radiation effect tissues and wound healing. Clinics in Plastic Surgery 20 (3): 435–53.

Berrouschot J, Oeken J, Steniger L, Schneider D (1997) Perioperative complication of percutaneous dilational tracheostomy. Laryngoscope 107 (11Pt1): 1538–44.

Berthong M (1986) Pathologic changes secondary to radiation. World Journal of Surgery 10: 155–170.

Beumer J III, Harrison R, Sanders et al (1983a) Preradiation dental extractions and the incidence of bone necrosis. Head Neck Surgery 5: 514–21.

Beumer J III, Harrison R, Sanders et al (1983b) Postradiation dental extractions: a review of the literature and a report of 72 episodes. Head Neck Surgery 6: 581–6.

Billy ML, Snow NJ, Haug RH (1994) Tracheocarotid fistula with life threatening haemorrhage; report of a case. Journal of Oral and Maxillofacial Surgery 52 (12): 1331–4.

Bjordal K, Kaasa S (1992) Psychometric validation of the EORTC Quality of Life Questionnaire, 30-item version and a diagnosis specific module for head and neck cancer patients. Acta Oncologica 31 (3): 311–21.

Bjordal K, Kaasa S (1995) Psychological distress in head and neck cancer patients 7–11 years after curative treatment. British Journal of Cancer 71: 592–7.

Bjordal K, Ahlner-Elmqvist M, Tollesson E et al (1994a) Development of a European organisation for research and treatment of cancer (EORTC) questionnaire module to be used in quality of life assessments in head and neck cancer patients. Acta Oncologica 33 (8): 879–85.

Bjordal K, Kaasa S, Mastekaasa A (1994b) Quality of life in patients treated for head and neck cancer: a follow-up study 7 to 11 years after radiotherapy. International Journal of Radiation Oncology Biology Physics 28 (4): 847–56.

Bjordal K, Freng A, Thorvik J, Kaasa S (1995) Patient self-reported and clinician-rated quality of life in head and neck cancer patients: a cross-sectional study. European Journal of Cancer 31B (4): 235–41.

Black FO, Shupert CL, Peterka RJ, Nasher LM (1989) Effects of unilateral loss of vestibular function on the vestibulo-ocular reflex and postural control. Annals of Otology Rhinology Laryngology 98 (11): 884–9.

Blackburn C (1994) Low income, inequality and health promotion. Nursing Times 90 (39): 42–3.

Blakley BW, Gupta AK, Myers SF, Scwan S (1994) Archives of Otolaryngology Head and Neck Surgery 120 (5): 541–6.

Blessing R, Mann W, Beck C (1986) How important is preservation of the accessory nerve in neck dissection? Laryngology Rhinology Otology 65(7): 403–5.

Blom ED (1995) Tracheoesophageal speech. Seminars in Speech and Language 16 (3): 191–204.

Blom ED (1996). Leakage around a tracheoesophageal voice prosthesis. Clinical Insights Newsletter (Fall). Available from the International Center for Post-Laryngectomy Voice Restoration, 7440 North Shadeland, Suite 200, Indianapolis, Indiana 42650, USA.

Blom ED, Hamaker RC (1996) Tracheoesophageal voice restoration following total laryngectomy. In Myers EN, Suen J (eds) Cancer of the Head and Neck. London: WB Saunders.

Blood GW, Simpson KC, Dineen M et al (1994) Spouses of individuals with laryngeal cancer: caregiver strain and burden. Journal of Communication Disorders 27: 19–35.

Bloom B, Gift HC, Jack SS (1992) Dental Services and Oral Health. Washington DC Government Printing Office: Department of Health and Human Services, National Centre for Cancer statistics — DHHS Publication no (PHS) 93–1511 Vital and Health Statistics Series 10, no 83.

Blot WJ, McLaughlin JK, Winn DM et al (1988) Smoking and drinking in relation to oral and pharyngeal cancer. Cancer Research 48: 3282–7.

Bocca E, Pignataro O (1967) A conservation technique in radical neck dissection. Annals of Otology Rhinology Laryngology 76: 975–87.

Bofetta P et al (1992) Carcinogenic effect of tobacco smoke and alcohol drinking on anatomic sites of the oral cavity and oropharynx. International Journal of Cancer 52: 530–33.

Bonanno PC (1971) Swallowing dysfunction after tracheostomy. Annals of Surgery 174: 29–33.

Bottomley A (1997) Cancer support groups — are they effective? European Journal of Cancer Care 6: 11–17.

Bottomley A, Jones L (1997) Social support and the cancer patient — a need for clarity. European Journal of Cancer Care 6: 72–7.

Bowlby J (1969) Attachment. Volume 1 of Attachment and Loss. London: Hogarth.

Boyd KJ, Beeken L (1994) Tube feeding in palliative care: benefits and problems. Palliative Medicine 8: 156–8.

Boyle P, Veronesi U, Tubiana M et al (1995) European School of Oncology advisory report to the European Commission for the Europe Against Cancer Programme: European Code Against Cancer. European Journal of Cancer 31A (9): 1395–1405.

Boys L, Peat SJ, Manna MH, Burn K (1993) Audit of neural blockade for palliative care patients in an acute unit. Palliative Medicine 7: 205–11.

Brady L, Davis L (1988) Treatment of head and neck cancer by radiation therapy. Seminars in Oncology 15 (1): 29–37.

Breitbart W, Holland J (1988) Psychosocial aspects of head and neck cancer. Seminars in Oncology 15 (1): 61–9.

Brennan MJ, Weitz J (1992) Lymphoedema 30 years after radical mastectomy. American Journal of Physical Medicine and Rehabilitation 71: 12–14.

Brimelow M, Wilson J (1982) Ourselves alone. Social Work Today 13: 12–13.

British Medical Association and Royal Pharmaceutical Association of Great Britain (1994) British National Formulary (Number 27). London: BMA/RPSGB.

British Pharmacopoeia (1995) Addendum for Alginate Dressings.

Brock TD, Madigan MT (1991) Normal flora of the oral cavity. In Biology of Micro-organisms 6th edn. New Jersey: Prentice-Hall, pp 389–92

Brotherston TM, Lawrence JC (1993) Dressings for donor sites. Journal of Wound Care 2(2): 84–8.

Browman GP, Wong G, Hodson I et al (1993a) Influence of cigarette smoking on the efficacy of radiation therapy in head and neck cancer. New England Journal of Medicine 328 (3): 159–63.

Browman GP, Levine MN, Hodson DI et al (1993b) The Head and Neck Radiotherapy Questionnaire: a morbidity/quality of life instrument for clinical trials of radiation therapy in locally advanced head and neck cancer. Journal of Clinical Oncology 11 (5): 863–72.

Brown DG, Schatzle KC, Richter DK (1975) Distilled water and saline bottles: important reservoirs of nosocomial infection. Paper presented at American Society for Microbiology 75th Annual Meeting, New York.

Bruera E (1997) ABC of palliative care: anorexia, cachexia and nutrition. British Medical Journal 315: 1219–22.

Brunt LM, Wells SA Jr (1987) Advances in diagnosis and treatment of medullary thyroid carcinoma. Surgical Clinics of North America 67:263–79.

Bryant LR, Kent Trinkle J, Dublier L (1971) Reappraisal of tracheal injury from cuffed tracheostomy tubes. Journal of the American Medical Association 215: 4.

Bryn MR, Younger D (1988) Neurological disorders and aspirations. Otolaryngologic Clinics of North America. 22(4): 691–9.

Buchmann WF (1997) Adherence: a matter of self-efficacy and power. Journal of Advanced Nursing 26: 132–7.

Buchwalter JA, Sasaki CT (1984) Effects of tracheotomy on laryngeal function. Otolaryngologic Clinics of North America 17: 41–8.

Buckman R (1992) How to Break Bad News. Baltimore: The Johns Hopkins University Press.

Bukowski RM (1996) Amifostine (Ethyol): dosing, administration and patient management guidelines. European Journal of Cancer 32A(Supplement 4): 546–9.

Bull R, Rumsey N (1988) The Social Psychology of Facial Appearance. Berlin: Springer-Verlag.

Bunston T, Mings D, Mackie A, Jones D (1995) Facilitating hopefulness: the determinants of hope. Journal of Psychosocial Oncology 13 (4): 79–103.

Burns SL, Adams M (1997) Alcohol history taking by nurses and doctors — how accurate are they? Journal of Advanced Nursing 25: 509–13.

Burns SM, Spilman M, Wilmouth D et al (1998) Are frequent inner cannula changes necessary?: a pilot study. Heart and Lung 27 (1): 58–62.

Bushkin E (1995) Signposts of survivorship. Mara Mogensen Flaherty Lectures: Excellence in the psychosocial care of the patient with cancer. Oncology Nursing Forum 22 (3): 537–43.

Buxton V (1996) Global action. Nursing Times 92 (12): 28–31.

Byers RM, Jesse RH, Guillamondequi OM (1973) Malignant tumors of the submaxillary gland. American Journal of Surgery 126(4): 458–63.

Byrne A, Walsh M, Farrelly M, O'Driscoll K (1993) Depression following laryngectomy. British Journal of Psychiatry 163: 173–6.

Calman K, Hine D (1994) A Policy Framework for Commissioning Cancer Services. London: Department Of Health.

Campbell I, Illingworth M (1992) Can patients wash during radiotherapy to the breast or chest wall? A randomised controlled trial. Clinical Oncology 4: 78–82.

Cancerlink (1988) Starting a Cancer Support and Self-help Group. London: Cancerlink.

Candela FC, Shah J, Jacques DP, Shah JP (1994) Patterns of cervical node metastases from squamous carcinoma of the larynx. Archives of Otolaryngology Head and Neck Surgery 116: 432–5.

Cannon CR (1994) Hypothyroidism in head and neck cancer patients: experimental and clinical observations Laryngoscope 104: 1–21.

Carew JF, Shah JP (1998) Advances in multimodality therapy for laryngeal cancer. CA — A Cancer Journal for Clinicians 48 (4): 211–28.

Carl W, Emrich LS (1991) Management of oral mucositis during local radiation and systemic chemotherapy: a study of 98 patients. The Journal of Prosthetic Dentistry 66 (3): 361–9.

Carnevali D, Reiner A (1990) The Cancer Experience. Nursing Diagnosis and Management. Philadelphia: Lippincott.

Carr DB, Jacox AK, Chapman CR et al (1992) Acute pain management: operative or medical procedures and trauma. Clinical Practice Guideline No. 1. Rockville MD: Agency for Health Care Policy and Research, US Department of Health and Human Services.

Carr EJ (1997) Evaluating the use of a pain assessment tool and care plan: a pilot study. Journal of Advanced Nursing 26: 1073–9.

Carrillo EH, Spain DA, Bumpous JM (1997) Percutaneous dilational tracheostomy for airway control. The American Journal of Surgery 174: 469–73.

Carroll P (1989) Safe suctioning. Nursing 89: 48–51.

Carroll D, Bowsher D (1993) Pain Management and Nursing Care. Oxford: Butterworth-Heinemann Ltd.

Carter RL, Pittam MR, Tanner NSB (1982) Pain and dysphagia in patients with squamous carcinomas of the head and neck: the role of perineural spread. Journal of the Royal Society of Medicine 75: 598–606.

Casey D (1988) Carotid 'blow-out'. Nursing Standard 2(47): 30.

Casley-Smith JR, Morgan RG, Piller NB (1993) Treatment of lymphoedema of the arms and legs with 5,6-benzopyrone. New England Journal of Medicine 329: 1158–63.

Casper JK, Colton RH (1993a) Medical/surgical examination, diagnosis, and treatment. In Clinical Manual for Laryngectomy and Head and Neck Cancer Rehabilitation 1st edn. Clinical Competence Series. San Diego: Singular Publishing Group.

Casper JK, Colton RH (1993b) Oral cavity rehabilitation. In Clinical Manual for Laryngectomy and Head and Neck Cancer Rehabilitation 1st edn. Clinical Competence Series. San Diego: Singular Publishing Group.

Castel O, Agius G, Grignon B (1991) Evaluation of closed sterile prefilled humidification. Journal of Hospital Infection 17: 53–9.

Castelijns JA, Becker M, Hermans R (1996) Impact of cartilage invasion on treatment and prognosis of laryngeal cancer. European Radiology 6: 156–69.

Cervellino JC, Aranjo CE, Pirisi C et al (1991) Ifosfamide and mesna for the treatment of advanced squamous head and neck cancer: a Getlac study. Oncology 48: 89–92.

Chamberlain J (1993) Evaluation of screening for cancer. Community Dental Health 10 (Supplement 1): 5–11.

Chambers P, Harris L, Mitchell DA, Corrigan AM (1997) Comparative study of the ipsilateral full thickness forearm skin graft in closure of radial forearm flap donor site defects. Journal of Cranio-Maxillofacial Surgery 25: 245–8.

Chambers PA, Worral SF (1994) Closure of large orocutaneous fistulas in end-stage malignant disease. British Journal of Oral and Maxillofacial Surgery 32: 314–15.

Chang JT, See LC, Tang SG (1996) The role of brachytherapy in early stage nasopharyngeal carcinoma. International Journal of Radiation Oncology Biology Physics 36 (5): 1019–24.

Changing Faces (1996) The Psychology of Facial Disfigurement. London: Changing Faces.

Chaturvedi SK, Shenoy A, Prasad KMR et al (1996) Concerns, coping and quality of life in head and neck cancer patients. Supportive Care in Cancer 4: 186–90.

Cheeseman AD, Lund VJ (1986) Craniofacial resection for tumours of the nasal cavity and paranasal sinuses. Head Neck Surgery 8:429–35.

Chencharick J, Mossman KL (1983) Nutritional consequences of the radiotherapy of head and neck cancers. Cancer 51: 811–15.

Chernecky C, Berger B (1998) Airway obstruction. Chapter 5 in Advanced and Critical Care Oncology Nursing. Managing Primary Complications. Philadelphia: WB Saunders Company.

Chi DD, Moley JF (1998) Medullary thyroid carcinoma: genetic advances, treatment recommendations, and the approach to the patient with persistent hypercalcitonaemia. Surgical Oncology Clinics of North America 7 (4): 681–706.

Clark D (1995) Advising your client on nicotine replacement aids. Professional Care of Mother and Child 5 (3): 72–4.

Clarke A (1998) What happened to your face? Managing facial disfigurement. British Journal of Community Nursing 3 (1): 13–16.

Clarke L (1992) Caring for fungating tumours. Nursing Times (Journal of Wound Care) 88 (12): 66–70.

Clarke L (1995) A critical event in tracheostomy care. British Journal of Nursing 4 (12): 676–81.

Coates D, Death JE (1982) Use of buffered hypochlorite solution for disinfecting fibrescopes. Journal of Clinical Pathology 35 (3): 296–303.

Cohen B, Powswillo DE, Woods DA (1971) The effect of exposure to chewing tobacco on the oral mucosa of monkey and man. Annals of the Royal College of Surgeons of England 48: 255–73.

Cohen F, Lazarus RS (1979) Coping with the stresses of illness. In Stone G et al (Eds) Health Psychology. San Francisco: Jossey-Bass, pp. 217–55.

Cohen H (1994) Vestibular rehabilitation improves daily life function. American Journal of Occupational Therapy 48 (10): 919–25.

Colacchio TA, LoGerfo P, Colacchio DA, Feind C (1982) Radioiodine total body scan versus serum thyroglobulin levels in follow-up of patients with thyroid cancer. Surgery 91(1): 42–5.

Colevas AD, Busse PM, Norris CM et al (1998) Induction chemotherapy with docetaxel, cisplatin, fluorouracil, and leucovorin for squamous cell carcinoma of the head and neck: a phase i/ii trial. Journal of Clinical Oncology 16 (4): 1331–9.

Collier M (1997a) The assessment of patients with malignant fungating wounds — a holistic approach: Part 1. Nursing Times 93 (44): NT Professional Update insert.

Collier M (1997b) The assessment of patients with malignant fungating wounds — a holistic approach: Part 2. Nursing Times 93 (45): NT Professional Update insert.

Conger AD (1973) Loss and recovery of taste acuity in patients irradiated to the oral cavity. Radiation Research 53: 338–47.

Conkling V (1989) Continuity of care issues for cancer patients and families. Cancer 64 (1): 290–94.

Cooper D (1994a) Problem drinking. Nursing Times 90 (14): 36–9.

Cooper D (1994b) Alcohol Home Detoxification and Assessment. Oxford: Radcliffe Medical Press.

Copp G, Dunn V (1993) Frequent and difficult problems perceived by nurses caring for the dying in the community, hospice and acute care settings. Palliative Medicine 7: 19–25.

Coull A (1992) Making sense of surgical flaps. Nursing Times 88(1): 32–43.

Coull A, Wylie C (1990) Regular monitoring: the way to ensure flap healing. Professional Nurse 6(1): 18–21.

Cowan T (1997) Patient-controlled analgesia devices. Professional Nurse 13 (2): 119–24.

Coyle N, Cherny N, Portenoy RK (1995) Pharmacologic management of cancer pain. Chapter 5 in McGuire DB, Yarbro HC, Ferrell BR (eds) Cancer Pain Management, 2nd edn. London: Jones & Bartlett.

Craddock C (1993) Head and neck cancer prevention: the new challenge. Seminars in Oncology Nursing 9 (3): 169–73.

Craven A, West R (1987) Counselling and care of laryngectomees: a preliminary study. British Journal of Communication Disorders 22: 237–43.

Crile G (1906) Excision of cancer of the head and neck. Journal of the American Medical Association 47: 1780.

Crimlisk JT, Horn MH, Wilson DJ, Marino B (1996) Artificial airways: a survey of cuff management practices. Heart Lung 25 (3): 225–35.

Critchley D, Roulsten J (1993) Nurses' knowledge of nebulised therapy. Nursing Standard 8 (10): 37–9.

Cronin CJ, Maklebust J (1989) Case-managed care: capitalizing on the CNS. Nursing Management 20: 41–7.

Crosby LJ, Parsons LC (1974) Measurements of lateral wall pressure exerted by tracheostomy and endotracheal tube cuffs. Heart and Lung 3: 5.

Crosher R, Baldie C, Mitchell R (1997) Selective use of tracheostomy in surgery for head and neck cancer: an audit. British Journal of Maxillofacial Surgery 35 (1): 43–5.

Crow S, Carroll PF (1985) Changing the suction catheter each time you enter a tracheostomy; necessity or waste? Nursing Life 5 (3): 44–5.

Crumley, RL (1990) Teflon versus thyroplasty versus nerve transfer: a comparison. Annals of Otology Rhinology Laryngology 99:759–63.

CSG (1998) Improving Clinical Communications. Wetherby: Department of Health, Two Ten Communications Ltd.

Cullen N (1998) Getting to grips with the research evidence. Nursing Times 94 (21): 60–1.

Cummings CW (1974) Incidence of nodal metastases in T2 supraglottic carcinoma. Archives of Otolaryngology 99: 268–9.

Cunningham AJ, Lockwood GA, Cunningham JA (1991) A relationship between perceived self-efficacy and quality of life in cancer patients. Patient Education and Counselling 17: 71–8.

Cutting K (1997) Wounds and evidence of infection. Nursing Standard 11 (25): 49–51.

Czarnik RE, Stone KS, Everhart CC et al (1991) Differential effects of continuous versus intermittent suction on tracheal tissue. Heart and Lung 20 (2): 144–51.

Daeffler R (1980) Oral hygiene measures for patients with cancer II. Cancer Nursing 3: 427–32.

Daeffler R (1981) Oral hygiene measures for patients with cancer III. Cancer Nursing 4: 29–35.

Daly JM, Hoffman K, Lieberman M et al (1990) Nutritional support in the cancer patient. Journal of Parenteral and Enteral Nutrition 14 (6): Supplement; 2445–85.

D'Antonio LL, Zimmerman GJ, Cella DF, Long SA (1996) Quality of life and functional status measures in patients with head and neck cancer. Archives of Otolaryngology Head and Neck Surgery 122: 482–7.

D'Antonio LL, Long SA, Zimmerman GJ et al (1998) Relationship between quality of life and depression in patients with head and neck cancer. Laryngoscope 108: 806–11.

Dattatreya A, Nuijen MS, Van Swaaij AC, Klopper PJ (1991) Evaluation of boiled potato peel as a wound dressing. Burns 17(4): 323–8.

Davies ADM, Davies C, Delpo MC (1986) Depression and anxiety in patients undergoing diagnostic investigations for head and neck cancers. British Journal of Psychiatry 149: 491–3.

Davis JW (1989). Prosthodontic management of swallowing disorders. Dysphagia 3: 199–205.

Davison C (1994) Conflicts of interest. Nursing Times 90 (13): 40–2.

Dear S (1995) Breaking bad news: caring for the family. Nursing Standard 10 (11): 31–3.

De Boer MF, Pruyn JF, Van den Borne B et al (1995) Rehabilitation outcomes of long-term survivors treated for head and neck cancer. Head and Neck 17: 503–15.

Deems DA, Doty RL, Settle RG et al (1991) Smell and taste disorders, a study of 750 patients from the University of Pennsylvania smell and taste centre. Archives of Otolarngology Head and Neck Surgery 117: 519–28.

Deleyiannis FW, Weymuller EA, Coltrera MD (1997) Quality of life of disease free survivors of advanced (stage III or IV) oropharyngeal cancer. Head and Neck 19: 466–73.

Demers RR, Saklad M (1976) The aetiology, pathophysiology and treatment of atelectasis. Respiratory Care 27: 234–9.

Department of Health and Social Security (1987) Restriction on the use of Crystal Violet. The Pharmaceutical Journal 239 (665).

Department of Health (1998) Nutritional aspects of the development of cancer. Report on Health and Social Subjects 48. Norwich: The Stationery Office.

Department of Veterans Affairs Laryngeal Cancer Study Group (1991) Induction chemotherapy plus radiation compared with surgery plus radiation in patients with advanced laryngeal cancer. New England Journal of Medicine 324: 1685–90.

Depondt J, Gehanno P (1995) Laryngectomised patients' education and follow-up. Patient Education and Counselling 26: 33–6.

De Santo LW (1985) Cancer of the supraglottic larynx: a review of 260 patients. Otolaryngology — Head and Neck Surgery 93: 705–11.

Dettelbach MA, Gross RD, Mahlmann J, Eibling DE (1995) Effect of the Passy Muir valve on aspiration in patients with tracheostomy. Head and Neck 17 (4): 297–302.

Deveney K (1990) Endoscopic gastrostomy and jejunostomy. In Rombeau JL, Caldwell MD (eds) Clinical Nutrition Enteral and Parenteral Feeding, 2nd edn. Philadelphia: WB Saunders Company.

Devine EC, Cook TD (1983) A meta-analytic analysis of effects of psychoeducational interventions on length of postsurgical hospital stay. Nursing Research 32 (5): 267–73.

Devins GM, Henderikus HJ, Koopmans JP (1994) Psychosocial impact of laryngectomy mediated by perceived stigma and illness intrusiveness. Canadian Journal of Psychiatry 39: 608–16.

DeWalt EM (1975) Effect of timed hygienic measures on oral mucosa in a group of elderly subjects. Nursing Research 24 (2): 104–8.

DeWalt EM, Haines AK (1969) The effects of specified stressors on healthy oral mucosa. Nursing Research 18 (1): 22–7.

Dhooper SS (1985) Social work with laryngectomees. Health and Social Work: 217–27.

DiClemente CC, Prochaska JO, Fairhurst SK et al (1991) The processes of smoking cessation: an analysis of precontemplation, contemplation and preparation stages of change. Journal of Consulting and Clinical Psychology 59: 295–304.

Dikeman KJ, Kazandjian MS (1995) Communication and swallowing management of tracheostomized and ventilator dependent adults. In Pathophysiology of Swallowing. San Diego: Singular Publishing Group.

Dinman S, Giovannone MK (1994) The care and feeding of microvascular flaps: how nurses can help prevent flap loss. Plastic Surgical Nursing 14(3): 154–64.

Dodd MJ (1987) Efficacy of proactive information on self-care in radiation therapy patients. Heart and Lung 16 (5): 538–44.

Dodd MJ, Larson PJ, Dibble SL (1996) Randomized clinical trial of chlorhexidine versus placebo for prevention of oral mucositis in patients receiving chemotherapy. Oncology Nursing Forum 23 (6): 921–7.

Doerr TD, Marunick MT (1997) Timing of edentulation and extraction in the management of oral cavity and oropharyngeal malignancies. Head and Neck 19: 426–30.

Doherty C, Lynch G, Noble S (1986) Granuflex hydrocolloid as a donor site dressing. Care of the Critically Ill 2: 5.

Donnelly MJ, O'Meara N, O'Dwyer TP (1995) Thyroid dysfunction following combined therapy for laryngeal cancer. Clinical Otolaryngology 20: 254–7.

Donner B, Zenz M, Strumpf M, Raber M (1998) Long-term treatment of cancer pain with transdermal fentanyl. Journal of Pain and Symptom Management 15 (3): 168–75.

Dow KH, Ferrel BR, Anello C (1997a) Balancing the demands of cancer surveillance among survivors of thyroid cancer. Cancer Practice 5 (5): 289–95.

Dow KH, Ferrel BR, Anello C (1997b) Quality of life changes in patients with thyroid cancer after withdrawal of thyroid hormone therapy. Thyroid 7 (4): 613–19.

Downer MC (1993) Patterns of disease and treatment and their implications for dental health services research. Community Dental Health 10 (2): 39–46.

Drettner B, Allbom A (1983) Quality of life and state of health for patients with cancer of the head and neck. Acta Otolaryngologica 96: 307–14.

Dropkin MJ (1979) Compliance in postoperative head and neck patients. Cancer Nursing October: 379–84.

Dropkin MJ (1989) Coping with disfigurement and dysfunction after head and neck cancer surgery: a conceptual framework. Seminars in Oncology Nursing 5 (3): 213–19.

Dropkin MJ, Scott DW (1983) Body image reintegration and coping effectiveness after head and neck surgery. Journal of the Society of Otorhinolaryngology Head and Neck Nursing 2: 7–16.

Dropkin MJ, Malgrady RG, Scott DW et al (1983) Scaling of disfigurement and dysfunction in postoperative head and neck patients. Head and Neck Surgery 6: 559–70.

Dudjak L (1987) Mouth care for mucositis due to radiation therapy. Cancer Nursing 10 (3): 131–40.

Duffy V (1996) The flavour of food? It's all in your head! Journal of the American Dietetic Association 96 (7): 655–6.

Duffy V, Backstrand J, Ferris A (1995) Olfactory dysfunction and related nutritional risk in free-living, elderly women. Journal of the American Dietetic Association 95 (8): 879–84.

Dukes MNG (1993) Meyler's Side Effects of Drugs: An Encyclopaedia of Adverse Reactions and Interactions, 12th edn. Amsterdam: Elsevier.

Dunlop RJ, Ellershaw JE, Baines MJ et al (1995) On withholding nutrition and hydration in the terminally ill: has palliative medicine gone too far? A reply. Journal of Medical Ethics 21 (3): 141–3.

Duxbury AJ, Thakker NS, Wastell DG (1989) A double blind cross over trial of a mucin-containing artificial saliva. British Dental Journal 166 (4): 115–20.

Dzurec LC (1997) Experiences of fatigue and depression before and after low dose l-thyroxine supplementation in essentially euthyroid individuals. Research in Nursing and Health 20: 389–98.

Edels Y (1979) Some Aspects Relevant to the Successful Acquisition of Pseudo-Voice. Laryngectomy Rehabilitation Seminars. A Macmillan Report. London: The National Association of Laryngectomy Clubs.

Edwards D (1997) Face to Face. Patient, Family and Professional Perspectives of Head and Neck Cancer Care. London: King's Fund Publishing.

Edwards G, Gross MM (1976) Alcohol dependence; provisional description of a clinical syndrome. British Medical Journal 1: 1058–61.

Edwards J (1998) Plastic surgery: a community perspective. Journal of Community Nursing 12(10): 22–6.

EEC Directive (1993) Class 11A, Rule 7 Council directive concerning medical devices 93/42.

Eilers J, Berger AM, Petersen MC (1988) Development, testing, and application of the oral assessment guide. Oncology Nursing Forum 15 (3): 325–30.

Einfeldt H, Henkel M, Schmidt-Auffurth T, Lange G (1986) Therapeutic and palliative lymph drainage in the treatment of face and neck edema. HNO 34: 365–7 (German).

Ekberg O, Nylander G (1983). Webs and weblike formations in the pharynx and cervical oesophagus. Diagnostic Imaging 52: 10–18.

Elia M (1990) Artificial nutritional support. Medicine International 82: 3392–6.

El Kilany (1980) Complications of tracheostomy. Ear, Nose and Throat Journal 59: 123–8.

El-Sarraf M, LeBlanc M, Shanker Giri PG et al (1998) Chemoradiotherapy versus radiotherapy in patients with advanced nasopharyngeal cancer; Phase III randomised intergroup study 0099. Journal of Clinical Oncology 16 (4): 1310–17.

Enderby P, Crow E (1995) The effect of dairy products on the viscosity of saliva. Clincal Rehabilitation 9: 61–4.

Epstein JB, Stewart KH (1993) Radiation therapy and pain in patients with head and neck cancer. European Journal of Cancer 29B (3): 191–9.

Epstein JB, Jones CK (1993) Presenting signs and symptoms of nasopharyngeal carcinoma. Oral Surgery Oral Medicine Oral Pathology 75: 32–6.

Epstein JB, Stevenson-Moore P, Jackson S et al (1989) Prevention of oral mucositis in radiation therapy: a controlled study with benzydamine hydrochloride rinse. International Journal of Radiation Oncology Biology Physics 16: 1571–5.

Ernst E, Pittler MH (1998) The effectiveness of acupuncture in treating acute dental pain: a systematic review. British Dental Journal 184 (9): 443–7.

Essex B, Doig R, Renshaw J (1990) Pilot study of records shared care for people with mental illness. British Medical Journal 300: 1442–6.

Ethridge P, Lamb GS (1989) Professional nursing case management improves quality, access and cost. Nursing Management 20: 30–5.

Evans E (1990) Communication aids. In Evans E (ed) Working with Laryngectomees. Bicester: Winslow Press.

Eveson JW, Cawson RA (1985) Salivary gland tumours: a review of 2410 cases with particular reference to histological types, sites, age and sex distribution. Journal of Pathology 146: 51–8.

Faithfull S (1998) Fatigue in patients receiving radiotherapy. Professional Nurse 13 (7): 459–61.

Fajardo LF (1982) Salivary glands and pancreas. In Masson (ed) Pathology of radiation injury. New York: Springer-Verlag, pp 77–87.

Fallowfield L (1993) Giving sad or bad news. The Lancet 341: 476–8.

Fallowfield L, Baum M (1989) Psychological welfare of patients with breast cancer. Journal of the Royal Society of Medicine 82: 4–5.

Fallowfield LJ, Baum M, Maguire GP et al (1987) Addressing the psychological needs of the conservatively treated cancer patient. Journal of the Royal Society of Medicine 80: 696–700 .

Fallowfield L, Ford S, Lewis S (1995) No news is not good news: information preferences of patients with cancer. Psycho-Oncology 4: 197–202.

Farberow NL, Ganzler S, Cutter F et al (1971) An eight year survey of hospital suicides. Life Threatening Behaviour 1: 184–201.

Feber T (1995) Mouth care for patients receiving oral irradiation. Professional Nurse 10 (10): 666–70.

Feber T (1996) Management of mucositis in oral irradiation. Clinical Oncology 8: 106–11.

Feber T (1998) Design and evaluation of a strategy to provide support and information for people with cancer of the larynx. European Journal of Cancer Nursing 2 (2): 106–14.

Feldman SA, Deal CW, Urquhart W (1966) Disturbance of swallowing after tracheostomy. The Lancet 1: 954–5.

Fell H, Boehm M (1998) Easing the discomfort of oxygen therapy. Nursing Times 94 (38): 56–8.

Felton G, Huss K, Payne EA, Sric K (1976) Preoperative nursing intervention with the patient for surgery: outcomes of three alternative approaches. International Journal of Nursing Studies 13: 83–96.

Ferretti GA, Ash RC, Brown AT et al (1987) Chlorhexidine for prophylaxis against oral infections and associated complications in patients receiving bone marrow transplants. Journal of the American Dental Association 114: 461–7.

Fialka V, Vinzenz K (1988) Investigations into shoulder function after radical neck dissection. Journal of Craniomaxillofacial Surgery 16 (3): 143–7.

Fiegenbaum W (1981) A social training programme for clients with facial disfigurations: a contribution to the rehabilitation of cancer patients. International Journal of Rehabilitation Research 44: 501–9.

Fieler VK, Wlasowicz G, Mitchell ML et al (1996) Information preferences of patients undergoing radiation therapy. Oncology Nursing Forum 23 (10): 1603–8.

Finlay H (1995) Oral fungal infections. European Journal of Palliative Care 2 (2): Supplement 1; 4–7.

Finlay IG, Bowszyc J, Ramlau C, Gwiezdzinski Z (1996) The effect of topical 0.75% metronidazole gel on malodorous cutaneous ulcers. Journal of Pain and Symptom Management 11 (3): 158–62.

Fiorenti A (1992) Potential hazards of tracheobroncial suctioning. Intensive and Critical Care Nursing 8: 217–26.

Fisch U (1978) Infratemporal fossa approach to tumours of the temporal bone and base of skull. Journal of Laryngology and Otology 92: 949–67.

Fisch U (1982) Infratemporal fossa approach for glomus tumors of the temporal bone. Annals of Otology Rhinology Laryngology 91: 474–9.

Fisch U (1983) The infratemporal fossa approach for nasopharyngeal tumors. Laryngoscope 93: 36–44.

Fisher SG (1983) The psychosexual effects of cancer and cancer treatment. Oncology Nursing Forum 10 (2): 63–8.

Fitzpatrick PJ, Tepperman BS, Deboer G (1984) Multiple primary squamous cell carcinomas in the upper digestive tract. International Journal of Radiation Oncology, Biology, Physics 10(12): 2273–9.

Flannagan M (1997) Wound cleansing. Chapter 5 in Morison M, Moffat C, Bridel-Norton J, Bale S (eds) Nursing Management of Chronic Wounds, 2nd edn. London: Mosby.

Fletcher CDM (1995) Diagnostic Histopathology of Tumours, Volume 1. Edinburgh: Churchill Livingstone.

Flotra L, Gjermo P, Rolla G, Waerhaug J (1971) A 4-month study on the effect of chlorhexidine mouth washes on 50 soldiers. Scandinavian Journal of Dental Research 80: 10–17.

Foldi E, Foldi M, Clodius L (1989) The lymphedema chaos: a lancet. Annals of Plastic Surgery 22: 505–15.

Foltz AT (1980) Nursing care of ulcerating metastatic lesions. Oncology Nursing Forum 7 (2): 8–13.

Foote RL, Loprinzi CL, Frank AR et al (1994) Randomized trial of a chlorhexidine mouthwash for alleviation of radiation-induced mucositis. Journal of Clinical Oncology 12 (12): 2630–3.

Forbes K (1997) Palliative care in head and neck cancer. Clinical Otolaryngology 22: 117–22.

Ford P, Walsh M (1989) Nursing Rituals, Research and Rational Actions. Oxford: Butterworth-Heinemann.

Ford S, Fallowfield L, Hall A, Lewis S (1995) The influence of audiotapes on patient participation in the cancer consultation. European Journal of Cancer 31A (13/14): 2264–9.

Forastiere AA (1993) Use of paclitaxel (Taxol) in squamous cell carcinoma of the head and neck. Seminars in Oncology 20 (supplement 3): 56–60.

Forastiere AA (1994) Overview of platinum chemotherapy in head and neck cancer. Seminars in Oncology 21 (supplement 12): 20–7.

Fortunato L, Ridge JA (1995) Surgical palliation of head and neck cancer. Current Problems in Cancer 19(3): 153–65.

Fotheringham K (1998) And now a few words from our good friends the audiologists. ENT/Maxillofacial Nursing Forum Newsletter, Winter: 5–6.

Fountzilas G, Athanassiades A, Kalogera-Fountzila A (1997) Paclitaxel in combination with carboplatin or gemcitabine for the treatment of advanced head and neck cancer. Seminars in Oncology 24 (supplement 19): 28–32.

Fowler A (1994) Nursing management of a patient with burns. British Journal of Nursing 3 (21): 1105 –12.

Franchesci S, La Vecchia C, Bidoli E (1998) High incidence of thyroid cancer in central Italy. International Journal of Cancer 77 (3): 481–2.

Freeman JA, Nairne J (1995) Using a class setting to teach Cawthorne-Cooksey exercises as a means of vestibular rehabilitation. Physiotherapy 81 (7): 374–9.

Freedman HM, Kern EB (1979) Complications of intranasal ethmoidectomy. A review of 1000 consecutive operations. Laryngoscope 89: 421–34.

Frith B (1991) Giving information to radiotherapy patients. Nursing Standard 5 (34): 33–5.

Frye FD, Schwartz BS, Doty RL (1990) Chronic dose related influence of cigarette smoking on olfactory function. Journal of the American Medical Association 263: 1223–36.

Fu KK, Phillips TL (1991) Biologic rationale of combined radiotherapy and chemotherapy. Hematology Oncology Clinics of North America 5: 737–51.

Funk GF, Karnell LH, Dawson CJ et al (1997) Baseline and post-treatment assessment of the general health status of head and neck cancer patients compared with United States population norms. Head and Neck 19: 675–83.

Funk GF, Arcuri MR, Frodel JL (1998) Functional dental rehabilitation of massive palatomaxillary defects: cases requiring free tissue transfer and osseointegrated implants. Head and Neck 20: 38–51.

Futran ND, Trotti A, Gwede C (1997) Pentoxifylline in the treatment of radiation related soft tissues injury: preliminary observations. Laryngoscope 107: 391–5.

Galanti MR, Sparen P, Karlsson A et al (1995) Is residence in areas of endemic goitre a risk factor for thyroid cancer? International Journal of Cancer 61: 615–21.

Gamba A, Romano M, Grosso IM et al (1992) Psychosocial adjustment of patients surgically treated for head and neck cancer. Head and Neck 14: 218–23.

Gammon J (1998) Analysis of the effects of hospitalisation and source isolation on coping and psychological constructs. International Journal of Nursing Practice 4(2): 84–96.

Ganley BJ (1996) Mouth care for the patient undergoing head and neck radiation therapy: a survey of radiation oncology nurses. Oncology Nursing Forum 23 (10): 1619–23.

Gardine RL, Kokal WA, Beatty D, Riitimati du Wagman LD (1988) Predicting the need for prolonged enteral supplementation in the patient with head and neck cancer. American Journal of Surgery 156: 63–5.

Gelder MG, Edwards G (1968) Metronidazole in the treatment of alcohol addiction: a controlled trial. British Journal of Psychiatry 114: 473–5.

Gelman JJ, Aro M, Weiss SM (1994) Tracheo-innominate artery fistula. Journal of the American College of Surgeons 179 (5): 626–34.

Gerbaulet AP, Haie-Meder CM, Habrand JL (1993) Clinical brachytherapy for head and neck cancer. Refresher course at the ESTRO Meeting New Orleans. In ESTRO (1998) Teaching Course on Modern Brachytherapy Techniques, Volume 2. Berlin: ESTRO.

Gharib H, Goellner JR, and Johnson DA (1993) Fine-needle aspiration cytology of the thyroid. A 12-year experience with 11,000 biopsies. Clinical Laboratory Medicine 13: 699–709.

Ghosh S, Eastwood MA (1994) Percutaneous endoscopic gastrostomy: a user's perspective. Journal of Human Nutrition and Dietetics 7: 2331–5.

Gill-Body KM, Popat RA, Parker SW, Krebs DE (1997) Rehabilitation of balance in two patients with cerebellar dysfunction. Physical Therapy 77 (5): 534–52.

Gillham L (1994) Lymphoedema and physiotherapists: control not cure. Physiotherapy 80 (12): 835–43.

Ginsberg MK (1961) A study of oral hygiene nursing care. The American Journal of Nursing 61 (10): 67–9.

Giovanni A, Robert D, Teston B et al (1996) Preliminary study of acoustic and aerodynamic parameters after Tucker frontal anterior laryngectomy. Annales d'Oto-Laryngologie et de Chirurgie Cervico- Faciale 113 (5): 277–84.

Giuliano J, Rudy S (1995) Nursing care of the patient with trismus. ORL—Head and Neck Nursing 13(1): 23–30.

Glanz H, Kimmich T, Eichhorn T, Kleinsasser O (1989) Results of treatment of 584 laryngeal cancers at the Ear-Nose-Throat Clinic of Marburg University. HNO 37: 1–10.

Gliklich RE, Goldsmith TA, Funk GF (1997) Are head and neck specific quality of life measures necessary? Head and Neck 19: 474–80.

Goffman E. (1963) Stigma. Notes on the Management of Spoiled Identity. London: Penguin.

Goldbold JH, Tompkins EA (1979) A long term mortality study of workers occupationally exposed to metallic nickel at the Oak Ridge Diffusion Plant. Journal of Occupational Medicine 21: 799–806.

Goldman JM, Goren EN, Cohen MH et al (1980) Anaplastic thyroid carcinoma: long-term survival after radical surgery. Journal of Surgical Oncology 14 (4): 389–94.

Goldman MS, Brown SA, Christiansen BA (1987) Expectancy theory: thinking about drinking. In Blane HT, Leonard KE (eds) Psychological Theories of Drinking and Alcoholism. New York: The Guilford Press.

Gotay CC, Moore TD (1992) Assessing quality of life in head and neck cancer. Quality of Life Research 1: 5–17.

Graham K, Pecoraro DA, Ventura M, Meyer CC (1993) Reducing the incidence of stomatitis using a quality assessment and improvement approach. Cancer Nursing 16 (2): 117–22.

Greenfield S, Kaplan S, Ware JE (1985) Expanding patient involvement in care. Annals of Internal Medicine 102: 520–8.

Griffiths J, Boyle S (1993) Colour Guide to Holistic Oral Care. A Practical Approach. London: Mosby-Year Book.

Grillo HC, Zannini PL (1986) Resectional management of airway invasion by thyroid carcinoma. Annals of Thoracic Surgery 42: 287–98.

Grillo HC, Donahue DM, Mathisen DJ et al (1995) Postintubation tracheal stenosis. Treatment and results. Journal of Thoracic and Cardiovascular Surgery 109 (3): 486–92.

Greenspan FS (1997) The role of fine needle aspiration biopsy in the management of palpable thyroid nodules. American Journal of Clinical Pathology 108 (4): Supplement 1; S26–S30.

Grindel CG, Whitmer K, Barsevice A (1996) Quality of life and nutritional support in patients with cancer. Cancer Practice 4 (2): 81–7.

Grocott P (1992) The latest on latex. Nursing Times 88 (12): 61–2.

Grocott P (1995) The palliative management of fungating malignant wounds. Journal of Wound Care 4 (5): 239–42.

Grocott P (1997) Evaluation of a tool used to assess the management of fungating wounds. Journal of Wound Care 6 (9): 421–4.

Groher M (1997) Neurologic disorders of swallowing. In Dysphagia: Diagnosis and Management, 3rd edn. Newton MA: Butterworth-Heinemann.

Grolman W, Schouwenburg PF, de Boer MF (1995). First results with the Blom-Singer adjustable tracheostoma valve. Oto-Rhino-Laryngology 57: 165–70.

Grond S, Zech D, Lynch J et al (1993) Validation of World Health Organisation guidelines for pain relief in head and neck cancer. A prospective study. Annals of Otology Rhinology Laryngology 102: 342–8.

Grunow JE, Christenson JC, Moutos D (1989) Contamination of enteral nutrition systems during prolonged intermittent use. Journal of Enteral and Parenteral Nutrition 13: 23–5.

Gupta SC, Ahluwalia H (1996) Fractured tracheostomy tube: an overlooked foreign body. Journal of Laryngology and Otology 110 (11): 1069–71.

Guthrie TH, Brubaker LHJ, Porubsky ES et al (1990) Circadian cisplatin, bleomycin, and 5-FU in advanced squamous cell carcinoma of the head and neck. Proceedings of the American Society of Clinical Oncology 9: 175.

Gutt LN, Held S, Paolucci V, Encke A (1996) Experiences with percutaneous endoscopic gastrostomy. World Journal of Surgery 20 (8): 1006–8. Discussion 1108–9.

Guyton D, Banner MJ, Kirby RR (1991) High volume low pressure cuffs. Are they always low pressure? Chest 100: 1076–81.

Haas CD, Coltman CA, Gottlieb JA et al (1976) Phase II evaluation of bleomycin. Seminars in Oncology 38 (8): 8–12.

Haddock J, Burrows C (1997) The role of the nurse in health promotion: an evaluation of a smoking cessation programme in surgical pre-admission clinics. Journal of Advanced Nursing 26: 1098–110.

Hagopian G (1996) The effects of informational audiotapes on knowledge and self-care behaviours of patients undergoing radiation therapy. Oncology Nursing Forum 23 (4): 697–700.

Haisfield-Wolfe ME (1997) Malignant cutaneous wounds: a management protocol. Ostomy/Wound Management 43 (1): 56–66.

Hakaim AG, Esselstyn CB (1993) Parathyroid carcinoma: a 50 year experience at the Cleveland Clinic Foundation. Cleveland Clinic Journal of Medicine 60: 331–5.

Halbreich U (1974) Tegretol dependency and diversion of the sense of taste. Israel Annals of Psychiatry 12: 328–32, cited in Mott AE (1992) General medical evaluation of chemosensory dysfunction. Journal of Head Trauma and Rehabilitation 7 (1): 25–41.

Hall B, Waterman H (1997) The psychosocial aspects of visual impairment in diabetes. Nursing Standard 11 (39): 40–46.

Hall P, Holm LE (1998) Radiation-associated thyroid cancer — facts and fiction. Acta Oncologia 37 (4): 325–30.

Hallquist A, Hardell L, Degerman A et al (1994) Medical diagnostic and therapeutic radiation and the risk of thyroid cancer. A case control study. European Journal of Cancer Prevention 3: 259–67.

Hamaker RC, Hamaker RA (1995) Surgical treatment of laryngeal cancer. Seminars in Speech and Language 16 (3): 221–31.

Hamlar D, Schuller D, Reinhard A et al (1996) Determination of the efficacy of topical oral pilocarpine for postirradiation xerostomia in patients with head and neck carcinoma. Laryngoscope 106: 972–6.

Hammerlid E, Bjordal K, Ahlner-Elmquist M et al (1997) Prospective, longitudinal quality of life study of patients with head and neck cancer: a feasibility study including the EORTC QLQ-C30. Otolaryngology—Head and Neck Surgery 116 (6): 666–73.

Hammerlid E, Wirblad B, Sandin C et al (1998) Malnutrition and food intake in relation to quality of life in head and neck cancer patients. Head and Neck 20: 540–48.

Hampson JP (1996) The use of metronidazole in treatment of malodorous wounds. Journal of Wound Care 5 (9): 421–6.

Hanks JB, Fisher ST, Myers WC et al. (1981) Effect of total laryngectomy on oesophageal motility. Annals of Otology Rhinology Laryngology 90: 331–4.

Hanley MV, Rudd T, Butler J (1978) What happens to intratracheal saline instillations? American Review of Respiratory Disease 117: 124.

Hansky J (1973) The use of oesophageal motility studies in the diagnosis of dysphagia. Australian New Zealand Journal of Surgery 42: 360–1.

Hanucharurnkul S (1989) Predictors of self-care in cancer patients receiving radiotherapy. Cancer Nursing 12 (1): 21–7.

Harari P (1997) Why has induction chemotherapy for head and neck cancer become a United States community standard practice? Journal of Clinical Oncology 15 (5): 2050–5.

Hard GC (1998) Recent developments in the investigation of thyroid regulation and thyroid carcinogenesis. Environmental Health Perspectives 106 (8): 427–36.

Hardy JR, Baum M (1991) Lymphoedema. Prevention rather than cure. Annals of Oncology 2: 532–3.

Har-El G, Krepsi YP, Har-El R (1990) Physical rehabilitation after mycutaneous flaps. Head and Neck 12: 218–24.

Harkin H (1998) Tracheostomy management. Nursing Times 94 (21): 56–8.

Harris A, Komray R (1993) Cost effective management of pharyngocutaneous fistulas following laryngectomy. Ostomy Wound Management 39 (8): 36–42.

Harris D (1997) Types, causes and physical treatment of visible differences. Chapter 17 in Lansdown R, Rumsey N, Bradbury E et al (eds) Visibly Different. Coping with Disfigurement. Oxford: Butterworth-Heinemann.

Harrison DFN, Lund VJ (1993) Tumours of the Upper Jaw. Edinburgh: Churchill Livingstone, p 78.

Harrison DH (1985) The pectoralis minor vascularized muscle graft for the treatment of unilateral facial palsy. Plastic Reconstructive Surgery 75: 206–12.

Harrison J, Haddad P, Maguire P (1995) The impact of cancer on key relatives: a comparison of relative and patient concerns. European Journal of Cancer 31A (11): 1736–40.

Harrison LB (1997) Applications of brachytherapy in head and neck cancer. Seminars in Surgical Oncology 13 (3): 177–84.

Harrison LB, Zelefsky MJ, Sessions RB et al (1992) Base-of-tongue cancer treated with external beam irradiation plus brachytherapy: oncologic and functional outcome. Radiology 184 (1): 267–70.

Harrison LB, Zelefsky MJ, Armstrong JG (1994) Performance status after treatment for squamous cell cancer of the base of tongue — a comparison of primary radiation therapy versus primary surgery. International Journal of Radiation Oncology Biology Physics 30 (4): 953–7.

Harrison LB, Zelefsky MJ, Pfister DG (1997) Detailed quality of life assessment in patients treated with primary radiotherapy for squamous cell cancer of the base of the tongue. Head and Neck 19: 169–75.

Hart GH, Mainous EG (1976) The treatment of radiation necrosis with hyperbaric oxygen. Cancer 37: 2580–5.

Hassan SJ, Weymuller EA (1993) Assessment of quality of life in head and neck cancer patients. Head and Neck 15: 485–96.

Hathaway D (1986) Effect of preoperative instruction on postoperative outcomes: a meta-analysis. Nursing Research 35 (5): 269–75.

Haydock DA, Hill GL (1986) Impaired wound healing in surgical patients with varying degrees of malnutrition. Journal of Parenteral and Enteral Nutrition 10: 550–4.

Hayward J (1975) Information: A Prescription Against Pain. London: Royal College of Nursing.

Heals D (1993) A key to wellbeing. Oral hygiene in patients with advanced cancer. Professional Nurse 8 (6): 391–8.

Health Devices (1977) Suction catheters evaluation. Health Devices 6 (4): 132–41.

Health Education Authority (1996a) News. Nursing Times 92 (2): 9.

Health Education Authority (1996b) Health Update: Smoking, 3rd edn. London: Health Education Authority.

Health Education Authority (1997) Health Update: Alcohol. London: Health Education Authority.

Heather N (1992) Why alcoholism is not a disease. Medical Journal of Australia 156: 212–15.

Heather N, Robinson I (1983) Controlled Drinking, 2nd edn. London: Methuen.

Heffner JE (1995) The technique of weaning from a tracheostomy. Journal of Critical Illness 10 (10): 729–73.

Heller KS, Strong EW (1979) Carotid arterial haemorrhage after radical head and neck surgery. American Journal of Surgery 138: 607–10.

Henderson JM, Ord RA (1997) Suicide in head and neck cancer patients. Journal of Oral and Maxillofacial Surgery 55: 1217–21.

Herdman SJ, Clendaniel RA, Mattox DE et al (1995) Vestibular rehabilitation exercises and recovery: acute stage after acoustic neuroma resection. Otolarngology Head and Neck Surgery 113 (1): 77–87.

Herndon DN, Ziegler ST (1993) Bacterial translocation after thermal injury. Critical Care Medicine 21 (supplement): S50–S54.

Herth K (1998) Integrating hearing loss into one's life. Qualitative Health Research 8: 207–23.

Herzon FS, Boshier M (1979) Head and neck cancer — emotional management. Head and Neck Surgery 2: 112–18.

Hidderley M, Weinel E (1997) Effects of TENS applied to acupuncture points distal to a pain site. International Journal of Palliative Nursing 3 (4): 185–91.

Higgins DM, Maclean JC (1997) Dysphagia in the patient with a tracheostomy: six cases of inappropriate cuff deflation or removal. Heart and Lung 26 (3): 215–20.

Higgs JD (1987) Pressure sores — is there a place for nutritional support? Physiotherapy 73: 457–9.

Hilderley L (1983) Skin care in radiation therapy. Oncology Nursing Forum 10 (1): 51–6.

Hildmann H, Kosberg RD, Tiedjen KU (1987) Lymphoscintigraphic studies on lymphatic drainage in patients with head and neck cancer. HNO 35: 31–3 (German).

Hilgers F, Aaronson NK, Ackerstaff A et al (1991) The influence of a heat/moisture exchanger on the respiratory symptoms after total laryngectomy. Clinical Otolaryngology 16: 152–6.

Hillel AD, Kroll H, Dorman J, Medieros J (1989) Radical neck dissection: a subjective and objective evaluation of postoperative disability. Journal of Otolaryngology 18 (1): 53–61.

Hinds C, Streater A, Mood D (1995) Functions and preferred methods of recieving information related to radiotherapy. Cancer Nursing 18 (5): 374–84.

Hodder SC, Edwards MJ, Brickley MR, Shepherd JP (1997) Multiattribute assessment of outcomes of treatment for head and neck cancer. British Journal of Cancer 75 (6): 898–902.

Holdgaard HO, Pedersen J, Jensen RH et al (1998) Percutaneous dilational tracheostomy versus conventional surgical tracheostomy. A clinical randomised study. Acta Anaesthesiologica Scandanavica 42 (5): 545–50.

Holland JC, Massie MJ (1987) Psychosocial aspects of cancer in the elderly. Clinics in Geriatric Medicine 3 (3): 533–9.

Hollis LJ, Almeyda JS, Mochloulis G, Patel KS (1996) An in vitro study of tracheostomy tube cuff herniation and inflation characteristics. Journal of Laryngology and Otology 110 (12): 1142–4.

Hollo G (1993) Bilateral intraocular pressure elevation and decrease of facility of aqueous humour outflow as a consequence of regional lymphoedema of head and neck. Acta Opthalmologica 71: 415–18.

Hooper M (1996) Nursing care of the patient with a tracheostomy. Nursing Standard 10 (34): 40–3.

Horn-Ross PL, Ljung BM, Morrow M (1997) Environmental factors and the risk of salivary gland cancer. Epidemiology 8 (4): 414–19.

Horowitz AM, Goodman HS, Yellowitz JA, Nourjal PA (1996) The need for health promotion in oral cancer prevention and early detection. Journal of Public Health and Dentistry 56 (6): 319–30.

Horowitz SW, Leonetti JP, Azar-Kia B et al (1994) CT and MR of temporal bone malignancies primary and secondary to parotid carcinoma. American Journal of Neuroradiology 15: 755–62.

Horwitz EM, Frazier AJ, Martinez AA et al (1996) Excellent functional outcome in patients with squamous cell carcinoma of the base of tongue treated with external irradiation and interstitial iodine-125 boost. Cancer 78 (5): 948–57.

Horwitz EM, Frazier AJ, Vicini FA et al (1997) The impact of temporary iodine-125 interstitial implant boost in the primary management of squamous cell carcinoma of the oropharynx. Head and Neck 19 (3): 219–26.

Hwang JM, Fu KK, Phillips TL (1998) Results and prognostic factors in the treatment of locally recurrent nasopharyngeal carcinoma. International Journal of Radiation, Biology, Oncology, Physics 41 (5): 1099–111.

Hotter AM, Warfield K (1997) Technique for promoting healing of complex tracheostomy wounds. Otolaryngology—Head and Neck Surgery 116 (6): 693–5.

Howarth H (1977) Mouthcare procedures for the very ill. Nursing Times 73: 354–5.

Hsu TC, Furlong C (1991) The role of ethanol in oncogenesis of the upper aerodigestive tract: inhibition of DNA repair. Anti Cancer Research 11: 1995–8.

Hughes RS, Frenkel EP (1997) The role of chemotherapy in head and neck cancer. American Journal of Clinical Oncology 20 (5): 449–61.

Hughes-Lamb B (1981) Caring for the visually handicapped. Nursing 28: 1221–4.

Huldij A, Giesbers A, Everdien H, Poelhuis K, Hart A, Hulshof, Bruning P (1986) Alterations in taste perception in cancer patients during treatment. Cancer Nursing 9 (1): 38–42.

Humble CA (1995) Lymphedema: incidence, pathophysiology, management, and nursing care. Oncology Nursing Forum 22 (10): 1503–9.

Humfleet G, Hall S, Reus V et al (1997) The efficacy of nortriptyline as an adjunct to the psychological treatment of smokers with and without depressive history. In Harris ES (ed) Problems of Drug Dependence: Proceedings of the 57th Annual Scientific Meeting The College of Problems of Drug Dependence, Inc. NIDA Research Monograph 162. Washington DC: Government Printing Office.

Humphrey GM, Zimpher DG (1996) Counselling for Grief and Bereavement. London: Sage Publications.

Hurt RD, Sachs PL, Elbert DG et al (1997) A comparison of sustained-release bupropion and placebo for smoking cessation. The New England Journal of Medicine 337 (17): 1195–201.

Huskisson EC (1994) Non narcotic analgesics. Chapter 3 in Wall PD, Melzack R (eds) Textbook of Pain. Edinburgh: Churchill Livingstone.

Huvos AG, Leaming RH, Moore OS (1973) Clinicopathologic study of causative factors and protective methods in carotid artery rupture. Archives of Otolaryngology Head and Neck Surgery 99: 235–41.

Ichimura K, Sugasawa M, Nibu K, et al (1997) The significance of arytenoid oedema following radiotherapy of laryngeal carcinoma with respect to residual and recurrent tumour. Auris, Nasus, Larynx 24 (4): 391–7.

Idris AM, Prokopczyck B, Hoffman D (1994) Toombak: a major risk factor for cancer of the oral cavity in Sudan. Preventive Medicine 23 (6): 832–9.

Imai S, Michi K (1992) Articulatory function after resection of the tongue and floor of mouth: palatometric and perceptual evaluation. Journal of Speech and Hearing Research 35: 68–78.

Imperial Cancer Research Fund (1994) Mortality from smoking in developed countries 1950–2000. London: Imperial Cancer Research Fund.

Inoue T, Chatani M, Teshima T (1992) Irradiated volume and arytenoid oedema after radiotherapy for T1 glottic carcinoma. Strahlentherapie und Onkologie 168 (1): 23–6.

Ivetic O, Lyne PA (1990) Fungating and ulcerating malignant lesions: a review of the literature. Journal of Advanced Nursing 15: 83–8.

Izquierdo JN, Rozier RG (1996) Oral and pharyngeal cancer research, prevention and control: Quo Vademus? Journal of Public Health Dentistry 56 (6): 303–5.

Jackson C (1996) Humidification in the upper respiratory tract: a physiological overview. Intensive and Critical Care Nursing 12: 27–31.

Jacob C, Goffinet DR, Giffinet L et al (1987) Chemotherapy as a substitute for surgery in the treatment of advanced resectable head and neck cancer. A report from the Northern California Oncology Group. Cancer 60: 1178–83.

Janecka IP (1988) Microvascular reconstruction in head and neck surgery. Advances in Otolaryngology Head and Neck Surgery 91: 205–26.

Janecka IP, Sen CN, Sekhar LN, Arriaga MA (1990) Facial translocation: a new approach to the cranial base. Otolaryngology Head and Neck Surgery 103: 413–19.

Jani RM, Schaaf NG (1978) An evaluation of facial prostheses. Journal of Prosthetic Dentistry 39 (5): 546–50.

Janjan NA, Weissman DE, Pahule A (1992) Improved pain management with daily nursing intervention during radiation therapy for head and neck carcinoma. International Journal of Radiation Oncology Biology Physics 23: 647–52.

Jansma J, Vissink A, Spijkervet F et al (1992) Protocol for the prevention and treatment of oral sequelae resulting from head and neck radiation therapy. Cancer 70 (8): 2171–3.

Janssen-Cilag Ltd (1996) Durogesic Product Monograph. Janssen-Cilag, High Wycombe, Bucks HP14 4HJ.

Jay S, Ruddy J, Cullen RJ (1991) Laryngectomy: the patient's view. Journal of Laryngology and Otology 105: 934–8.

Jeffs E (1993) The effect of acute inflammatory episodes (cellulitis) on the treatment of lymphoedema. Journal of Tissue Viability 3 (4): 51–5.

Jenkins P, Logemann JA, Lazarus C (1981) Functional Changes after Hemilaryngectomy. Paper presented at the American Speech Language Hearing Association Annual Meeting, Los Angeles.

Johantgen MA (1998) Carotid artery rupture. In Chernecky C, Berger BJ (eds) Advanced and Critical Care Oncology Nursing. Managing Primary Complications. Philadelphia: WB Saunders Company.

Johnson JE, Fieler VK, Wlasowicz GS et al (1997) The effects of nursing care guided by self-regulation theory on coping with radiation therapy. Oncology Nursing Forum 24 (6): 1041–50.

Johnson JT, Casper J, Lesswing NJ (1979) Toward the total rehabilitation of the alaryngeal patient. Laryngoscope 89: 1813–19.

Johnson JT, Ferretti GA, Nethery WJ et al (1993) Oral pilocarpine for post irradiation xerostomia in patients with head and neck cancer. The New England Journal of Medicine 329 (6): 390–5.

Johnson NW, Warnakulasuriya PK (1993) Epidemiology and aetiology or oral cancer in the United Kingdom. Community Dental Health 10 (Supplement 1): 13–29.

Jones A (1964) Transient radiation myelopathy (with reference to Lhermittes' sign of electrical parathesia. British Journal of Radiology 37: 727–44.

Jones AS, Beasley NJ, Houghton DJ et al (1998) Tumours of the minor salivary glands. Clinical Otolaryngology 23: 27–33.

Jones B, Donner MW (1989) How I do it: examination of the patient with dysphagia. Dysphagia 4: 162–72.

Jones B, Donner MW (1991) Normal and abnormal swallowing. In Imaging in Diagnosis and Therapy. New York: Springer-Verlag.

Jones E, Lund VJ, Howard DJ et al (1992) Quality of life of patients treated surgically for head and neck cancer. Journal of Laryngology and Otology 106: 238–42.

Jones J, Diner J (1992) A Different Dimension. Adapting to Monocular Vision. Available from Mr C Laycock, Oral Surgery Unit, West Middlesex University Hospital, Twickenham Road, Isleworth, Middlesex TW7 6AF.

Joseph RR (1988) Aggressive management of cancer in the elderly. Clinics in Geriatric Medicine 4 (1): 29–41.

Joyston-Bechal S (1992) Management of oral complications following radiotherapy. Oral Medicine: Dental Update August: 232–7.

Joyston-Bechal S, Kidd EAM (1987) The effect of three commercially available saliva substitutes on enamel in vitro. British Dental Journal 163 (6): 187–90.

Joyston-Bechal S, Hayes K, Davenport ES, Hardie JM (1992) Caries incidence, mutans streptococci and lactobacilli in irradiated patients during a 12 month preventative programme using chlorhexidine and fluoride. Caries Research 26: 384–90.

Jung RC, Gottlieb LS (1976) Comparison of tracheobroncial suction catheters in humans. Chest 69: 179–81.

Jurd SM (1992) Why alcoholism is a disease. Medical Journal of Australia 156: 215–17.

Kaplan M (1990) Progress in thyroid cancer. Endocrinology and Metabolic Clinics of North America 19: 469–78.

Karlan MS, Cady B, Dunkelman D et al (1984) A safe technique for thyroidectomy with complete nerve dissection and parathyroid preservation. Head and Neck 6: 1014–19.

Karnofsky DA, Burchenall JH (1949) The clinical evaluation of chemotherapeutic agents in cancer. In Macleod CM (ed) Evaluation of Chemotherapeutic Agents. New York: Columbia University Press.

Kaut K, Turcott JC, Lavery M (1996) Passy Muir speaking valve. Dimensions in Critical Care Nursing 15 (6): 298–306.

Keceligil HT, Erk MK, Kolbakir F (1995) Tracheinnominate artery fistula following tracheostomy. Cardiovascular Surgery 3 (5): 509–10.

Keefe FJ, Brantley A, Manuel G, Crisson J (1985) Behavioural assessment of head and neck cancer pain. Pain 23: 327–36.

Keefe FJ, Manuel G, Brantley A, Crisson J (1986) Pain in the head and neck cancer patient: changes over treatment. Head and Neck Surgery 8: 169–76.

Keith RL, Darley FL (1979) Laryngectomy Rehabilitation. Houston: College-Hill Press.

Keith RL, Shane HC, Coates HLC, Devine KD (1977) Looking Forward ... A Guidebook for the Laryngectomee. Produced by The National Association of Laryngectomy Clubs. Mayo Foundation.

Kelley DJ, Spiro RH (1996) Management of the neck in parotid cancer. American Journal of Surgery 172: 695–7.

Kennedy J, Faugier J (1989) Drug and Alcohol Dependency Nursing. Oxford: Heinemann Nursing.

Ketcham AS, Wilkins RH, Van Buren JM et al (1963) A combined intracranial facial approach to the paranasal sinuses. American Journal of Surgery 10: 698–703.

Khafif A, Schantz SP, Al-Rawi MA et al (1998) Green tea regulates cell cycle progression in oral leukoplakia. Head and Neck 20: 528–34.

Kim JH, Chu F, Lakshmi V, Houde R (1985) A clinical study of benzydamine for the treatment of radiotherapy induced mucositis of the oropharynx. International Journal of Tissue Reaction 7 (3): 215–18.

King GE, Scheetz J, Jacob RF, Martin JW (1989) Electrotherapy and hyperbaric oxygen: promising treatments for postradiation complications. Journal of Prosthetic Dentistry 62 (3): 331–4.

King VMF, Jacob PA (1993) Special procedures. Chapter 15 in Carroll D, Bowsher D (eds) Pain Management and Nursing Care. Oxford: Butterworth-Heinemann.

Kirchner JA (1975) Pyriform sinus cancer: a clinical and laboratory study. Annals of Otology 84: 793–804.

Kirchner JA, Satcliffe JH, Dey FL et al (1963). The pharynx after laryngectomy; changes in its structure and function. Laryngoscope 73: 18–33.

Kite K, Pearson L (1995) A rationale for mouth care: the integration of theory with practice. Intensive and Critical Care Nursing 11: 71–6.

Koka VN, Deo K, Lusinchi A et al (1990) Osteoradionecrosis of the mandible. Journal of Laryngology and Otology 104: 305–7.

Koster META, Bergsma J (1990) Problems and coping behaviour of facial cancer patients. Social Science Medicine 30 (5): 569–78.

Kouba J (1988) Nutritional care of the individual with cancer. Nutritional Clinical Practice 3: 175–82.

Kowalski et al (1994) Lateness of diagnosis of oral and oropharyngeal carcinoma : factors related to the tumour, the patient and health professionals. Oral Oncology, European Journal Cancer 30B (3): 167–73.

Kraus DH, Lanzieri CF, Wanamaker JR et al (1992) Complementary use of computed tomography and magnetic resonance imaging in assessing skull base lesions. Laryngoscope 102: 623–9.

Kronenberger MB, Meyers AD (1994) Dysphagia following head and neck cancer surgery. Dysphagia 9: 236–44.

Krouse JH, Krouse HJ, Fabian RL (1989) Adaptation to surgery for head and neck cancer. Laryngoscope 99: 789–94.

Kumar BN, Walsh RM, Courteney-Harris RG (1997) Laryngeal foreign body: an unusual complication of percutaneous tracheostomy. Journal of Laryngology and Otology 111 (7): 652–3.

Kumasaka LM, Dungan JM (1993) Nursing strategy for initial emotional response to cancer diagnosis. Cancer Nursing 16 (4): 296–303.

Kurtz ME et al (1994) Promotion of breast cancer screening in a work site population. Health Care for Women International 15 (1): 31–42.

Kusler DL, Rambur BA (1992) Treatment for radiation-induced xerostomia. An innovative remedy. Cancer Nursing 15 (3): 191–5.

Kuten A, Ben-Aryeh H, Berdicevsky I, Ore L et al (1986) Oral side effects of head and neck irradiation: correlation between clinical manifestations and laboratory data. International Journal of Radiation Oncology Biology Physics 12: 401–5.

Kwong DL, Wei WI, Sham JS et al (1996) Sensorineural hearing loss in patients treated for nasopharyngeal carcinoma: a prospective study of the effect of radiation and cisplatin treatment. International Journal of Radiation Oncology Biology Physics 36 (2): 281–9.

Labar B, Mrsic M, Pavletic Z et al (1993) Prostaglandin E2 for prophylaxis of oral mucositis following BMT. Bone Marrow Transplantation 11: 379–82.

Laccourreye H, Laccourreye O, Weinstein G et al (1990) Supracricoid laryngectomy with cricohyoidopexy: a partial laryngeal procedure for selected supraglottic and transglottic carcinomas. Laryngoscope 100: 735–41.

Laccourreye O, Brasnu D, Laccourreye H, Trotoux J (1989) Local extension of epithe-
lioma of the glottic floor; anatomo-clinical correlations and study of local failure.
Apropos of 432 patients treated by partial laryngeal surgery. Annals of
Otolaryngologie Chirugie Cervicofaciale 106: 322–9.

Lamey PJ (1993) Management options in potentially malignant and malignant oral
epithelial lesions. Community Dental Health 10 (Supplement 1): 53–62.

Lang NP, Brecx MC (1986) Chlorhexidine digluconate — an agent for chemical plaque
control and prevention of gingival inflammation. Journal of Periodontal Research
Supplement: 74–89.

Languis A (1997) Quality of life aspects in cases of oral cancer. Clinical Effectiveness in
Nursing 1: 212–19.

Languis A, Lind MG (1995) Well-being and coping in oral and pharyngeal cancer
patients. European Journal of Cancer 31B (4): 242–9.

Languis A, Bjorvell H, Lind M (1993) Oral and pharyngeal cancer patients' perceived
symptoms and health. Cancer Nursing 16 (3): 214–21.

Latham J (1983) Complications of nerve blocks. Nursing Times, May 11: 36–8.

Lauder E (1996–7) Emotional aspects. In Self Help for the Laryngectomee. San
Antonio, Texas: Lauder Enterprises.

Laurence DR, Bennett PN, Brown MJ (1997a) Pain. Chapter 17 in Clinical
Pharmacology, 8th edn. New York: Churchill Livingstone.

Laurence DR, Bennett PN, Brown MJ (1997b) Vitamins, calcium, bone. Chapter 39 in
Clinical Pharmacology, 8th edn. New York: Churchill Livingstone.

Lavertu P, Bonafede JP, Adelstein DJ et al (1998) Comparison of surgical complications after organ-preservation therapy in patients with stage III or IV squamous
cell head and neck cancer. Archives of Otolaryngology Head and Neck Surgery
124: 401–6.

Lavery B A (1995) Skin care during radiotherapy : a survey of UK practice. Clinical
Oncology 7: 184–7.

Lawler J (1991) Behind the Screens. Nursing, Somology, and the Problem of the Body.
Melbourne: Churchill Livingstone.

Lazarus RS, Folkman S (1984) Stress, Appraisal and Coping. Springer: New York.

Leake GJ, King AS (1977) Effects of counsellor expectation on alcohol recovery. Alcohol
Health Research 1 (3): 16–22.

Lear CS (1965) The frequency of deglutition in man. Archives of Oral Biology 10: 88–9.

Leder SB, Tarro JM, Morton IB (1996) Effect of occlusion of a tracheotomy tube on
aspiration. Dysphagia 11: 254–8.

Lee AW, Foo W, Chappell R et al (1998) Effect of time, dose, and fractionation on temporal lobe necrosis following radiotherapy for nasopharyngeal carcinoma.
International Journal of Radiation Oncology Biology Physics 40 (1): 35–42.

Lee NK, Goepfort H, Wendt CD (1990) Supraglottic laryngectomy for intermediate-
stage cancer: UT MD Anderson Cancer Centre experience with combined therapy.
Laryngoscope 100: 831–6.

Lefebvre JL, Sahmoud T for the EORTC Head and Neck Cancer Cooperative Group
(1994) Larynx preservation in hypopharynx squamous cell carcinoma: preliminary
results of a randomised study (EORTC 24891). Proceedings of the American
Society of Clinical Oncology 13: 199.

Lehman W, Krebs H (1991) Interdisciplinary rehabilitation of the laryngectomee.
Recent Results in Cancer Research 121: 442–9.

Lenander-Lumikari M, Tenovuo J, Mikola H (1993) Effects of a lactoperoxidase system-containing toothpaste on levels of hypothiocyanite and bacteria in saliva. Caries Research 27: 285–91.

Lepke RA, Lipshitz HI (1983) Radiation induced injury of the oesophagus. Radiology 148: 375–8.

Lesage C (1986) Carotid artery rupture. Predication, prevention, and preparation. Cancer Nursing 9 (1): 1–7.

Letheren MJ, Parry N, Slater RM (1997) A complication of percutaneous tracheostomy whilst using the Combitube for airway control. European Journal of Anaesthesiology 14 (4): 464–6.

Levendag PC, Schmitz PI, Jansen PP et al (1998) Fractionated high-dose-rate brachytherapy in primary carcinoma of the nasopharynx. Journal of Clinical Oncology 16 (6): 2213–20.

LeVeque F, Montgomery M, Potter D (1993) A multicenter randomised double blind placebo controlled dose titration study of oral pilocarpine for the treatment of radiation induced xerostomia in head and neck cancer patients. Journal of Clinical Oncology 11(6): 1124–31.

Leverstein H, Castelijns JA, Snow GB (1995) The value of magnetic resonance imaging in the differential diagnosis of parapharyngeal space tumours. Clinical Otolaryngology 20: 428–33.

Levine PA, Sasaki CT, Kirchner JA (1978) The long tracheostomy tube. Alternative management of distal tracheal stenosis. Archives of Otolaryngology 104 (2): 108–10.

Lewis CE, O'Sullivan C, Barraclough J (1994) The Psychoimmunology of Cancer. Mind, Body and Spirit in the Fight for Survival. Oxford: Oxford Medical Publications.

Liening DA, Duncan NO, Blakeslee DB et al (1990) Hypothyroidism following radiotherapy for head and neck cancer. Otolaryngology, Head and Neck Surgery 103: 10–13.

Lilly Oncology (1993) Cytotoxic Chemotherapy, 4th edn. Eli Lilly and Company Ltd, Basingstoke, Hampshire.

Lin JD, Tsang NM, Huang MJ, Weng HF (1997) Results of external beam radiotherapy in patients with well differentiated thyroid carcinoma. Japanese Journal of Clinical Oncology 27 (4): 244–7.

Lindberg R (1972) Distribution of cervical lymph node metastases from squamous cell carcinoma of the upper respiratory and digestive tracts. Cancer 29: 1446–9.

Lindenfield G (1995) Self Esteem. London: Thorsons.

Lippman SM, Spitz MR (1991) Intervention in the premalignant process. Cancer Bulletin 43: 473–4.

Lips CJM, Landsvater RM, Hoppener JWM et al (1994) Clinical screening as compared with DNA analysis in families with multiple endocrine neoplasia type 2a. New England Journal of Medicine 331: 828–35.

List MA, Ritter-Sterr C, Lansky SB (1990) A performance status scale for head and neck cancer patients. Cancer 66: 564–9.

List MA, D'Antonio LL, Cella DF et al (1996a) The performance status scale for head and neck cancer patients and the functional assessment of cancer therapy head and neck scale. Cancer 77: 2294–301.

List MA, Ritter-Sterr CA, Baker TM et al (1996b) Longitudinal assessment of quality of life in laryngeal cancer patients. Head and Neck 18: 1–10.

List MA, Mumby P, Haraf A et al (1997) Performance and quality of life in patients completing concomitant chemoradiotherapy protocols for head and neck cancer. Quality of Life Research 6: 274–84.

Littlefield N A, Blackwell B, Hewit C, Gaylor D W (1985) Chronic toxicity and carcinogenicity studies of Gentian Violet in mice. Fundamental and Applied Toxicology 5: 902–12.

Liu FF, Keane TJ, Davidson J (1993) Primary carcinoma involving the petrous temporal bone. Head and Neck 15: 39–43.

Lloyd GAS, Lund VJ, Phelps PD, Howard DJ (1987) Magnetic resonance imaging in the evaluation of nose and paranasal sinus disease. British Journal of Radiology 60: 957–68.

Loe H, Schiott CR (1970) The effect of mouthrinses and topical application of chlorhexidine on the development of dental plaque and gingivitis in man. Journal of Periodontal Research 5: 79–83.

Loeb EM (1987) Special problems of cancer care in the elderly. Primary Care Clinics in Office Practice 14 (2): 281–91.

Logemann JA (1983) Evaluation and Treatment of Swallowing Disorders. Austin, Texas: Pro-ed.

Logemann JA (1985) Aspiration in head and neck surgical patients. Annals of Otology Rhinology Laryngology 94: 373–6.

Logemann JA (1989) Swallowing and communication rehabilitation. Seminars in Oncology Nursing 5 (3): 205–12.

Logemann JA, Gibbons P, Rademaker AW, et al (1994) Mechanisms of recovery of swallow after supraglottic laryngectomy. Journal of Speech and Hearing Research 37: 965–74.

Logemann JA, Pauloski BR, Colangelo L (1998) Light digital occlusion of the tracheostomy tube: a pilot study of effects on aspiration and biomechanics of the swallow. Head and Neck 20: 52–7.

Long SA, D'Antonio LL, Robinson EB (1996) Factors related to quality of life and functional status in 50 patients with head and neck cancer. Laryngoscope 106: 1084–8.

Loprinzi CL, Cianflore SG, Dose AM et al (1990) A controlled evaluation of an allopurinol mouthwash as prophylaxis against 5-fluorouracil induced stomatitis. Cancer 65: 1879–82.

Lotan R, Lippman SM, Hong WK (1991) Retinoid modulation of squamous cell differentiation and carcinogenesis. Cancer Bulletin 43: 490–8.

Low WK, Fong KW (1998) Long-term hearing status after radiotherapy for nasopharyngeal carcinoma. Auris Nasus Larynx 25 (1): 21–4.

Lozza L, Cerrotta A, Gardani G et al (1997) Analysis of risk factors for mandibular bone necrosis after exclusive low dose rate brachytherapy for oral cancer. Radiotherapy Oncology 44 (2): 143–7.

Lucot J (1998) Pharmacology of motion sickness. Journal of Vestibular Research 8 (1): 61–6.

Lysons K (1978) How to Cope with Hearing Loss. London: Granada Publishing Ltd.

Mackay L (1997) Communication is the key. Macmillan Nurse 6 (6): 15.

Mackenzie CF (1983) Compromise in the choice of orotracheal or nasotracheal intubation and tracheostomy. Heart and Lung 12: 5.

MacLellan K (1997) A chart audit reviewing the prescription and administration of analgesia and the documentation of pain after surgery. Journal of Advanced Nursing 26: 345–50.

Macleod CM (ed) Evaluation of Chemotherapeutic Agents. New York: Columbia University Press.

McCann RM, Hall WJ, Groth-Juncter A (1994) Comfort care for terminally ill patients; the appropriate use of nutrition and hydration. Journal of the American Medical Association 272 (16): 1263–5.

McConnel FMS, Logemann JA (1990) Diagnosis and treatment of swallowing disorders. In Cummings CW (ed) Otolaryngology, Head and Neck Surgery (update 2). St. Louis: Mosby.

McConnel FMS, Mendelsohn MS (1987) The effects of surgery on pharyngeal deglutition. Dysphagia 1: 145–51.

McConnel FMS, Mendelsohn MS, Logemann JA (1986) Examination of the swallow after total laryngology using manofluorography. Head and Neck Surgery 9: 3.

McCoy G, Barsocchini LM (1968) Experiences in carotid artery occlusion. Laryngoscope 78: 1195–210.

McCready RA, Hyde GL, Bivins BA et al (1983) Radiation induced arterial injuries. Surgery 93: 306–12.

McCulloch TM, Niels FJ, Douglas AG et al (1997) Risk factors for pulmonary complications in the postoperative head and neck surgery patient. Head and Neck 19: 372–7.

McCusker K (1992) Mechanisms of respiratory tissues injury from cigarette smoking. The American Journal of Medicine 93 (Supplement 1A): 18–21.

McDonough ER, Vavares MA, Dunphy FR et al (1996) Changes in quality of life scores in a population of patients treated for squamous cell carcinoma of the head and neck. Head and Neck 18: 487–93.

McDonough EM, Boyd JH, Varvares MA, Maves MD (1996) Relationship between psychological status and compliance in a sample of patients treated for cancer of the head and neck. Head and Neck 18: 269–76.

McDougall IR (1997) [131]I treatment of ^{131}I negative whole body scan, and positive thyroglobulin in differentiated thyroid carcinoma; what is being treated? Thyroid 7 (4): 669–72.

McEleney M (1996) Radical support. Nursing Times 92 (20): 29–30.

McGarry J (1993) Hypnotic interventions in psychological and physiological aspects of amputation. The Australian Journal of Clinical Hypnotherapy and Hypnosis 14 (1): 7–12.

McGavran MH, Bauer WC, Ogura JH (1961) The incidence of cervical lymph node metastases from epidermoid carcinoma of the larynx and their relationship to certain characteristics of the primary tumour. Cancer 14: 55–66.

McGhee MA, Stern SJ, Callan D et al (1997) Osseointegrated implants in the head and neck cancer patient. Head and Neck 19: 659–65.

McGowan K L (1983) Radiation therapy: saving your patient's skin. Registered Nurse June: 24–26.

McGregor AD, MacDonald DG (1988) Routes of entry of squamous carcinoma to the mandible. Head and Neck Surgery 10: 294–301.

McGregor IA, MacDonald DG (1983) Mandibular osteotomy in the approach to the oral cavity. Head and Neck Surgery 5: 457.

McGregor I (1991) Fundamental Techniques of Plastic Surgery. London: Churchill Livingstone.

McGuire DB, Sheidler VR (1997) Pain. Chapter 20 in Groenwald SL, Hansen Frogge M, Goodman M, Henke Yarbro C (eds) Cancer Nursing. Principles and Practice, 4th edn. Boston: Jones & Bartlett.

McGuirt WF (1982) Panendoscopy as a screening examination for simultaneous primary tumors in head and neck cancer: a prospective sequential study and review of the literature. Laryngoscope 92 (5): 569–76.

McHenry CR, Raeburn CD, Lange RL, Priebe PP (1997) Percutaneous tracheostomy: a cost-effective alternative to standard open tracheosotmy. American Surgeon 63 (7): 646–51.

McKenzie MR, Wong FLW, Epstein KB, Lepawsky M (1993) Hyperbaric oxygen and postradiation osteonecrosis of the mandible. European Journal of Cancer 29B (3): 201–7.

McMinn RMH, HutchingsRT, Logan BM (1994) Color Atlas of Head and Neck Anatomy, 2nd edn. London: Mosby-Wolfe.

McMurran M (1994) The Psychology of Addiction. London: Taylor & Francis.

McNeill R (1981) Surgical management of carcinoma of the posterior pharyngeal wall. Head and Neck Surgery 3: 380–84.

McRae D, Jones A, Young P, Hamilton J (1995) Resistance, humidity and temperature of the tracheal airway. Clinical Otolaryngology 20: 355–6.

McRae D, Young P, Hamilton J, Jones A (1996) Raising airway resistance in laryngectomees increases tissue oxygen saturation. Clinical Otolaryngology 21: 366–8.Madeya ML (1996) Oral complications from cancer therapy: Part 1 — Pathophysiology and secondary complications. Oncology Nursing Forum 23 (5): 801–7.

Madeya ML (1996) Oral complications from cancer therapy: Part 1 — Pathophysiology and secondary complications. Oncology Nursing Forum 23 (5): 801–7.

Maguire P, Selby P (1989) Assessing quality if life in cancer patients. British Journal of Cancer 60: 437–40.

Maguire P, Faulkner A, Booth K, Elliott C, Hillier V (1996) Helping cancer patients disclose their concerns. European Journal of Cancer Care 32A (1): 78–81.

Mah MA, Johnston C (1993) Concerns of families in which one member has head and neck cancer. Cancer Nursing 16 (5): 382–7.

Maier H, Dietz A, Gewelke U, Heller WD (1991) Occupational exposure to hazardous substances and risk of cancer in the area of the mouth cavity, oropharynx, hypopharynx and larynx. A case control study. Journal Laryngorhinootologie 70: 93–6.

Mair RG, Doty RL, Kelly KM et al (1986) Multi modal sensory discrimination deficits in Korsakoff's psychosis. Neuropsychology 24: 831–9.

Makkonen TA, Bostrom P, Vilja P, Joensuu H (1994) Sucrulfate mouth washing in the prevention of radiation-induced mucositis: a placebo-controlled double blind randomised study. International Journal of Radiation Oncology Biology Physics 30 (1): 177–82.

Maksud DP (1992) Nursing management of patients following combined free flap mandible reconstruction. Plastic Surgical Nursing 12 (3): 95–105.

Mallinckrodt Medical Inc. (1993) Airway management. Catalogue of Anaesthesia Division. Mallinckrodt Medical Inc.: Northampton.

Maniglia AJ (1986) Indications and techniques of midfacial degloving. A 15 year experience. Archives of Otolaryngology Head Neck Surgery 112: 750–2.

Mann W, Beck C, Freudenberg N, Leupe M (1981) The effect of irradiation on the inner laryngeal lymphatics HNO 29 (11): 381–7 (German).

Mapp CS (1988) Trach care. Are you aware of all the dangers? Nursing (18) 7: 34–42.

Maran AG, MacKenzie IJ, Stanley RE (1984) Recurrent pleomorphic adenomas of the parotid gland. Archives of Otolaryngology 110: 167–71.

Maran AGD, Gaze M, Wilson JA et al (1993) Head and Neck Surgery. Oxford: Butterworth-Heinemann.

Marks JE, Davis CC, Gottsman VL, Purdy JE et al (1981) The effects of radiation on parotid salivary function. International Journal of Radiation Oncology Biology Physics 7: 283–8.

Martin J, Austin J, Chambers M et al (1994) Postoperative care of the maxillectomy patient. ORL—Head and Neck Nursing 12(3): 14–20

Martin L (1989) Management of the altered airway in the head and neck cancer patient. Seminars in Oncology Nursing 5 (3): 182–90.

Martini F (1992a) Fundamentals of Anatomy and Physiology Chapter 23, 2nd edn. New Jersey: Prentice Hall.

Martini F (1992b) Chapter 17 in Fundamentals of Anatomy and Physiology, 2nd edn. New Jersey: Prentice Hall.

Martini F (1992c) Chapter 13 in Fundamentals of Anatomy and Physiology, 2nd edn. New Jersey: Prentice Hall.

Martini F (1992d) Chapter 18 in Fundamentals of Anatomy and Physiology, 2nd edn. New Jersey: Prentice Hall.

Marunick MT, Seyedsadr M, Ahmad K, Klein B (1991) The effect of head and neck cancer treatment on whole salivary flow. Journal of Surgical Oncology 48: 81–8.

Matejka M, Nell A, Kment G et al (1990) Local benefit of prostaglandin E2 in radiotherapy induced oral mucositis. British Journal of Oral and Maxillofacial Surgery 28: 89–91.

Mathieson CM, Stam HJ, Scott JP (1992) The impact of a laryngectomy on the spouse: who is better off? Psychology and Health 5: 153–63.

Mathog RH, Shibuya T, Leider J, Marinick M (1997) Rehabilitation of patients with extended facial and craniofacial resection. Laryngoscope 107 (1): 30–9.

Mattes RD, Curran WJ, Lan J et al (1992) Clinical implications of learned food aversions in patients with cancer treated with chemotherapy and radiotherapy. Cancer 70 (1): 192–200.

Matthewson K (1995) Percutaneous endoscopic gastrostomy. Care of the Critically Ill 11(2): March/April.

Maurer I (1985) Hospital Hygiene. London: Edward Arnold.

Mayou RA, Smith KA (1997) Post traumatic symptoms following medical illness and treatment. Journal of Psychosomatic Research 43 (2): 121–3.

Mazzon D, Paolin A, Vigneri M (1998) Peristomal infection after translaryngeal tracheostomy: a risk linked to colonisation of the oropharynx? Intensive Care Medicine 24 (3): 278–9.

Meier C, Braverman L, Ebner S et al (1994) Diagnostic use of recombinant human thyrotropin in patients with thyroid carcinoma (Phase 1/11 study). Journal of Endocrinology and Metabolism 76: 188–96.

Melzack R, Wall PD (1991a) Sensory modulation of pain. In The Challenge of Pain. London: Penguin Books.

Melzack R, Wall PD (1991b) Acupuncture and other forms of folk medicine. In The Challenge of Pain. London: Penguin Books.

Mendenhall WM, Parsons JT, Stringer SP et al (1989) Radiotherapy after excisional biopsy of carcinoma of the oral tongue/floor of mouth. Head and Neck 11: 129–31.

Mendenhall WM, Parsons JT, Mancuso AA et al (1996) Radiotherapy for carcinoma of the supraglottic larynx: an alternative to surgery. Head and Neck 18: 24–35.

Mennie A (1997) An essential and ancient oil. Nursing Times 93 (47): 31–2.

Mercadante S, Dardanoni G, Salvaggio L et al (1997) Monitoring opioid therapy in advanced cancer pain patients. Journal of Pain and Symptom Management 13 (4): 204–12.

Merlano M, Vitale V, Rosso R et al (1992) Treatment of advanced squamous cell carcinoma of the head and neck with alternating chemotherapy and radiotherapy. New England Journal of Medicine 327: 1115–21.

Merriman GR, Szechter A, Focht EF (1972) The effects of ionising radiation on the eye. Frontiers of Radiation Therapy Oncology 6: 346–85.

Mesters I, Van Den Borne H, McCormick L et al (1997) Openness to discuss cancer in the nuclear family: scale, development, and validation. Psychosomatic Medicine 59: 269–79.

Metcalfe MC, Fischman SH (1985) Factors affecting the sexuality of patients with head and neck cancer. Oncology Nursing Forum 12 (2): 21–5.

Meyers AD, Aarons B, Suzuki B, Pilcher L (1980) Sexual behaviour following laryngectomy. Ear, Nose and Throat Journal 59: 35–9.

Miller NH, Smith PM, DeBusk RF et al (1997) Smoking cessation in hospitalised patients. Archives of Internal Medicine 157: 409–15.

Miller WR (1983) Motivational interviewing with problem drinkers. Behavioural Psychotherapy 16: 251–68.

Milligan F (1998) The iatrogenic epidemic. Nursing Standard 13 (2): 46–7.

Million RR, Cassisi NJ (1994) Management of Head and Neck Cancer. A Multidisciplinary Approach, 2nd edn. Philadelphia: JB Lippincott Company.

Milne AA (1957) The World of Pooh. New York: EP Dutton.

Milner QJ, Allen JG, Abdy S (1997) Management of severe tracheal obstruction with helium/oxygen and a laryngeal mask airway. Anaesthesia 52 (11): 1087–9.

Minear D, Lucente MD (1979) Current attitudes of laryngectomy patients. Laryngoscope 89: 1061–5.

Mistiaen P, Duijnhouwer E, Wijkel D (1997) The problems of elderly people at home one week after discharge from an acute care setting. Journal of Advanced Nursing 25: 1233–40.

Mitxelena J, Aguirre A, Bilbao I et al (1998) Contact dermatitis in a tracheostomised patient due to a rubber disc. Contact Dermatitis 38 (3): 181–2.

Miura M, Takeda M, Sasaki T et al (1998) Factors affecting mandibular complications in low dose rate brachytherapy for oral tongue carcinoma with special reference to spacer. International Journal of Radiation Oncology Biology Physics 41 (4): 763–70.

Mohr RM, Quenelle DJ, Shumrick DA (1983) Vertico-frontolateral laryngectomy (hemilaryngectomy). Indications, technique, and results. Archives of Otolaryngology 109: 384–95.

Monga U, Tan G, Osterman HJ, Monga TN (1997) Sexuality in head and neck cancer patients. Archives of Physical Medicine and Rehabilitation 78: 298–304.

Moody M (1998) Metrotop: a topical antimicrobial agent for malodorous wounds. International Journal of Palliative Nursing 4 (3): product focus insert.

Moody M, Grocott P (1993) Let us extend our knowledge base. Assessment and management of fungating malignant wounds. Professional Nurse 8 (9): 586–90.

Moore GJ, Parsons JT, Mendenhall WM (1996) Quality of life outcomes after primary radiotherapy for squamous cell carcinoma of the base of tongue. International Journal of Radiation Oncology Biology Physics 36 (2): 351–4.

Morgan D (1994) Establishing a dressing formulary. British Journal of Nursing 3 (8): 387–92.

Morris J (1991) Outcome following treatment for head and neck cancer: beyond clinical assessment. European Journal of Cancer Care 27 (5): 675.

Morrison P (1994) Understanding Patients. London: Ballière Tindall.

Morton RP (1995a) Life-satisfaction in patients with head and neck cancer. Clinical Otolaryngology 20: 499–503.

Morton RP (1995b) Evolution of quality of life assessment in head and neck cancer. The Journal of Laryngology and Otology 109: 1029–35.

Mossman KL (1983) Quantitative radiation dose response relationships for normal tissues in man II. Response of the salivary glands during radiotherapy. Radiation Research 95: 392–8.

Mossman KL, Shatzman AR, Chencharick JD (1982) Longterm effects of radiotherapy on taste and salivary function in man. International Journal of Radiation Oncology Biology Physics 8: 991–7.

Mott AE (1992) General medical evaluation of chemosensory dysfunction. Journal of Head Trauma and Rehabilitation 7 (1): 25–41.

Mulvaney D (1976) Maintaining minimal occluding volume or use cuffs with care. Journal of American Nursing 2 (5): 17–18.

Munro AJ (1995) An overview of randomised controlled trials of adjuvant chemotherapy in head and neck cancer. British Journal of Cancer 71: 83–91.

Murphy C, Davidson TM (1992) Geriatric issues: special considerations. Journal of Head Trauma Rehabilitation 7 (1): 76–82.

Murray Parkes C (1972) Components of the reaction to loss of a limb, spouse or home. Journal of Psychosomatic Research 16: 343–9.

Murray Parkes C (1975) Bereavement: Studies of Grief in Adult life. Harmondsworth: Penguin Books.

Murry T, Madasu R, Martin A, Robbins KT (1998) Acute and chronic changes in swallowing and quality of life following intraarterial chemoradiation for organ preservation in patients with advanced head and neck cancer. Head and Neck 20: 31–7.

Muscat JE, Wynder EL (1998) A case control study of risk factors for major salivary gland cancer. Otolaryngology Head and Neck Surgery 118 (2): 195–8.

Muz J, Mathog RH, Nelson R, Jones LA (1989) Aspiration in patients with head and neck cancer and tracheostomy. American Journal Otolaryngology 10: 282–6.

Muz J, Hamlet S, Mathog R, Farris R (1994) Scintigraphic assessment of aspiration in head and neck cancer patients with tracheostomy. Head and Neck 16: 17–20.

Nakao, MA, Killam D, Wilson R (1983) Pneumothorax secondary to inadvertent nasotracheal placement of a naso-enteric tube past a cuffed endotracheal tube. Cancer Care Medicine 11: 210–11.

Nakhla V (1997) A home-made modification of a spacer device for delivery of bronchodilator or steroid therapy in patients with tracheotomies. Journal of Laryngology and Otology 111 (4): 363–5.

Nash M (1988) Swallowing problems in the tracheotomized patient. Otolaryngologic Clinics of North America 21: 701–9.

National Association of Laryngectomy Clubs (1991) Handbook for Laryngectomy Patients. London: NALC.

Natvig K (1983) Laryngectomees in Norway: Study no. 2 Preoperative counselling and postoperative training evaluated by the patients and their spouses. Journal of Otolaryngology 12: 155–62.

Naylor M (1990) Comprehensive discharge planning for hospitalised elderly: a pilot study. Nursing Research 3 (3): 1156–61.

Nazarko L (1997) Improving hospital discharge arrangements for older people. Nursing Standard 11 (40): 44–7.

Neal A, Hoskin P (1994) Clinical Oncology. A Textbook for Students. London: Edward Arnold.

Needham PR, Hoskin PJ (1994) Radiotherapy for painful bone metastases. Palliative Medicine 8: 95–104.

Nelson G (1998) Biology of taste buds and the clinical problem of taste loss. The Anatomical Record (New Anatomy) 253: 70–8.

Neovius EB, Lind MG, Lind FG (1997) Hyperbaric oxygen therapy for wound complications after surgery in the irradiated head and neck: a review of the literature and a report of 15 consecutive patients. Head and Neck 19: 315–22.

Nerenz DR, Levanthal H, Easterling DV, Love RR (1986) Anxiety and drug taste as predicators of anticipatory nausea in cancer chemotherapy. Journal of Clinical Oncology 4(2): 224–33.

Netscher DT, Clamon J (1994) Methods of reconstruction. Nursing Clinics of North America 29(4): 725–39.

Netterville JL, Civantos FJ (1993) Rehabilitation of cranial nerve deficits after neurologic skull base surgery. Laryngoscope 103: 45–54.

Neufeld KR, Degner LF, Dick JA (1993) A nursing intervention strategy to foster patient involvement in treatment decisions. Oncology Nursing Forum 20: 631–5.

Neufmann S, Gudrun B, Buchholz D (1995) Swallowing therapy of neurologic patients: correlation of outcome therapy, pre-treatment variables and therapeutic methods. Dysphagia 10: 1–5.

Newman V, Allwood M, Oakes RA (1989) The use of metronidazole gel to control the smell of malodorous lesions. Palliative Medicine 3: 303–5.

Oberst MT, Hughes SH, Chang AS, McCubbin MA (1991) Self-care burden, stress appraisal, and mood among persons receiving radiotherapy. Cancer Nursing 14 (2): 71–8.

O'Doherty MJ, Coakley AJ (1998) Drug therapy alternatives in the treatment of thyroid cancer. Drugs 55 (6): 801–12.

O' Donnell I (1996) Stressing the point. Nursing Standard 10 (16): 22–3.

Oermann M, McHugh N, Deitrich J et al (1983) After a tracheostomy: patients describe their sensations. Cancer Nursing Oct: 361–6.

Office for National Statistics (1997) Census, Population, and Health Group. 1 Drummond Gate London SW1V 2QQ.

Oguchi M, Shikama N, Sasaki S et al (1998) Mucosa-adhesive water-soluble polymer film for treatment of acute radiation-induced oral mucositis. International Journal of Radiation Oncology Biology Physics 40(5): 1033–7.

Oken MM, Creech RH, Tormey DC et al (1982) Toxicity and response criteria of the Eastern European Cooperative Oncology Group. American Journal of Clinical Oncology 5: 649–55.

Ophir D, Guterman A, Gross-Isseroff R (1988) Changes in smell acuity induced by radiation exposure of the olfactory mucosa. Archives of Otolaryngology Head and Neck Surgery 114: 853–5.

Ostroff JS, Jacobsen PB, Moadel AB et al (1995) Prevalence and predictors of continued tobacco use after treatment of patients with head and neck cancer. Cancer 75 (2): 569–76.

Overgaard J, Hansen HS, Overgaard M et al (1997) Conventional radiotherapy as pri-
    mary treatment of sqauamous cell carcinoma of the head and neck. A randomised
    multicentre study of 5 versus 6 fractions per week — report from the DAHANCA 7
    trial. International Journal of Radiation Oncology Biology Physics 39 (2): 188.

Palmer C (1984) The team approach to the care of the patient with head and neck
    cancer. Enteral nutrition (Part 8). The American Journal of Intravenous Therapy
    and Clinical Nutrition 8: 12–18.

Panje WR, Scher N et al (1989) Transoral carbon dioxide ablation for cancer, tumours
    and other diseases. Archives of Otolaryngology Head and Neck Surgery 115: 681–8.

Pappas CJ, O'Donnell TF (1992) Long term results of compression treatment for lym-
    phoedema. Journal of Vascular Surgery 16: 555–64.

Park RI, Liberman FZ, Lee DJ et al (1991) Iodine-125 seed implantations as an adjunct
    to surgery in advanced recurrent squamous cell cancer of the head and neck.
    Laryngoscope 101 (4 Part 1): 405–10.

Parsons JT (1994) The effect of radiation on normal tissues of the head and neck. In
    Million RR, Cassisi NJ (eds) Management of Head and Neck Cancer. A
    Multidisciplinary Approach, 2nd edn. Philadelphia: JB Lippincott Company.

Partridge MR, Flood-Page P (1997) Multiple tracheal strictures following mechanical
    ventilation. Respiratory Medicine 91 (8): 503–4.

Parving A, Tos M, Thomsen J et al (1992) Some aspects of quality of life after surgery for
    acoustic neuroma. Archives of Otolaryngology Head and Neck Surgery 118 (10):
    1061–4.

Passos J, Brand L (1966) Effects of agents used for oral hygiene. Nursing Research 15:
    196–202.

Pauloski BR, Blom ED, Logemann JA, Hamaker RC (1995) Functional outcome after
    surgery for prevention of pharyngospasms in tracheosophageal speakers. Part two.
    Swallow characteristics. Laryngoscope 105 (10): 1104–10.

Payne JJ, Grimble CR, Silk D (eds) (1995) Artificial Nutrition Support in Clinical
    Practice. London: Edward Arnold.

Pearson L (1996) A comparison of the ability of foam swabs and toothbrushes to remove
    dental plaque: implications for nursing practice. Journal of Advanced Nursing 23:
    62–9.

Pearson BW, Woods RW, Hartman D (1980) Extended hemilaryngectomy for T3 glottic
    carcinoma with preservation of speech and swallowing. Laryngoscope 90: 1950–61.

Peckham S, Winters M (1996) Unequal approach. Nursing Times 92 (12): 31–5.

Pelikan DM, Lion HL, Hermans J, Gaslings BM (1997) The role of radioactive iodine in
    the treatment of advanced differentiated thyroid carcinoma. Clinical Endocrinology
    (Oxford) 47 (6): 713–20.

Pembroke L (1998) Echoes of me. Nursing Times 94 (9): 30–1.

Perlman AL, Schulze-Delrieu K (1997) Diseases and operations of head and neck. In
    Deglutition and its Disorders. Anatomy, Physiology, Clinical Diagnosis and
    Management. San Diego: Singular Publishing Group.

Pernot M, Hoffstetter S, Peiffert D (1996) Role of interstitial brachytherapy in oral and
    pharyngeal carcinoma: a reflection of a series of 1344 patients treated at the time of
    initial presentation. Otolaryngology Head and Neck Surgery 115 (6): 519–26.

Pernot M, Luporsi E, Hoffstetter S et al (1997) Complications following definitive irradi-
    ation for cancers of the oral cavity and the oropharynx (in a series of 1134 patients).
    International Journal of Radiation Oncology Biology Physics 37 (3): 577–85.

Pettifer A (1992) Oral candidiasis and HIV infection. Nursing Standard 6 (42): 34–5.

Pfeiffer P, Hansen O, Madsen EL, May O (1990) A prospective pilot study on the effect of sucrulfate mouth swishing in reducing stomatitis during radiotherapy of the oral cavity. Acta Oncologica 29 (4): 471–3.

Platt AJ, Phipps A, Judkins K (1996) A comparative study of silicone net dressing and paraffin gauze dressing in skin grafted sites. Burns 22 (7): 543–5.

Platt S, Tannahill A, Watson J, Fraser E (1997) Effectiveness of antismoking telephone helpline: follow up survey. British Medical Journal 314: 1371–5.

Poroch D (1995) The effect of preparatory patient education on the anxiety and satisfaction of patients receiving radiation therapy. Cancer Nursing 18 (3): 206–14.

Powaser MM et al (1976) The effectiveness of hourly cuff deflation in minimising tracheal damage. Heart and Lung 5: 5.

Ponzoli V (1968). Zenkers diverticulum. Southern Medical Journal 61: 817–21.

Preisler VK, Hagen R, Hoppe F (1998) Pros and cons of the manual lymph drainage treatment for secondary lymphoedema of the head and neck. Larnygo-Rhino-Otologie 77: 207–12 (German)

Prescott CA (1992) Peristomal complications of paediatric tracheostomy. International Journal of Pediatric Otorhinolaryngology 23 (2): 141–9.

Price B (1990) Body image. In Nursing Concepts and Care. Hemel Hempstead: Prentice-Hall.

Price B (1995) Assessing altered body image. Journal of Psychiatric and Mental Health Nursing 2: 169–75.

Price B (1998) Cancer: altered body image. Nursing Standard 12 (21): 49–55.

Price E (1996) The stigma of smell. Nursing Times 92 (20): 70–1.

Prinsley P (1992) Ballooned trachea as a consequence of intubation. Journal of Laryngology and Otology 106: 561–2.

Prochaska JO, de Clemente C (1985) Common processes of change for smoking, weight loss and psychological distress. In Schiffman S, Wills T (eds) Coping and Substance Abuse. New York: Academic Press.

Prochaska JO, DiClemente CC, Norcross JC (1992) In search of how people change: applications to addictive behaviours. American Psychologist 47: 1102–14.

Prochaska JO, DiClemente CC, Velicer WF, Rossi JS (1993) Standardised, individualised, interactive and personalised self help programs for smoking cessation. Health Psychology 12 (5): 399–405.

Prout MN, Heeren TC, Barber CE et al (1990) Use of health services before diagnosis of head and neck cancer among Boston residents. American Journal of Preventive Medicine 6 (2): 77–83.

Prout MN, Sidaris JN, Witzburg RA et al (1992) A multidisciplinary educational program to promote head and neck screening. Journal Cancer Education 7 (2): 139–46.

Prout MN, Sidaris JN, Witzburg RA et al (1997) Head and neck cancer screening among 4611 tobacco users older than 40 years. Otolaryngology Head and Neck Surgery 116: 201–8.

Ptok M, Maddalena H (1990) Subjective and objective voice assessment following partial resection of the larynx. Laryngo-Rhino-Otologie 69(7): 356–9.

Purandare L (1997) Attitudes to cancer may create a barrier to communication between the patient and caregiver. European Journal of Cancer Care 6: 92–9.

Quick A (1994) Dressing choices. Nursing Times 90 (45) 71–2.

Rachlis M, Kusner C (1989) Second Opinion: What's Wrong with Canada's Health Care System and How to Fix It. Toronto: Harper and Collins.

Ransier A, Epstein JB, Lunn R, Spinelli J (1995) A combined analysis of a toothbrush, foam brush and a chlorhexidine soaked foam brush in maintaining oral hygiene. Cancer Nursing 18 (5): 393–6.

Rapoport Y, Kreitler S, Chaitchik S et al (1993) Psychosocial problems in head and neck cancer patients and their change with time since diagnosis. Annals of Oncology 4: 69–73.

Rathmell AJ, Ash DV, Howes M, Nicholls J (1991) Assessing quality of life in patients treated for advanced head and neck cancer. Clinical Oncology 3: 10–16.

Raufman JP (1988) Odynophagia/dysphagia in AIDS. Gastroenterology Clinics of North America 17 (3): 599.

Raybould T, Carpenter AD, Ferretti GA et al (1994) Emergence of Gram-negative bacilli in the mouths of bone marrow transplant recipients using chlorhexidine mouthrinse. Oncology Nursing Forum 2 (4): 691–6.

Reding DJ, Huber JA, Lappe KA (1995). Results of a rural health education demonstration project. Cancer Practice : A Multidisciplinary Journal of Cancer Care 3 (5): 295–301.

Reese JL (1990) Nursing interventions for wound healing in plastic and reconstructive surgery. Nursing Clinics of North America 25 (1): 223–33.

Regan M (1988) Tracheal mucosal injury — the nurse's role. Nursing 29: 1064–6.

Remmler D, Byers R, Scheetz J et al (1986) A prospective study of shoulder disability resulting from radical and modified neck dissections. Head and Neck Surgery 8: 280–86.

Reuler DUB, Balazs JAR (1991) Portable medical record for the homeless mentally ill. British Medical Journal 303: 446.

Richardson JL, Graham JW, Shelton DR (1989) Social environment and adjustment after laryngectomy. Health and Social Work November: 283–92.

Rickman J (1998) Percutaneous endoscopic gastrostomy: psychological effects. British Journal of Nursing 7 (12): 723–9.

Rigrodsky S, Lerman J, Morrison EB (1971) Diagnostic techniques for determining methods and potential for teaching alaryngeal speech. In Therapy for the Laryngectomized Patient. A Speech Clinician's Manual. Columbia University: Teachers College Press.

Riley AJ (1996) Perceived carer attitudes to alcohol dependent patients. Nursing Standard 10 (27): 39–44.

Ripamonti C, Zecca E, Brunelli C (1997) A randomised controlled clinical trial to evaluate the effects of zinc sulphate on cancer patients with taste alterations caused by head and neck irradiation. Cancer 82 (10): 1938–45.

Robbins KT, Davidson W, Peters LJ, Goepfort H (1988) Conservation surgery for T2 and T3 carcinomas of the supraglottic larynx. Archives of Otolaryngology Head and Neck Surgery 114: 421–6.

Robbins KT, Medina JE, Wolf GT, Levine PA, Sessions RB, Pruet CW (1991) Standardising neck dissection terminology. Official report of the Academy's Committee for Head and Neck Surgery and Oncology. Archives of Otolaryngology Head and Neck Surgery 117: 601–6.

Robertson AG, Robertson C, Boyle et al (1993) The effect of differing radiotherapeutic schedules on the response of glottic carcinoma of the larynx. European Journal of Cancer 4: 501–10.

Robinson E, Rumsey N, Partridge J (1996) An evaluation of the impact of social interaction skills training for facially disfigured people. British Journal of Plastic Surgery 49: 281–9.

Robinson L, Cawthorne J, Parys H, Howells B (1983) The use of beeswax as a dressing. Nursing Mirror November 9: 25–6.

Rodrigues M, Havlik E, Peskar B, Sinzinger H (1997) Prostaglandins as biochemical markers of radiation injury to the salivary glands after iodine-131 therapy? European Journal of Nuclear Medicine 25: 265–9.

Rodzwic D, Donnard J (1986) The use of myocutaneous flaps in reconstructive surgery for head and neck cancer: guidelines for nursing care. Oncology Nursing Forum 13: 29–35.

Rogers M (1990) Nursing: science of unitary, irreducible, human beings. In Barret EAM (ed) Visions of Rogers Science Based Nursing. New York: National League for Nursing.

Rogers SN, Humphris G, Lowe D et al (1998) The impact of surgery for oral cancer on quality of life as measured by the medical outcomes short form 36. Oral Oncology 34: 171–9.

Rollnick S, Miller WR (1995) What is motivational interviewing? Cognitive Behavioural Psychotherapy 23: 325–34.

Rollnick S, Butler C, Stott N (1997) Helping smokers make decisions: the enhancement of brief intervention for general medical practice. Patient Education and Counselling 31: 191–203.

Rombeau JL, Camilo Palacio (1990) Feeding by tube enterostomy. In Rombeau JL, Caldwell MD (eds) Clinical Nutrition Enteral and Parenteral Feeding, 2nd edn. Philadelphia: WB Saunders Company.

Roncetti P (1998) Cleaning up your practice. Nursing Times 94 (28): 70–1.

Rosen IB, Azadian A, Walfish PG et al (1993) Ultrasound guided fine needle aspiration biopsy in the management of thyroid disease. American Journal of Surgery 166: 346–9.

Rosenberg B, Katz Y (1997) Airway obstruction with a minitracheostomy tube. Journal of Cardiothoracic Vascular Anaesthesia 11 (5): 613–14.

Rossing MA, Voigt LF, Wicklund KG et al (1998) Use of exogenous hormones and risk of papillary thyroid cancer. Cancer Causes and Control 9 (3): 341–9.

Ross Russel RW, Wiles CM (1985) Intracranial tumours. In McNicol GP (ed) Neurology: Integrated Clinical Science. Chicago: Year Book Medical Publishers.

Roter DL (1984) Patient question asking in physician–patient interaction. Health Psychology 3: 395–409.

Rothman KJ et al (1980) Epidemiology of laryngeal cancer. Epidemiology Review 2: 195–209.

Rovirosa A, Ferre J, Biete A (1998) Granulocyte macrophage-colony-stimulating factor mouthwashes heal oral ulcers during head and neck radiotherapy. International Journal of Radiation Oncology Biology Physiology 41 (4): 747–54.

Rowe BH, Rampton J, Bota GW (1996) Life threatening luminal obstruction due to mucous plugging in chronic tracheostomies: three case reports and a review of the literature. Journal of Emergency Medicine 14 (5): 565–7.

Rugg T, Saunders MI, Dische S (1990) Smoking and mucosal reactions to radiotherapy. British Journal of Radiology 63: 554–6.

Ruhl CM, Gleich LL, Gluckman JL (1997) Survival, function, and quality of life after total glossectomy. Laryngoscope 107: 1316–21.

Rumsey N (1997) Historical and anthropological perspectives on appearance. Chapter 15 in Lansdown R, Rumsey N, Bradbury E et al (eds) Visibly Different. Coping with Disfigurement. Oxford: Butterworth-Heinemann.

Rumsey N, Bull R (1986) The effects of facial disfigurement on social interaction. Human Learning 5: 203–8.

Rumsey N, Bull R, Gahagan D (1982) The effect of facial disfigurement in the proxemic behaviour of the general public. Journal of Applied Social Psychology 12 (2): 137–50.

Rumsey N, Bull R, Gahagan D (1986) A preliminary study of the potential skills for improving the quality of social interaction for the facially disfigured. Social Behaviour 1: 143–5.

Rush KL (1997) Health promotion ideology and nursing education. Journal of Advanced Nursing 25: 1292–8.

Rushworth C (1994) Making a Difference in Cancer Care. London: Human Horizons Series, Souvenir Press.

Saah D, Braverman I, Sichel JY et al (1996) An unusual bronchial foreign body: a fragment of a tracheostomy tube. Harefuah 130 (8): 519–20.

Sagar SM, Thomas RJ, Lovercock LT, Spittle MF (1991) Olfactory sensations produced by high energy photon irradiation of the olfactory receptor mucosa in humans. International Journal of Radiation Oncology Biology Physics 20: 771–6.

Sakabu S, Levine JH, Trottier SJ et al (1997) Airway obstruction with percutaneous tracheostomy. Chest 111 (5): 1468.

Salmon SJ (1979a) Methods of air intake for oesophageal speech and their associated problems. In Keith RL, Darley FL (eds) Laryngectomy Rehabilitation. Houston: College Hill Press.

Salmon SJ (1979b) Pre and postoperative conferences with laryngectomized patients and their spouses. In Keith RL, Darley FL (eds) Laryngectomy Rehabilitation. Houston: College Hill Press.

Salter M (1988) Altered Body Image. The Nurse's Role. Chichester: J. Wiley & Sons.

Sanchez-Salazar V, Stark A (1972) The use of crisis intervention in the rehabilitation of laryngectomees. Journal of Speech and Hearing Disorders 37 (3): 323–8.

Sasaki CT, Suzuki M, Homuchi M, Kirchner JA (1977) The effect of tracheostomy on the laryngeal closure reflex. Laryngoscope 87: 1428–33.

Sataloff RT, Myers DL, Lowry LD, Spiegel JR (1987) Total temporal bone resection for squamous cell carcinoma. Otolaryngology Head Neck Surgery 96: 3–14.

Saunders C (1990) Hospice and Palliative Care, An Interdisciplinary Approach. London: Edward Arnold.

Saunders MI, Dische S, Hong A et al (1989) Continuous hyperfractionated accelerated radiotherapy in locally advanced carcinoma of the head and neck region. International Journal of Radiation Oncology Biology Physics 17: 1287–93.

Saunders WH, Johnson EW (1975) Rehabilitation of the shoulder after radical neck dissection. Annals of Otology 84: 812–16.

Sawyer N (1997) Back from the twilight zone. Nursing Times 93 (7): 28–9.

Schafer U, Schmilowski GM, Micke O et al (1996) A method of brachytherapeutic treatment of tracheal stoma recurrence in head and neck cancer. The British Journal of Radiology 69: 348–50.

Schierhout G, Roberts I (1998) Fluid resuscitation with colloid or crystalloid solutions in critically ill patients: a systematic review of randomised trials. British Medical Journal 316: 961–4.

Schiffman S (1983a) Taste and smell in disease. New England Journal of Medicine 308 (21): 1275–9.

Schiffman S (1983b) Taste and smell in disease. New England Journal of Medicine 308 (22): 1337–43.

Schleper JR (1989) Prevention, direction and diagnosis of head and neck cancers. Seminars in Oncology Nursing 5 (3): 139–49.

Schmidt W, Popham RE (1981) The role of drinking and smoking in mortality from cancer and other causes in male alcoholics. Cancer 47: 1031–41.

Schnetler JFC (1992) Oral cancer diagnosis and delays in referral. British Journal of Oral and Maxillofacial Surgery 30: 210–13.

Schultheiss TE, Stephens LC (1992) Radiation myelopathy. British Journal of Radiology 65: 737–53.

Schutheiss TE, Stephens LC, Peters LJ (1986) Survival in radiation myelopathy. International Journal of Radiation Oncology Biology Physics 12:1765–9.

Schwarz R, Chan NH, MacFarlane JK (1990) Fine needle aspiration cytology in the evaluation of head and neck masses. American Journal of Surgery 159: 482–5.

Schweiger JL et al (1980) Oral assessment: how to do it. American Journal of Nursing 80: 654–7.

Scott E, Cowen B (1997) Multidisciplinary collaborative care planning. Nursing Standard 12 (1): 39–42.

Scully C, Malamos D et al (1986) Sources and patterns of referrals of oral cancer: role of general practitioners. British Medical Journal Clinical Research 293 (6547): 599–601.

Seifert G, Sobin LH (1992) The World Health Organization's histological classification of salivary gland tumors: a commentary on the second edition. Cancer 70(2): 379–85.

Sekhar LN, Schramm VL Jr, Jones NF (1987) Subtemporal-preauricular infratemporal fossa approach to large lateral and posterior cranial base neoplasms. Journal of Neurosurgery 67: 488–99.

Selecky P (1974) Tracheostomy: a review of present day indications, complications and care. Heart and Lung 3 (2): 272–82.

Seymour J (1997) Alginate dressings in wound care. Nursing Times 93 (44): 49–51.

Shaari CM, Buchbinder D, Constantino PD et al (1998) Complication of microvascular head and neck surgery in the elderly. Archives of Otolaryngology Head and Neck Surgery 124: 407–11.

Shah JP (1986) Management of regional metastases in salivary and thyroid cancer. In Larson DL, Ballantyne AJ, Guillamondegui OM (eds) Cancer in the Neck — Evaluation and Treatment. New York: MacMillan.

Shah JP (1990) Patterns of cervical lymph node metastases from squamous carcinomas of the upper aerodigestive tract. American Journal of Surgery 160: 405–9.

Shah JP, Candella FC, Poddar AK (1990) The patterns of cervical lymph node metastases from squamous carcinoma of the oral cavity. Cancer 66: 109–13.

Shah JP, Loree T, Dharker D et al (1992) Lobectomy vs. total thyroidectomy for differentiated carcinoma of the thyroid. A matched pair analysis. American Journal of Surgery 166: 331–5.

Shaha AR, Jaffe BM (1998) Parathyroid preservation during thyroid surgery. American Journal of Otolaryngology 19 (2): 113–17.

Shaha AR, Shah JP, Loree TR (1997) Differentiated thyroid cancer presenting initially with distant metastasis. American Journal of Surgery 174 (5): 474–6.

Shane E (1994) Parathyroid carcinoma. In Bilezikian JP, Marcus R, Levine MA (eds) The Parathyroids: Basic and Clinical Concepts. New York: Raven Press.

Shanks J (1979) Development of the feminine voice and refinement of oesophageal voice. In Keith R, Darley F (eds) Laryngectomee Rehabilitation. Houston, Texas: College Hill Press (cited by Stam et al, 1991).

Shapsay SM, Scott RM, McCann CF, Stoelting I (1980) Pain control in advanced and recurrent head and neck cancer. Otolaryngologic Clinics of North America 13 (3): 551–60.

Shaw JH (1987) Causes and control of dental caries. New England Journal of Medicine 317: 996–1004.

Shedd DP, Carl A, Shedd C (1980) Problems of terminal head and neck cancer patients. Head and Neck Surgery 2: 476–82.

Shell JA (1995) Do you like the things that life is showing you? The sensitive self-image of the person with cancer. Oncology Nursing Forum 22 (6): 907–11.

Shelley MP, Lloyd GM, Park GR (1988) A review of the mechanisms and methods of humidification of inspired gases. Intensive Care Medicine 14: 1–9.

Shepherd G et al (1987) The mouthtrap. Nursing Times 83: 19: 25–7.

Shike M, Berner Y, Gerdes H et al (1989) Percutaneous endoscopic gastrostomy and jejunostomy. Otolaryngology — Head and Neck Surgery 101(Supplement): 549–54.

Shillitoe EJ (1987) Viruses in the aetiology of head and neck cancer. Cancer Bulletin 39: 82–5.

Shils ME (1979) Principles of nutritional therapy. Cancer 43: 2093–102.

Short SO, Kaplan JN, Laramore GE, Cummings CW (1984) Shoulder pain and function after neck dissection with or without preservation of the spinal accessory nerve. American Journal of Surgery 148: 478–82.

Shumrick DA (1973) Carotid artery rupture. Laryngoscope 83: 1051–61.

Sibbald WJ, Keenan SP (1997) Show me the evidence: a critical appraisal of the pulmonary artery catheter consensus conference and other musings on how critical care practitioners need to improve the way we conduct business (editorial). Critical Care Medicine 25: 2060–3.

Silverstein P (1992) Smoking and wound healing. The American Journal of Medicine 93 (Supplement 1A): 22–4.

Simons D, Kidd EAM, Beighton D, Jones B (1997) The effect of chlorhexidine/xylitol chewing gum on cariogenic salivary microflora: a clinical trial in elderly patients. Caries Research 31: 91–6.

Sims R, Fitzgerald V (1985) Community nursing management of patients with ulcerating/fungating malignant breast disease. London: RCN Oncology Nursing Society.

Singer MI, Blom ED (1980) An endoscopic technique for restoration of voice after laryngectomy. Annals of Otology Rhinology Laryngology 89: 529–33.

Singh B, Balwally AN, Shaha AR, Rosenfeld RM, Har - El G, Lucente FE 1996 Upper aerodigestive tract squamous cell carcinoma. The human immunodeficiency virus connection. Archives of Otolaryngology Head and Neck Surgery 122 (6): 639–43.

Siston AK, List MA, Schleser R, Vokes E (1997) Sexual functioning and head and neck cancer. Journal of Psychosocial Oncology 15 (3/4): 107–22.

Slevin ML, Plant H, Lynch D et al (1988) Who should measure quality of life, the doctor or the patient? British Journal of Cancer 57: 109–12.

Smale BF, Mullen JL, Buzby GP, Rossaro EF (1981) The efficiency of nutritional assessment and support in cancer surgery. Cancer 47: 2375–81.

Soren M Bentzen & Jens Overgaard (1996) Clinical normal-tissue radiobiology. In Tobias JS, Thomas PRM (eds) Current Radiation Oncology, Volume 2. London: Arnold.

Souhami S, Tobias J (1995) Cancer and Its Management, 2nd edn. Oxford: Blackwell Science.

Soutar DS, Scheker LR, Tanner NSB, McGregor IA (1983) The radial forearm flap: a versatile method of intraoral reconstruction. British Journal of Plastic Surgery 36: 1–8.

Soylu L, Kiroglu M, Aydogan B et al (1998) Pharyngocutaneous fistula following laryngectomy. Head and Neck 20: 22–5.

Smith AM (1994) Emergencies in palliative care. Annals of Academy Medicine of Singapore 23(2): 186–90.

Smith JW, Aston SJ (eds) (1991) Grabb & Smith's Plastic Surgery. 4th edn. Boston: Little Brown & Co. Cited in Edwards J (1998) Plastic surgery: a community perspective. Journal of Community Nursing 12(10): 22–6.

Speigel D, Bloom J, Kraemer H, Gottheil E (1989) The beneficial effect of psychosocial treatment on survival of metastatic breast cancer patients: a randomised prospective outcome study. The Lancet 340: 888–91.

Spencer T (1988) Dry skin and skin moisturisers. Clinics in Dermatology 6: 3.

Spijkervet FKL, Saene HKF van, Saene JJM van, Panders AK et al (1990) Effect of selective elimination of the oral flora on mucositis in irradiated head and neck cancer patients. Journal Oral Pathology Medicine 19: 486–9.

Spiro RH (1986) Salivary neoplasms: overview of a 35-year experience with 2,807 patients. Head and Neck Surgery 8(3): 177–84.

Spiro RH, Huvos AG, Wong GY et al (1986) Predictive value of tumor thickness in squamous cell cancer confined to the tongue and floor of mouth. American Journal of Surgery 152: 345–50.

Spitz MR (1994) Epidemiology and risk factors for head and neck cancer. Seminars in Oncology 21(3): 281–8.

Spitz MR, Sider JG, Newell GR, Batsakis JG (1988) Incidence of salivary gland cancer in the United States relative to ultraviolet radiation exposure. Head and Neck 12 (3): 254–6.

Spross JA, McGuire DB, Schmitt RM (1990) Oncology Nursing Society position paper on cancer pain. Oncology Nursing Forum 17 (4): 595–613.

Stachler RJ, Hamlet SL, Choi J, Fleming S (1996) Scintigraphic quantification of aspiration reduction with the Passy Muir valve. Laryngoscope 106 (2 Pt1): 231–4.

Stafford A, Hannigan B (1997) Client-held records in community mental health. Nursing Times 93 (7): 50–1.

Stafford N, Samaranayake LP, Robertson AG, Macfarlane TW et al (1988) The effect of chlorhexidine and benzydamine mouthwashes on mucositis induced by therapeutic irradiation. Clinical Radiology 39: 291–4.

Stafford N, Walsh-Waring G, Munro A (1989) Tumours of the tonsil and retromolar trigone.

Stam HJ, Koopmans JP, Mathieson CM (1991) The psychosocial impact of laryngectomy: a comprehensive assessment. Journal of Psychosocial Oncology 9 (3): 37–59.

Steiner W (1993) Results of curative laser microsurgery of laryngeal carcinomas. American Journal of Otolaryngology 14(2): 116–21.

Stockley IH (1991) Drug Interactions. Oxford: Blackwell Scientific Publications cited in Hampson JP (1996) The use of metronidazole in treatment of malodorous wounds. Journal of Wound Care 5 (9): 421–6.

Strauss M, Bushey MJ, Chung C, Baum S (1982) Fracture of the clavicle following radical neck dissection and postoperative radiotherapy: a case report and review of the literature. Laryngoscope 92 (11): 1304–7.

Strauss RP (1989) Psychosocial responses to oral and maxillofacial surgery for head and neck cancer. Journal of Oral and Maxillofacial Surgery 47: 343–8.

Strohl, R. (1998) The nursing role in radiation oncology. Oncology Nursing Forum 15 (4): 429–34.

Stucchi F, Bertoni F, Bignardi M et al (1987) Proposed evaluation scale for damage to healthy tissues as a result of radiotherapy of chest, head and neck cancers. International Journal of Tissue Reaction 6: 509–13.

Suarez O (1963) El problema de al metastasis linfaticas y alejudas del cancer de alringe e hipofaringe. Revista Otorinolaringogica 23: 83–99.

Swain RE, Biller HF, Ogura JH (1974) An experimental analysis of causative factors and protective methods in carotid artery rupture. Archives of Otolaryngology Head and Neck Surgery 99: 235–41.

Swanson GM, Burns PB (1997) Cancers of the salivary gland: workplace risks among women and men. Annals of Epidemiology 7 (6): 369–74.

Swanson M (1995) The use of patient complaints to improve service delivery. Nursing Times 91 (41): 29.

Swerdlow M, Cundill JF (1981) Anti-convulsant drugs used in the treatment of lancinating pain: a comparison. Anaesthesiology 36: 1129–32.

Symonds RP, McIlroy P, Khourami J et al (1996) The reduction of radiation mucosis by selective decontamination antiobiotic pastilles: a placebo-controlled double blind trial. British Journal of Cancer 74: 312–17.

Talmi YP, Waller A, Bercovici M (1997) Pain experienced by patients with terminal head and neck carcinoma. Cancer 80: 1117–23.

Tami TA, Gomez P, Parker GS, et al (1991) Thyroid dysfunction following radiation therapy in the head and neck cancer patient. Presented at the 33rd annual meeting of the American Society for Head and Neck Surgery, Waikoloa, Hawaii.

Tapazoglon E, Fish J, Emsley J et al (1986) The activity of single agent 5-fluorouracil infusion in advanced and recurrent head and neck cancer. Cancer 57: 1105–9.

Tatchell RH, Lerman JW, Watt J (1985) Olfactory ability as a function of nasal airflow volume in laryngectomees. American Journal of Otolaryngology 6: 426–32.

Taylor S, Goodinson-McLaren S (1992) Nutritional Support : A Team Approach. London: Wolfe Publishing Ltd.

Telfer MR, Shepherd JP (1993) Psychological distress in patients attending an oncology clinic after definitive treatment for maxillofacial malignant neoplasia. International Journal of Oral and Maxillofacial Surgery 22: 347–9.

Tell R, Sjodin H, Lundell G (1997) Hypothyroidism after external radiotherapy for head and neck cancer. International Journal of Radiation Oncology Biology Physics 39 (2): 303–8.

Teoh N, Parr MJ, Finfer SR (1997) Bacteraemia following percutaneous dilational tracheostomy. Anaesthesia and Intensive Care 25 (4): 354–7.

Terrell JE, Nanavati KA, Esclamado RM et al (1997) Head and neck cancer specific quality of life. Archives of Otolaryngology Head and Neck Surgery 123: 1125–32.

The Health of the Nation (1992) A Strategy for Health in England. London: HMSO.

Theologies A (1978) Origins of anorexia in neoplastic disease. American Journal of Clinical Nutrition 31: 1104–7.

Theriault C, Fitzpatrick PJ (1986) Malignant parotid tumors: prognostic factors and optimum treatment. American Journal of Clinical Oncology 9(6): 510–16.

Thomas S (1990) Wound Management and Dressings. London: Pharmaceutical Press.

Thomas S (1992) Current Practices in the Management of Fungating Lesions and Radiation Damaged Skin. Bridgend General Hospital: The Surgical Materials Testing Laboratory.

Tippetts D, Siebens A (1991) Speaking and swallowing on a ventilator. Dysphagia 6: 94–9.

Tiwari RM (1985) Reconstruction after subtotal temporal bone resection. Journal of Laryngology and Otology 99: 143–6.

Toljanic JA, Siddiqui AA, Patterson GL, Irwin ME (1996) An evaluation of a dentrifice containing salivary peroxidase elements for the control of gingival disease in patients with irradiated head and neck cancer. The Journal of Prosthetic Dentistry 76 (3): 292–6.

Toljanic JA, Ali M, Haraf DJ, Vokes EE et al (1998) Osteoradionecrosis of the jaws as a risk factor in radiotherapy: a report of an eight year retrospective review. Oncology Reports 5 (2): 345–9.

Tombes BT, Gallucci B (1993) The effects of hydrogen peroxide rinses on the normal oral mucosa. Nursing Research 42 (6): 332–7.

Tonge H (1997) The management of infected wounds. Nursing Standard 12 (12): 49–53.

Toursarkissian B, Zweng TN, Kearney PA et al (1994) Percutaneous dilational tracheostomy: report of 141 cases. Annals of Thoracic Surgery 57 (4): 862–7.

Trenter Roth P, Creason N (1986) Nurse administered oral hygiene: is there a scientific basis? Journal of Advanced Nursing 11: 323–31.

Trotti A, Johnson DJ, Gwede C et al (1998) Development of a head and neck companion module for the quality of life-radiation therapy instrument (QOL-RTI) International Journal of Radiation Oncology Biology Physics 42 (2): 257–61.

Truelson JM, Pearce AN (1997) Tongue reconstruction procedures for treatment of cancer. AORN Journal 65(3): 528–51.

Tucker SL, Chan K (1990) The selection of patient for accelerated radiotherapy on the basis of tumour growth kinetics and intrinsic radiosensitivity. Radiotherapy Oncology 18: 197–211.

Twycross R (1994) Pain Relief in Advanced Cancer. Edinburgh: Churchill Livingstone.

Twycross R (1997) Pain Relief. Chapter 2 in Symptom Management in Advanced Cancer, 2nd edn. Abingdon: Radcliffe Medical Press.

Twycross R, Wilcock A, Thorp S (1998) Palliative Care Formulary. Abingdon: Radcliffe Medical Press.

UICC International Union Against Cancer (1997) In Sobin LH, Witteknid Ch (eds) TNM Classification of Malignant Tumours, 5th edn. New York: Wiley-Liss.

Ulbricht GF (1986) Laryngectomy rehabilitation: a woman's viewpoint. Women and Health 11 (314): 131–6.

Urken ML, Biller MF (1994) A new design for the sensate radial forearm free flap to preserve tongue mobility following significant glossectomy. Archives of Otolaryngology Head and Neck Surgery 120: 126–31.

Urken ML, Moscoso JF, Lawson W, Biller MF (1994a) A systematic approach to functional reconstruction of the oral cavity following partial and total glossectomy. Archives of Otolaryngology Head and Neck Surgery 120: 589–601.

Urken ML, Vickery C, Wienberg H, Biller MF (1994b) The neurofasciocutaneous radial forearm flap in head and neck reconstruction; a preliminary report. Laryngoscope 100: 161–73.

US Department of Health and Human Services (1986). The Health Consequences of Using Smokeless Tobacco; A report of the Advisory Committee to the Surgeon General NIH Publication 86–2874. Washington, DC: US Government Printing Office.

Van Bokhorst-de van der Schueren MAE, Van le Euwen PAM, Sauerwein HP et al

(1997) Assessment of malnutrition parameters in head and neck cancer and their relation to post-operative complications. Head and Neck 19: 419–25.

Van den Brekel M (1992) Assessment of lymph node metastases in the neck. A radiological and histopathological study. Academic Thesis, Drukkerij Elinkwijk bv, Utrecht.

Van den Brekel MW (1996) US-guided fine-needle aspiration cytology of neck nodes in patients with N0 disease. Radiology 201: 580–1.

Van Dusen W (1967) The natural depth in man. In Rogers CR, Stevens B (eds) Person to Person. The Problem of Being Human. London: Souvenir Press.

Van Harteveld JTM, Mistaen PJML, Dukkers van Emden D (1997) Home visits by community nurses for cancer patients after discharge from hospital: an evaluation study of the continuity visit. Cancer Nursing 20 (2): 105–14.

Van Wersch A, de Boer MF, van der Does E et al (1997) Continuity of information in cancer care: evaluation on a logbook. Patient Education and Counselling 31: 223–36.

Vecht CJ, Anneke MH, Kansen PJ (1992) Types and causes of pain in cancer of the head and neck. Cancer 70 (1): 178–84.

Velicer WF, Prochaska JO, Bellis JM et al (1993) An expert system intervention for smoking cessation. Addictive Behaviors 18: 269–90.

Verrill P (1994) Sympathetic ganglion lesions. Chapter 3.C.2 in Wall PD, Melzack R (eds) Textbook of Pain. Edinburgh: Churchill Livingstone.

Vissink A, 's-Gravenmade EJ, Panders AK et al (1983) A clinical comparison between commercially available mucin- and CMC- containing saliva substitutes. International Journal of Oral Surgery 12: 232–8.

Vlantis AC, Marres HA, van den Hoogen FJ (1998) A surgical technique to prevent tracheostomal stenosis after laryngectomy. Laryngoscope 108 (1 Pt1): 134–7.

Vloemans J, Bankras JH (1991) Fixation of split thickness skin grafts with Mepitel. An open non-comparative study in twenty children. Presented at the European Burns Congress, Barcelona. Cited in Williams C (1995) Mepitel. British Journal of Nursing 4 (1): Product focus insert.

Vloemans AFPM, Kreis RW (1994) Fixation of skin grafts with a new silicone rubber dressing (Mepital). Scandinavian Journal of Plastic Reconstructive Hand Surgery 28: 75–6.

Vokes EE, Haraf DJ, Weichselbaum RR et al (1992) Perspectives on combination chemotherapy with concomitant radiotherapy for poor prognosis head and neck cancer. Seminars in Oncology 19 (Supplement 11): 47–56.

Vrabec DP, and Heffron TJ (1981) Hypothyroidism following treatment for head and neck cancer. Annals of Otology Rhinology Laryngology 90: 440–53.

Waldron J (ed) Management of Oral Cancer Oxford: Oxford Medical Publications.

Waldron J, Padgham ND, Hurley SE (1990) Complications of emergency and elective tracheostomy. Annals of the Royal College of Surgeons of England 72: 218–20.

Walizer EM, Ephraim PM (1996) Clinical trial of vegetable oil versus Xerolube for xerostomia: an expanded study abstract. ORL—Head and Neck Nursing 14 (1): 11–12.

Wang WL, Hussain K, Chevretton E et al (1996) Validation and clinical application of computer-combined computed tomography and positron emission tomography with 2-(18F) fluoro-2-deoxy-D-glucose head and neck images. American Journal of Surgery 172: 628–32.

Ware JE, Sherbourne CD (1992) The MOS 36-item Short Form Health Survey (SF-36). I. Conceptual framework and item selection. Medical Care 30: 473–83.

Watt-Watson J, Graydon J (1995) Impact of surgery on head and neck cancer patients and their caregivers. Nursing Clinics of North America 30 (4): 659–71.

Webb P (1979) Nursing care of patients undergoing treatment by teletherapy. In Tifford R (ed) Cancer Nursing: Radiotherapy. London: Faber and Faber.

Weber M, Reimer M (1993) Laryngectomy: grieving disfigurement and dysfunction. The Canadian Nurse March: 31–4.

Weinrich SP, Weinrich MC (1986) Cancer knowledge among elderly individuals. Cancer Nursing 9 (6): 301–7.

Weintraub FN, Hagopian GA (1990) The effect of nursing consultation on anxiety, side effects, and self care of patients receiving radiation therapy. Oncology Nursing Forum 17 (3) (Supplement): 31–7.

Weissler MC (1997) Management of complications resulting form laryngeal cancer treatment. Otolaryngology Clinics of North America 30 (2): 269–78.

Weissler MC, Melin S, Sailer SL et al (1992) Simultaneous chemoradiation in the treatment of advanced head and neck cancer. Archives of Otolaryngology Head and Neck Surgery 118: 806–10.

Weissman DE, Janjan N, Byhardt RW (1989) Assessment of pain during head and neck irradiation. Journal of Pain and Symptom Management 4 (2): 90–5.

Welch LB (1982) Buttermilk and yoghurt odour control of open lesions. Critical Care Update 9 (11): 39–44.

Wells M (1998) The hidden experience of radiotherapy to the head and neck: a qualitative study of patients after completion of treatment. Journal of Advanced Nursing 28 (4): 840–8.

Wells SA, Chi DD, Toshima K et al (1994) Predictive DNA testing and prophylactic thyroidectomy in patients at risk for multiple endocrine neoplasia type 2a. Annals of Surgery 220: 237–50.

Wendt TG, Graenbauer GG, Rodel CM (1998) Simultaneous radiochemotherapy versus radiotherapy alone in advanced head and neck cancer: a randomised multicenter study. Journal of Clinical Oncology 16 (4): 318–24.

Western Consortium for Cancer Nursing Research (1991) Staging system for stomatitis. Cancer Nursing 14 (1): 6–12.

Westin T, Jamsson A, Zenckert C et al (1988) Mental depression is associated with malnutrition in patients with head and neck cancer. Archives of Otolaryngology Head and Neck Surgery 114: 1449–53.

Wetmore SJ, Krueger K, Wesson K, Blessing ML (1985) Long term results of the Blom-Singer speech rehabilitation procedure. Archives of Otolaryngology 111: 106–9.

White C (1998) Psychological management of stoma-related concerns. Nursing Standard 12 (36): 35–8.

Wickham R, Roham K (1997) Endocrine malignancies. Chapter 37 in Groenwald SL, Hansen Frogge M, Goodman M, Henke Yarbro C (eds) Cancer Nursing. Principles and Practice, 3rd edn. Boston: Jones & Bartlett.

Wiernik G et al (1990) Final report of the general clinical results of the British Institute of Radiology fraction study of 3F/wk versus 5F/wk in radiotherapy of carcinoma of the laryngo-pharynx. British Journal of Radiology 63: 169–80.

Wiley SB (1969) Why glycerol and lemon juice? American Journal of Nursing 69: 342–4.

Wilkes GM (1996) Toxicity to rapidly proliferating normal cell populations. Chapter 5 in Barton Burke M, Wilkes, GM, Ingwersen KC (eds) Cancer Chemotherapy. A Nursing Process Approach. Boston: Jones & Bartlett.

Wilkinson B (1997) Hard graft. Nursing Times 93 (16): 63–8.

Williams A (1997) Lymphoedema. Professional Nurse 12 (9): 645–8.

Williams A, Venables J (1995) Skin care in patients with uncomplicated lymphoedema. Journal of Wound Care 5 (5): 223–6.

Williams C (1995) Mepitel. British Journal of Nursing 4 (1), Product focus insert.

Williams PT et al (1994) In office cancer screening of primary care physicians. Journal of Cancer Education 9 (2): 90–5.

Wilson C, Bilodeau ML (1989) Current management for the patient with lymphoedema. Journal of Cardiovascular Nursing 4: 79–88.

Wilson PR, Herman J, Chubon SJ (1991) Eating strategies used by persons with head and neck cancer during and after radiotherapy. Cancer Nursing 14 (2): 98–104.

Wingren G, Hallquist A, Hardell L (1997) Diagnostic xray exposure and female papillary thyroid cancer: a pooled analysis of two Swedish studies. European Journal of Cancer Prevention 6 (6): 550–6.

Winn DM, Blot WJ, Shy CM et al (1981) Snuff dipping and oral cancer among women in southern United States. New England Journal of Medicine 304: 49–62.

Wong JK, Wood RE, McLean M (1998) Pain preceding recurrent head and neck cancer. Journal of Orofacial Pain 12: 52–9.

Wood DE, Mathiesen DJ (1991) Late complications of tracheostomy. Clinics in Chest Medicine 12 (3): 597–609.

Wood KM (1994) Peripheral nerve and root chemical lesions. Chapter 3.C.1 in Wall PD, Melzack R (eds) Textbook of Pain. Edinburgh: Churchill Livingstone.

Woods JE, Chong GC, Beahrs OH (1975) Experience with 1,360 primary parotid tumors. American Journal of Surgery 1075 (130): 460–2.

Woodtli MA, Ort SV (1991) Nursing diagnoses and functional health patterns in patients receiving external beam radiation therapy: cancer of the head and neck. Nursing Diagnosis 2 (4): 171–9.

World Health Organization (1984) Control of oral cancer in developing countries. Bulletin of the World Health Organization 62: 817–30.

World Health Organization (1986) Cancer Pain Relief. Geneva. Cited in Grond S, Zech D, Lynch J et al (1993) Validation of World Health Organization guidelines for pain relief in head and neck cancer. A prospective study. Annals of Otology Rhinology Laryngology 102: 342–8.

World Health Organization (1990) Cancer pain relief and palliative care. Geneva: WHO.

Wright B (1993) Caring in Crisis. A Handbook of Intervention Skills. Edinburgh: Churchill Livingstone.

Wright CD (1996) Management of tracheinnominate artery fistula. Chest Surgery Clinics of North America 6 (4): 865–73.

Wynder EL, Hoffman D (1982) Tobacco. In Scottenfield D, Fraumeni JF Jr (eds) Cancer Epidemiology and Prevention. Philadelphia: Saunders, pp 277–92.

Yang CS, Wang ZY (1993) Tea and cancer. Journal of the National Cancer Institute 85: 1038–49.

Yellowitz JA, Goodman HS (1995) Assessing physicians and dentists oral cancer knowledge, opinions and practices. Journal of the American Dental Association 126: 53–60.

Yokoyama M, Kaga K, Suzuki M, Ishimoto S (1995) Innominate artery erosion complication use of tracheal tube with adjustable flange. ORL Otorhinolaryngology and its Related Specialities 57 (5): 293–5.

Yorkshire Cancer Organisation (1994) Head and Neck Cancers Cancer Registry Special Report Series 2, Leeds: Yorkshire Cancer Organisation.

Yoshida K, Oshima H, Iwata K et al (1998) Rupture of the innominate artery following tracheostomy: report of a case. Surgery Today 28 (4): 433–4.

Young JS, Brady WJ, Kesser B, Mullins D (1996) A novel method for replacement of the dislodged tracheostomy tube: the nasogastric tube 'guidewire' technique. Journal of Emergency Medicine 14 (2): 205–8.

Young T, Fowler A (1998) Nursing management of skin grafts and donor sites. British Journal of Nursing 7(6): 324–34.

Yu E, Shenouda G, Beaudet MP, Black MJ (1997) Impact of radiation therapy fraction size on local control of early glottic carcinoma. International Journal of Radiation Oncology Biology Physics 37 (3): 587–91.

Yuska CM (1989) Introduction. Seminars in Oncology Nursing 5 (3): 137–8.

Yuska Bildstein C, Blendowski C (1997) Head and neck malignancies. In Groenwald SL, Hansen Frogge M, Goodman M, Henke Yarbro C (eds) Cancer Nursing. Principles and Practice, 4th edn. Boston: Jones & Bartlett.

Zanaret M, Giovanni A, Gras R, Cannoni M (1993) Near total laryngectomy with epiglottic reconstruction: long-term results in 57 patients. American Journal of Otolaryngology 14 (6): 419–25.

Zasler ND, McNeny R, Heywood PG (1992) Rehabilitative management of olfactory and gustatory dysfunction following brain injury. Journal of Head Trauma Rehabilitation 7 (1): 66–9.

Zeitels SM, Koufman JA, Davis RK, Vaughan CW (1994) Endoscopic treatment of supraglottic and hypopharynx cancer. Laryngoscope 104: 71–8.

Zemlin WR (1981) Speech and Hearing Science. Anatomy and Physiology, 2nd edn. Englewood Cliffs, New Jersey: Prentice Hall.

Zharen P, Becker M, Lang H (1997) Staging of laryngeal cancer: endoscopy, computed tomography and magnetic resonance versus histopathology. European Archives of Oto-Rhino-Laryngology 1 (Supplement): 117–22.

Zheng W, Shu XO, Ji BT, Gao YT (1996) Diet and other risk factors for cancer of the salivary glands: a population based case control study. International Journal of Cancer 67 (2): 194–8.

Zigmond AS, Snaith RP (1983) The hospital anxiety and depression scale. Acta Psychiatrica Scandinavica 67: 361–70.

Index